COMPLETE CARNIVORE

Achieving **Better Health** Through a **Meat-Based Diet**

JENNY MITICH

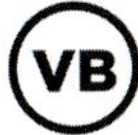

VICTORY BELT PUBLISHING INC.
LAS VEGAS

First published in 2025 by Victory Belt Publishing Inc.

ISBN-13: 978-1-628605-76-1

The author is not a licensed practitioner, physician, or medical professional and offers no medical diagnoses, treatments, suggestions, or counseling. The information presented herein has not been evaluated by the U.S. Food and Drug Administration, and it is not intended to diagnose, treat, cure, or prevent any disease. Full medical clearance from a licensed physician should be obtained before beginning or modifying any diet, exercise, or lifestyle program, and physicians should be informed of all nutritional changes.

The author/owner claims no responsibility to any person or entity for any liability, loss, or damage caused or alleged to be caused directly or indirectly as a result of the use, application, or interpretation of the information presented herein.

Cover design by Justin-Aaron Velasco

Interior design by Crizalie Olimpo

Author photos by Evan Sheehan and Alex Wallbaum

Illustrations by Elita San Juan and Alyanna Alcira

Printed in Canada

TC 0125

To my family—Mom, Dad, Karen, Kyle, Kayla, Kaylee, Aubrey, and Mimi: Thank you for standing by me through life's highs and lows. Your love and support mean everything, and I love you all more than words can say.

To my husband, Goran: Thank you for being my best friend, my partner in crime, and my unwavering support. I love you deeply and can't imagine life without you.

To Max and Harry, my stinky little babies: I love you to the ends of the universe and back. You are the lights of my life, and I am so happy to be your Mama.

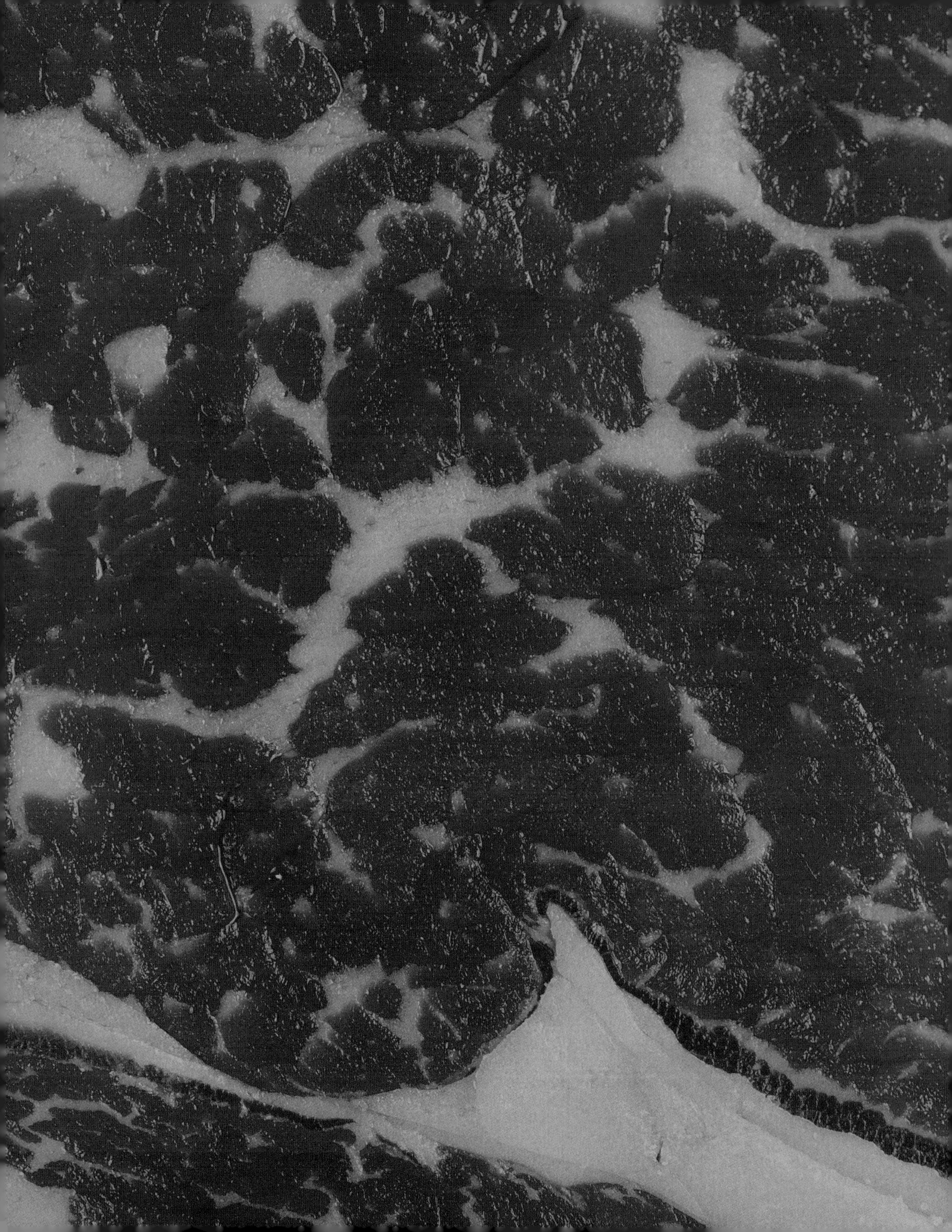

TABLE OF CONTENTS

Foreword *by Robert Kiltz, MD* 7

Introduction 8

My Story 15

PART 1: A COMPREHENSIVE GUIDE TO THE CARNIVORE DIET 28

Chapter 1: Carnivore 101 30

Chapter 2: In-Depth Guide 52

Chapter 3: Carnivore Timeline 83

Chapter 4: Beyond Carnivore: Other Important Metabolic Health Factors 101

Chapter 5: Troubleshooting Carnivore 115

Chapter 6: Carnivore FAQ 139

Chapter 7: Carnivore Myths 153

Chapter 8: Monitoring Your Progress 161

PART 2: RECIPES 190

Chapter 9: Carnivore Staples 193

Chapter 10: Breakfast 227

Chapter 11: Appetizers 245

Chapter 12: Soups and Sandwiches 261

Chapter 13: Replacement Recipes 275

Chapter 14: Holiday Meals 299

Chapter 15: Keto Cheat Meals 317

Chapter 16: Desserts 331

Chapter 17: Spice Mixes, Sauces, and Dressings 345

Chapter 18: Breads 363

Appendix A: How to Quickly Evaluate the Quality of a Scientific Paper 374

Appendix B: Recommended Reading 378

Index 384

FOREWORD

I first met Jenny several years ago when we attended a similar slate of carnivore events. We crossed paths every couple of months and bonded over our rocky upbringings, hers in Rockford, Illinois, and mine in Los Angeles. We had similar stories: difficult beginnings, hard lessons, and the tragic loss of loved ones. Those experiences fueled our passion for helping others find healing. And, like me, Jenny discovered that a high-fat, low-carb, meat-based lifestyle could quiet the chronic aches, fatigue, and struggles that steal joy from everyday living. Our friendship has been rooted in that shared transformation, and it's one I deeply cherish.

For decades, conventional wisdom told us to fill our plates with plants and push meat aside. But people are learning, experimenting, and realizing that health, energy, and vitality often require the opposite approach. In *Complete Carnivore*, Jenny shares her powerful story of reclaiming health through a meat-based diet. Her journey is both deeply personal and incredibly practical, showing how aligning with our biology can bring clarity, strength, and freedom from the confusion of modern nutrition advice.

As a fertility doctor, I've spent my career working with couples who are struggling to conceive. Time and again, I've witnessed how nutrition and the standard American diet can disrupt hormones, fuel inflammation, and stand in the way of new life. But I've also seen the opposite: how adopting the carnivore diet, rooted in simplicity and ancestral wisdom, can restore health, improve fertility, and bring hope where it once seemed lost.

Jenny's story is one of courage and clarity. She not only embraced the carnivore lifestyle but also mapped out a practical guide for anyone ready to reclaim their health. Her gift for guiding others makes this book so much more than a diet guide. It's a roadmap to possibility. It reminds us that our bodies are designed to thrive when we fuel them properly and that extraordinary change is always possible.

I am honored to introduce *Complete Carnivore*. May it inspire you, challenge you, and, most of all, remind you that better health—and in many cases, new life—begins with what we put on our plates.

—Robert Kiltz, MD
Founder and CEO
CNY Fertility and Kiltz Health

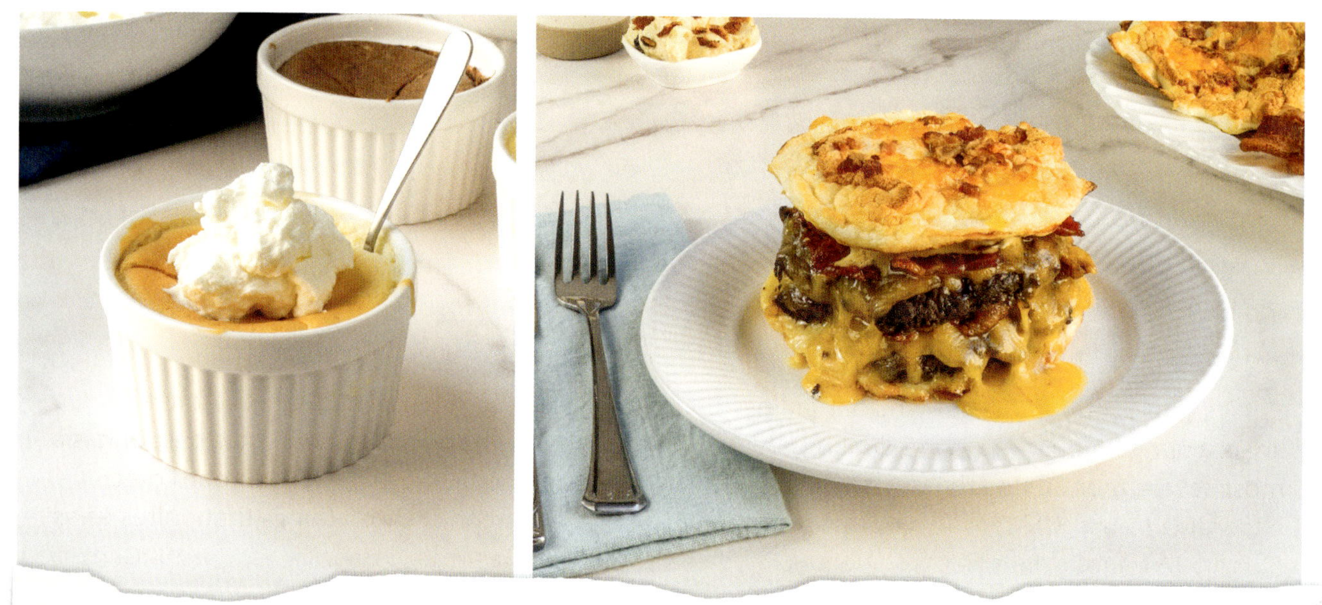

INTRODUCTION

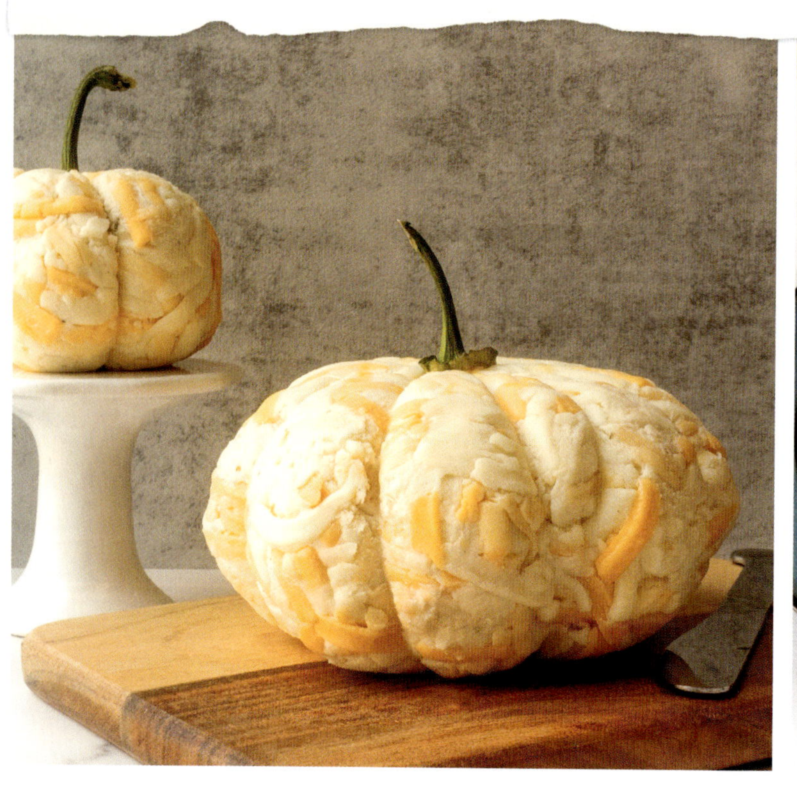

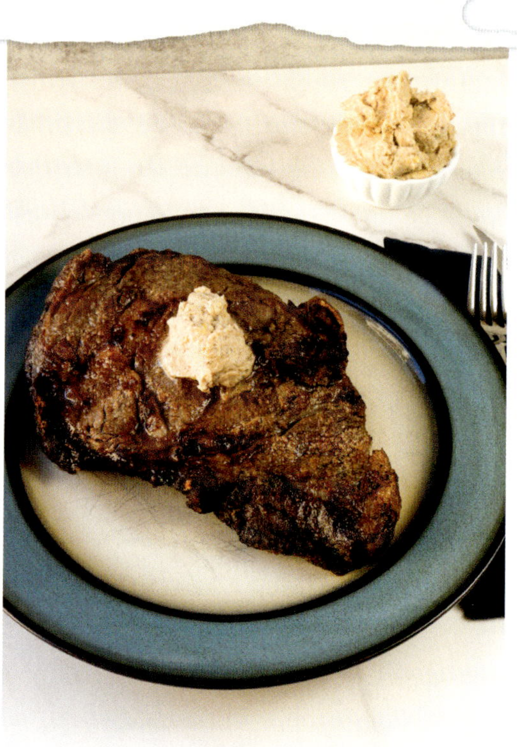

Over the last fifty years, we've been getting sicker and sicker. It's estimated that one in three Americans has metabolic syndrome.[1] Almost 12 percent of the US population has type 2 diabetes,[2] and almost 75 percent are overweight or obese.[3] It seems like as we age, our bodies fall apart. As I run my daily errands, I hear snippets of people's conversations, and it's always, "Oh, you know, I turned fifty, and my health went down the drain," or "Getting older sucks." We believe that as our bodies age, metabolic syndrome, diabetes, obesity, and a plethora of other conditions are inevitable.

But it's not just the older set who are falling apart. Younger generations are dealing with the most severe mental health issues ever seen. According to the *2022 National Healthcare Quality and Disparities Report*, "Nearly 20% of children and young people ages 3–17 in the United States have a mental, emotional, developmental, or behavioral disorder, and suicidal behaviors among high school students increased more than 40% in the decade before 2019."[4] Depression, anxiety, and suicide are rampant in the younger generations. And their physical health isn't great, either. There's something to be said when the US Army is having a hard time finding recruits because the pool of applicants does not have the physical health required to serve.[5]

So, what has happened over the past fifty or so years that has caused such a drastic decline in our health as a society? That is a complicated question with a multitude of interconnected answers, but a big part of it is a monumental change to our standard diet.

Food is one of those things that unites us as humans. Regardless of age, race, gender, sexual orientation, or political persuasion, we all need to eat! And most of us eat at least two or three times per day, plus snacks.

Over the last five decades, our diets have become overwhelmingly plant based. The 2020–2025 USDA Dietary Guidelines for Americans recommend that 45 to 65 percent of daily calories should come from carbohydrates or other plant sources.[6] Because of these recommendations, we've drastically increased our consumption of ultra-processed foods, vegetable seed oils, and added sugar. At the same time, we've decreased the amount of red meat, eggs, and butter we eat.

---

[1] "What is metabolic syndrome?" National Heart, Lung, and Blood Institute, https://www.nhlbi.nih.gov/health/metabolic-syndrome, accessed July 8, 2025.

[2] CDC, "National diabetes statistics report," May 15, 2024, https://www.cdc.gov/diabetes/php/data-research/index.html.

[3] CDC, "Obesity and overweight," National Center for Health Statistics, May 15, 2024, https://www.cdc.gov/nchs/fastats/obesity-overweight.htm.

[4] "Child and adolescent mental health," *2022 National Healthcare Quality and Disparities Report*, National Library of Medicine, Oct. 2022, https://www.ncbi.nlm.nih.gov/books/NBK587174.

[5] Mark Satter, "Military obesity rates soar, compounding recruitment challenges," Roll Call, October 18, 2023, https://rollcall.com/2023/10/18/military-obesity-rates-soar-compounding-recruitment-challenges/.

[6] "Dietary guidelines for Americans 2020–2025," USDA, https://www.dietaryguidelines.gov/sites/default/files/2020-12/Dietary_Guidelines_for_Americans_2020-2025.pdf.

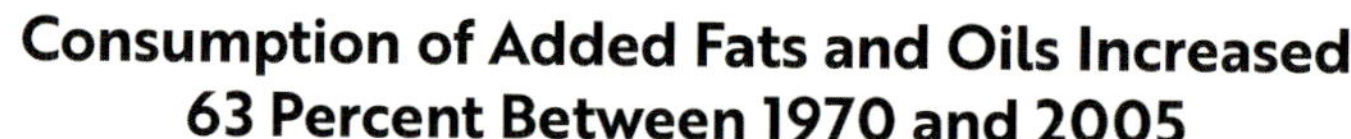

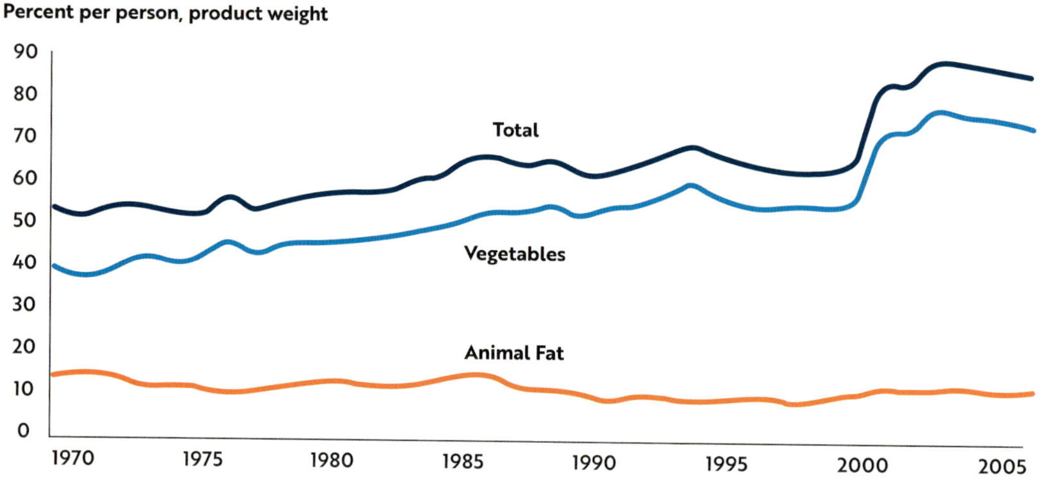

Note: In 2000, there was a dramatic increase in the number of firms reporting vegetable oil production to the U.S. Census Bureau.
Source: USDA, ERS Food Availability (Per Capita) Data System.

There are many reasons for this drastic shift, but the USDA dietary guidelines that were introduced in the 1970s (we all remember the food pyramid!) played a large part, along with the slow and steady demonization of animal-based foods in nutrition science and the media.

In the 1980s, Big Tobacco companies like Philip Morris and R.J. Reynolds purchased Big Food companies such as Kraft, General Foods, and Nabisco[7] because cigarettes were declining in popularity. Big Tobacco took its experience crafting habit-forming products and applied it to packaged foods. As a result, more and more low-fat, ultra-processed foods hit the shelves. Behind the scenes, food engineers designed these products to be highly addictive.[8] While ultra-processed foods have very few nutrients, they have a "perfect" mix of fat and carbohydrates that does not exist in nature. When you eat this stuff, your brain goes into overdrive, and you want more, more, more. That's a top priority for the food engineer: You are never fully satisfied and always coming back for seconds and thirds. Why do you think the Pringles container says, "Once you pop, you can't stop!"

[7] Anahad O'Connor, "Many of today's unhealthy foods were brought to you by Big Tobacco," *Washington Post*, September 19, 2023.
[8] "How the food industry helps engineer our cravings," *Here & Now*, NPR, December 16, 2015, https://www.npr.org/sections/thesalt/2015/12/16/459981099/how-the-food-industry-helps-engineer-our-cravings.

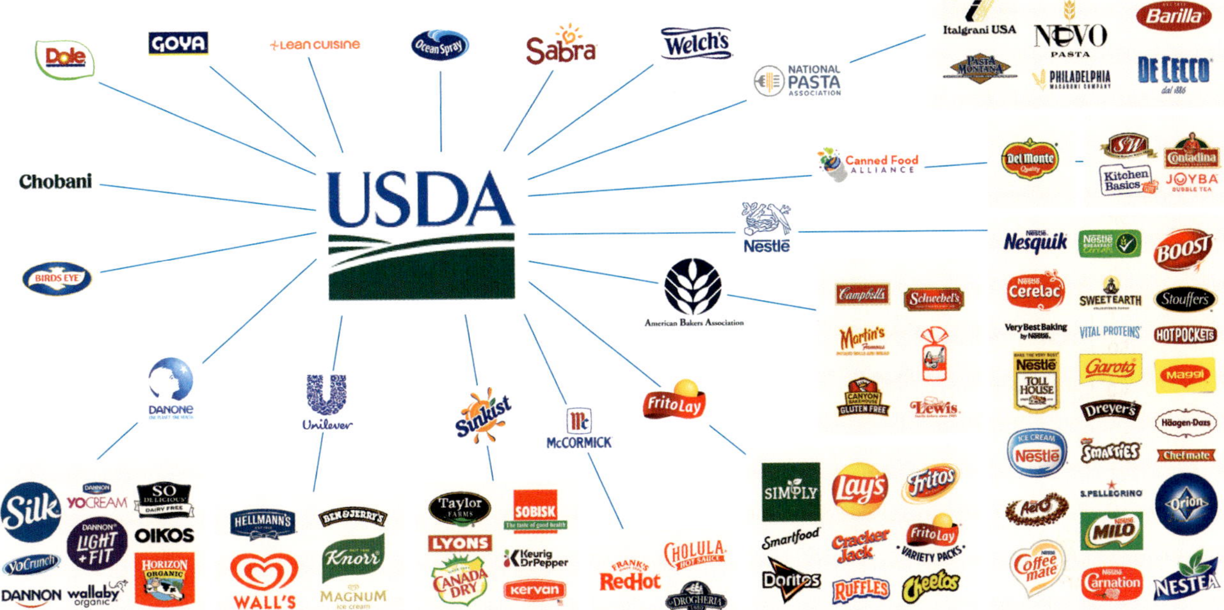

Based on new dietary recommendations in the 1970s, people largely stopped eating lard and butter and replaced them with vegetable oil and Crisco. Instead of a steak, we eat a microwaveable frozen dinner. Instead of eggs and bacon, we eat oatmeal or cereal and a banana for breakfast. Despite these dietary "improvements," we are consuming more calories than we did in the 1970s, and most of them are coming from refined carbohydrates and vegetable seed oils.[9] And we drink most of our liquids in the form of sugary sodas, juices, and coffees.

The Standard American Diet

Average daily calories consumed

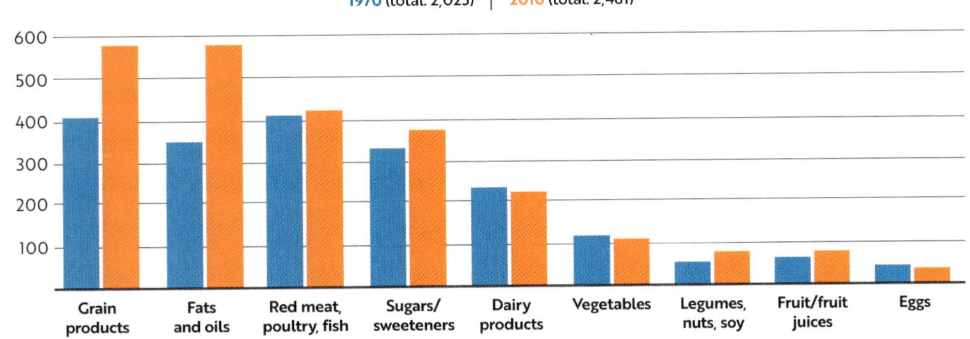

Note: "Fats and oils" includes butter, cream and other dairy fats. Figures adjusted for spoilage and other losses.
Source: USDA Economic Research Service; Pew Research Center analysis

---

[9] Drew Desilver, "What's on your table? How America's diet has changed over the decades," Pew Research Center, December 13, 2016.

We've increased our eating frequency to the point where most people eat every few hours. Sleep seems to be the only time we aren't eating or at least thinking about our next meal because we are hungry.

Slowly but surely, our average weight has increased, and our metabolic health has decreased. In the 1970s, it was estimated that about 14 percent of people were obese. In the 2020s, that number has ballooned to almost 40 percent.[10] Dialysis (a treatment for people with failing kidneys) used to be rare, and you would have to travel long distances to find a facility that could do it. Nowadays, there seems to be a dialysis clinic in every town, maybe even several of them, with over 557,000 people currently on dialysis in the US.[11] GLP-1 receptor agonists like Ozempic and Mounjaro are often promoted as miracle drugs, but the standard starting doses are very high and can trigger serious side effects, which can include severe stomach problems, pancreatitis, and a loss of lean mass and bone mass.[12] Without proper guidance on diet and exercise, patients risk losing up to 40 percent of their lean muscle mass. We've tried every fad diet, weight-loss drug, and even gastric bypass surgery to no avail. We may lose weight in the short term, but it always seems to come back. Sometimes, we gain back even more than we originally lost.

Add those dietary changes to the fact that we are more sedentary than we've been at any point in modern history.[13] We spend 95 percent of our time indoors watching screens, covering ourselves up from the sun. Our stress levels are through the roof, while our life satisfaction levels are plummeting. Environmental toxins and so-called forever chemicals permeate everything.[14] We are overmedicated; there is a pill for every malady that afflicts us. The results of all of these changes over the past fifty years? Staggering rates of diabetes, cancer, obesity, and mental health issues. People are sick, overworked, and unsatisfied with the status quo and are looking for an alternative.

---

[10] "Obesity in the U.S.," Food Research & Action Center, https://frac.org/obesity-health/obesity-u-s-2.

[11] "Quick kidney disease facts and stats," American Kidney Fund, https://www.kidneyfund.org/all-about-kidneys/quick-kidney-disease-facts-and-stats, last updated June 6, 2025.

[12] Berkeley Lovelace Jr., "Popular weight loss drugs linked to rare but severe stomach problems, study finds," NBC News, October 5, 2023.

[13] Charles E. Matthews et al., "Sedentary behavior in U.S. adults: fall 2019," *Medicine & Science in Sports & Exercise 53*, no. 12 (2021): 2512–2519.

[14] "PFAS—the 'forever chemicals,'" CHEM Trust, https://chemtrust.org/pfas/.

WHAT'S THE SOLUTION?
THE CARNIVORE DIET

There is no one simple answer to this complicated question, but I believe we must first address our diet. Eating is one of the few things we must do to stay alive, so nutrition is a low-hanging fruit that can improve our metabolic health quickly.

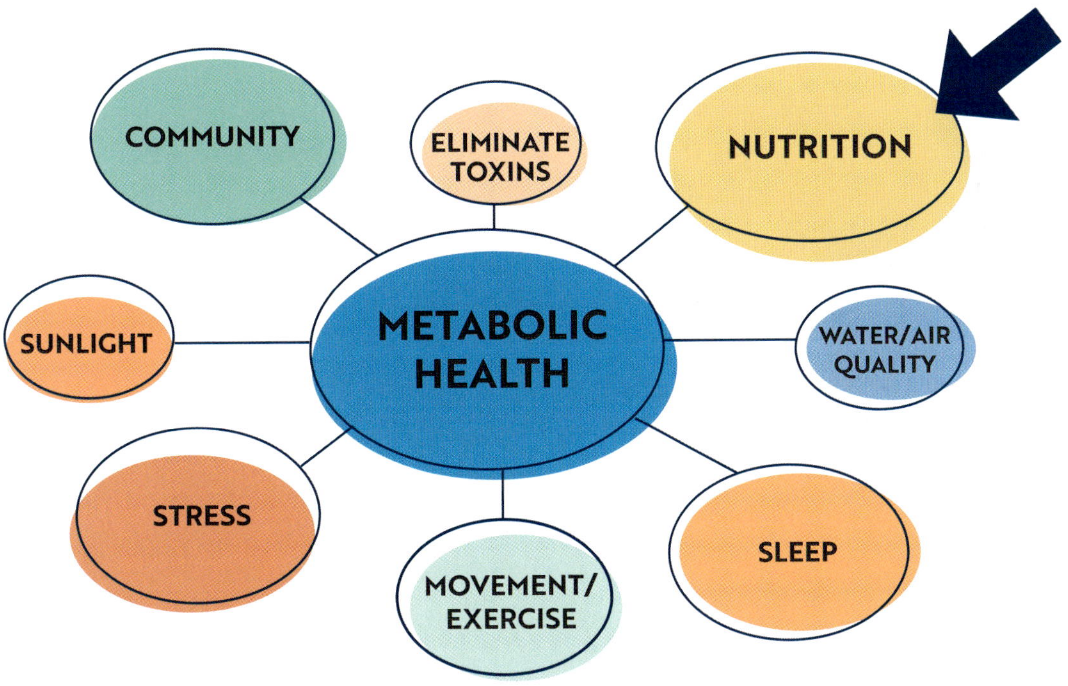

We need to get back to basics and revert to the way humans ate for hundreds of thousands (if not millions) of years. We need our ancestral food—the food that allowed humans to become the apex predator that dominates the globe. And that food is meat and animal products. We didn't evolve to consume 45 to 65 percent of our daily calories from carbohydrates! For most of history, the human diet was made up mainly of the proteins and fats from animals and their by-products. Depending on geography and availability, our ancient ancestors would have consumed plant material only in season, and sparingly. And while that ancestral knowledge may have been lost for some time, it has begun to bubble back up in our collective memory.

More and more people are regaining their metabolic health, getting back to a healthy weight, and improving their lives by trusting the innate knowledge that meat is a powerful and nourishing food. But some of us are not satisfied with eating meat based and still including some plant material. We are called carnivores.

The carnivore diet is a way of eating that includes only meat and animal by-products. While it may seem like a new and trendy diet, it has ancient roots. If you look back at cave paintings from over thirty thousand years ago, you'll notice that the subject was often a hunt of some kind.[15] Closer to modern times, many Indigenous tribes subsisted on meat almost year-round, including the Maasai and the Inuit.[16] An all-meat diet was used from the late 1700s to the 1900s to treat diabetes but faded from popularity after insulin was discovered.[17] Dr. Robert Atkins popularized a low-carb diet with his first book on the topic in 1972 and reached peak popularity in the early 2000s, but the meat-heavy Atkins diet did reintroduce carbohydrates after the induction phase.

True carnivore has always been around, though. In the late 1990s and early 2000s, a group of people gathered in an online forum called Zeroing In On Health and were doing what they called a zero-carb diet, which meant they did not consume any plant foods. A lot of the people in this forum were not having the success they thought they should using a low-carb diet, so they took it to the next level. Some long-term carnivores whose names you may recognize were members of this group: Kelly Hogan, Amber O'Hearn, Dr. Lisa Wiedeman, and many others.

But Zeroing In On Health was (and still is) a small and mostly unknown forum. It wasn't until 2017 that O'Hearn gave her first lectures on the carnivore diet, quickly followed by the first carnivore conference in 2019. These events mainly drew people in the low-carb space. Dr. Shawn Baker's appearance on the *Joe Rogan Experience* podcast in late 2017 brought carnivore back into the mainstream. He released his book, *The Carnivore Diet*, in late 2019, and carnivore has been gaining popularity ever since. Recently, it has exploded.

But a lot of questions have come up as more and more people have started going carnivore:

- How do I switch to carnivore from a standard American diet?
- Is carnivore safe?
- Can I stay carnivore long term, or is it just a short-term intervention?
- How will I get all of the vitamins and minerals I need from eating only meat?

I was asking all of these questions and more when I started carnivore. Like so many people out there, I had some weight to lose and wasn't feeling great. Carnivore has been a game changer for me, and in the next chapter, I'll share with you all of the ways it has made my life better. After that, I will guide you through all of these questions about getting started on carnivore and more.

---

[15] "Style in cave paintings," Royal Society of Chemistry, https://edu.rsc.org/resources/style-in-cave-paintings/1541.article, accessed July 8, 2025.
[16] Georgia Ede, "The history of all-meat diets," diagnosis:Diet, https://www.diagnosisdiet.com/full-article/all-meat-diets, accessed July 8, 2025.
[17] Gary Taubes, *Rethinking Diabetes* (New York: Vintage Books, 2024).

MY STORY

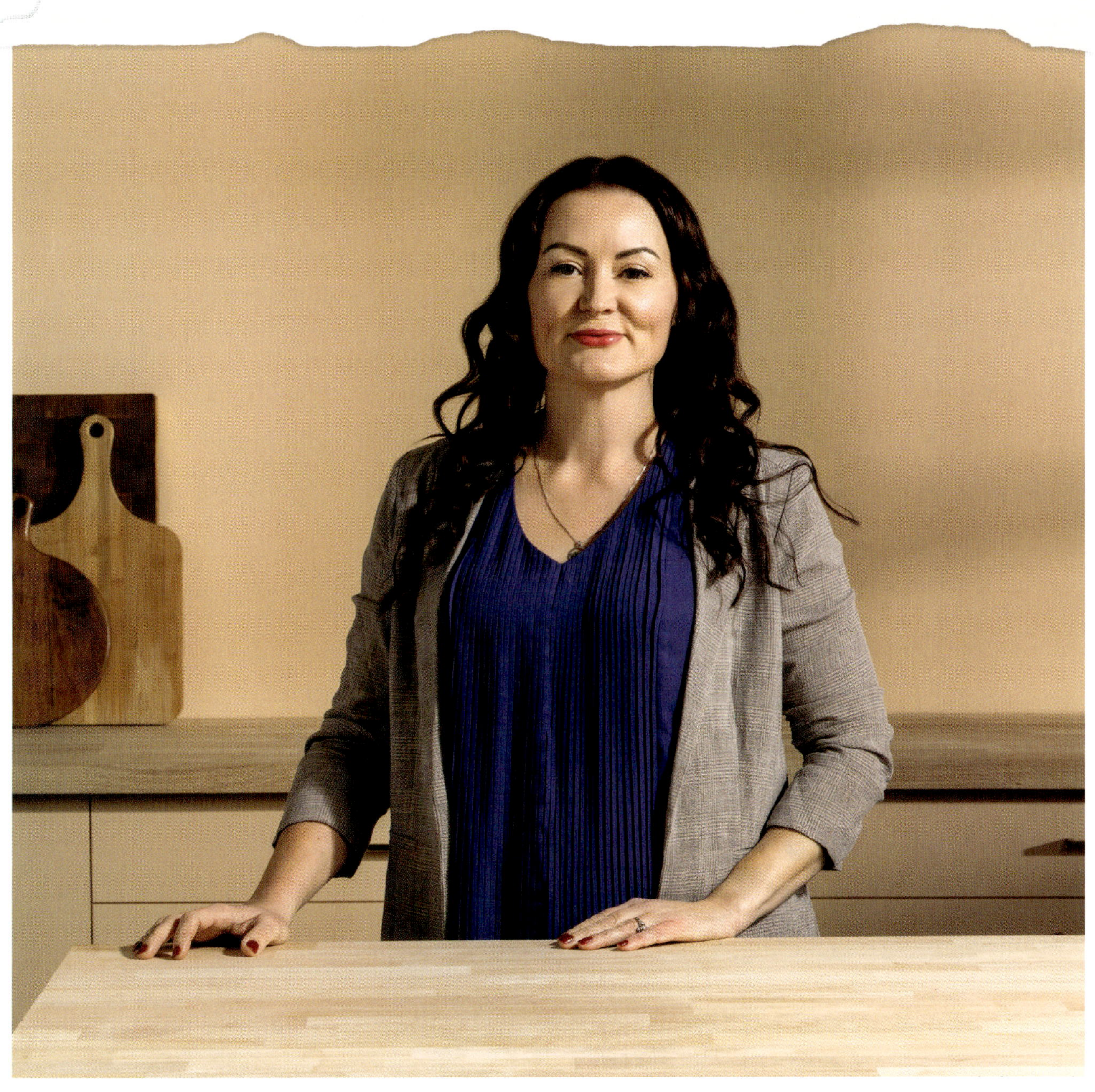

My path to the carnivore lifestyle was anything but quick or easy—I didn't discover it until I was nearly forty! I often wish I'd found it sooner, but it wasn't really on the radar until the 2000s, and even then, it stayed pretty fringe until the 2020s. I wanted to share my backstory with you so you can understand how I got here and why I now fully embrace this way of living. That said, if you'd rather skip ahead to the next chapter and dive straight into carnivore, I totally get it. But if you're up for it—hang on tight. This is one wild ride!

HOW IT ALL STARTED

I was a child of the 1980s and '90s, born and raised in Rockford, Illinois. My brother and I grew up on mac and cheese, fish sticks, and hot dogs. White-bread sandwiches slathered with Miracle Whip and filled with American cheese and Buddig lunchmeat, bags of potato chips, Little Debbie snack cakes, and Kool-Aid sweetened with a full cup of sugar were standard lunch fare. We were healthy, active kids, but as I came into puberty, I had an explosion of acne along with severe cramping with every menstrual cycle and some weight gain. The acne and weight gain drew some bullying in fifth and sixth grade. I was put on a few different medications for my skin issues, and they helped. I also thinned out as I grew a bit taller, but my mental health suffered because of the bullying.

At thirteen, I started drinking alcohol and smoking marijuana and cigarettes. That coincided with a depression and anxiety diagnosis. The experimentation and self-medicating evolved into alcoholism by fifteen (having a fake ID and going to bars on the weekends probably didn't help with that), cocaine use by sixteen, and full-blown heroin addiction by nineteen. I basically lived on candy, Coca-Cola, cigarettes, and heroin on and off for the next seven years. Sporadic homelessness, minor run-ins with the law, and a plethora of other traumatic experiences were par for the course for me during that time.

During my active heroin addiction, I did have periods of clean time. I was in and out of rehab, doing three stints in total. My final stay was a year long and involved intensive therapy and coursework. I relapsed a couple of times after leaving that facility, but eventually, in my mid-to-late twenties, I was able to get clean. I moved away from my hometown and started to get my life together, but I was still just sort of skating through life with no direction.

Everything changed in January 2011. I was home visiting family, and something happened that altered the course of my life forever. I got together with my best friend to hang out, and later that evening he overdosed and died in my father's basement. I was later charged in connection with his death because I was in the vehicle when he purchased the heroin that ended up killing him.

I spent four months in county jail awaiting a bond reduction hearing and had a lot of time to think about my life. How did I get here? Why did I find it "normal" to hang out with an active drug user? Was this the life I wanted to live? I decided then and there that when I was released from jail, I would do something different.

Eventually, I was released to fight the case on the outside. From that time on, I completely changed my life. I went back to school at the local community college. I ended up graduating valedictorian and gave the commencement speech. I also started volunteering at my grandmother's church. The church hired me first as the membership secretary and then as the director of youth development. I managed the junior and senior high youth groups, and it remains the most fulfilling job I have ever had.

As far as the court case, after about a year we came to an impasse. The judge met with my lawyer and the prosecutor and said that if I pleaded guilty to involuntary manslaughter, she would give me probation, and that would be the end of it. Otherwise, we would need to prepare to go to trial. That would have meant at least another one to two years of court dates and at least $10,000 to $20,000 more in legal fees, plus the intense stress. After discussing the options with my family, I decided to plead guilty to involuntary manslaughter and was sentenced to two and a half years' probation, which I successfully completed in August 2015.

I later earned my bachelor's degree in management and finance while working full-time at the church. In my senior year of college, I received a research grant to do a comparative analysis of the Nordic and American prison systems. I was able to tour Halden, a maximum-security prison outside of Oslo, Norway, as well as an open prison in Finland. My time in jail had ignited a passion for prison reform, and there is a lot to learn from Nordic philosophies on incarceration. They believe that incarceration should focus on rehabilitation over punishment. The key idea is that losing freedom is the punishment—not harsh treatment, poor conditions, or dehumanization. I later did a TEDx talk on my research. It was a full-circle moment for me: In six years I'd gone from active heroin addiction, a manslaughter charge, and a wreck of a life to graduating at the top of my class, conducting research on prison systems, and mentoring teens. A lot of it had to do with my best friend's death and my subsequent jail stay. Deciding to make a change was half the battle, but I had to put in the work, too. I learned a lot about grit and persistence during that period of my life.

A JOURNEY TO HEALTH

My journey to health was far from over, however, and getting off drugs was only one small piece. At that time, my idea of "healthy" food was juice, lots of salads, and chicken. I had zero experience with nutrition and just followed the same standard dietary advice that most people did: keep fat intake low, eat fruits and veggies, and avoid red meat. It wasn't until I heard Mark Sisson on the *Joe Rogan Experience* podcast in 2016 that I realized I was dead wrong. Sisson talked about the benefits of a low-carbohydrate, high-fat diet, which he called the "Primal Blueprint." I purchased all of Mark's books and binge-read them, receiving my first introduction into a whole, real-food diet with a focus on meat and animal fats.

I then learned about Paleo and keto, but I never fully took the plunge. Instead, I did a lot of weight training and cycling and ate a low-fat diet for years. I eventually cut gluten and began to reduce my intake of ultra-processed foods. That approach did work, for a time. But the minute I strayed from the diet, I would put on weight. And while I had been clean from drugs for a long time, I was still drinking alcohol almost every day, which wasn't helpful.

When I met my future husband in 2017, we did a lot of traveling and eating together. We considered ourselves foodies. I gained 20 pounds that first year of dating, but we were happy, and I didn't think it was a big deal.

Then the pandemic hit. Surprisingly, I had really slowed down my drinking by that point and actually lost some weight during 2020. My husband and I were contemplating having children, and I wanted to get down to a healthier weight before attempting to get pregnant. But I put it off, with the excuse of "I can start a diet next month; it's not a big deal."

We started trying for a baby in early 2021, and I ended up getting pregnant with twins in the spring. My starting weight was 173 pounds, and by the day I gave birth I had ballooned to 242 pounds—a total gain of almost 70 pounds. I was understandably miserable: Swollen hands, wrists, and feet. Back pain. Exhaustion. And I couldn't seem to eat enough food; I was always hungry. Unfortunately, I pretty much ate a standard American diet for the duration of my pregnancy, and I think that played a part in why I felt so crummy for the majority of it.

Upon giving birth, I lost about 25 pounds, what with 12 pounds of babies, placentas, and fluids being removed from my body. I felt better almost instantly. After three months of adjusting to life with newborn twins, I was finally ready to attempt to lose the remainder of the weight. I started on February 1, 2022, at 216 pounds. Over the next eleven months, I slowly lost some weight using Noom, a psychology-based app that preaches the high-carb, medium-protein, low-fat, and 1,200 calories per day approach that most conventional weight-loss programs start with. (This was pre-Ozempic; most weight-loss apps now prescribe GLP-1s in addition to whatever their "program" is.)

I dropped an average of 2 pounds per month following that program, losing a total of about 22 pounds, but I was constantly hungry. I started tracking my glucose levels with a (non-diabetic) continuous glucose monitor and discovered that they were in the high 90s to low 100s on average, with peaks as high as 176. (For reference, a desirable average would be between 75 and 95, with peaks of 140 or less. Turn to chapter 8 for details on these and other important numbers.) And while I had lost a bit of weight, from July through December 2022 I had been losing and regaining the same 5 pounds and remained stuck in the mid-190s. I was understandably frustrated.

That summer, my husband started researching the carnivore diet. He had lost over 130 pounds on keto before we met, but he wanted to take it to the next level because he still had about 70 pounds to lose. He found a YouTube channel from Dr. Ken Berry, a leading proponent of meat-based and ancestral diets, and tried to convince me to do carnivore with him. His rationale was that it's so much easier to stick to a way of eating if your significant other is doing it with you.

But I thought carnivore was crazy. I thought there was no way it could be good for you. How were you going to get all of your vitamins and minerals if you were only eating meat? And I may have said that Dr. Berry was a cult leader. But, over the next six months, I ended up watching a lot of Dr. Berry's videos with my husband, and some of what he was saying started to make sense to me.

Finally, in December 2022, I became so frustrated by my lack of progress that I decided to try carnivore for one month. I was interested to see how much weight I would lose. I had been wearing a continuous glucose monitor for three and a half months at that point, so I was also curious about how my blood glucose levels would change when I transitioned from Noom to carnivore.

It's funny, I actually started carnivore before my husband did. We decided to stagger our start dates so that we wouldn't be experiencing keto flu at the same time (our boys were only one year old at that point). My first day on carnivore was December 27, 2022, and in that first month I lost 8 pounds, which is the most weight I've ever lost in a single month of using any way of eating. Also, my average blood glucose dropped by 15 to 20 points.

I did not have an easy go of it, though. I had severe keto flu symptoms, with fatigue and diarrhea being the worst of them. While keto flu typically lasts only two to three weeks, I suffered for six. The symptoms were bad, but not bad enough for me to quit. I now know that I was likely dealing with oxalate dumping in addition to keto flu. Not being aware that oxalate dumping was a possibility when going into carnivore cold turkey was the first of many mistakes I made. (Don't worry, you don't have to make the same mistake; in chapter 2, you'll find everything you need to avoid the worst of the keto flu and oxalate dumping.)

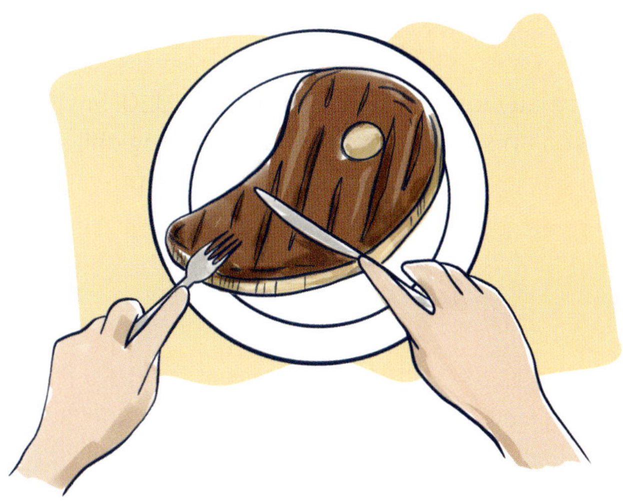

Over the next year, I lost a total of 35 pounds and improved my metabolic health across the board. In addition, I experienced vast improvements in mental health, oral health, strength, and stamina. I was getting to sleep much easier and feeling more refreshed upon waking. I no longer experienced sugar crashes and hangry feelings in the afternoon. And carnivore was so simple to follow! I was saving a ton of time in the kitchen and saving money at the grocery store because we were only eating meat and had eliminated a lot of items from our weekly shopping list. Not having to spend as much time cooking was a lifesaver for me as a mom to young children.

I began sharing my carnivore diet journey on my YouTube channel in June 2023, and two of my update videos exploded in popularity. My channel went from 1,600 to 8,600 subscribers in two weeks. By the following year, I had hit over 100,000 subscribers, and my channel is now solely focused on the carnivore diet. My health has improved so drastically that I had to share it with the world! I couldn't keep this information to myself.

A lot of the content I share on YouTube revolves around metabolic testing and data gathering. I believe that people should know their numbers and have access to a variety of ways to measure their health. I have been tracking my progress through weigh-ins, body measurements, DEXA scans, continuous glucose monitoring, blood work, and arterial scans and sharing my results to help dispel some of the myths and misconceptions about carnivore. And to think, it all started with tracking my blood glucose with a continuous glucose monitor!

Through my YouTube channel, I was able to talk to and help thousands of people get started on carnivore. But I kept getting the same questions over and over, and I realized that there was a deficit in the available materials on the topic.

What I was finding was that people needed a very detailed but easy-to-understand step-by-step guide to how to do carnivore correctly. With that in mind, I decided to pull together all of my knowledge into an almost hour-long how-to video. I released my "In-Depth Reference Guide to the Carnivore Diet" video in January 2024, and it has helped hundreds of thousands of people get started on carnivore. But there's only so much I could cover in video form. What was really needed was a single volume. A guidebook. Something people could hold in their hands that would answer every one of their questions while giving them the most accurate information out there. There are some fabulous books on the market that talk about carnivore by experts like Dr. Shawn Baker, Judy Cho, and Paul Saladino, but people still had questions. It was clear to me that I needed to translate and expand my video into book format.

This book is the fruit of that labor. Just like its title suggests, *Complete Carnivore* tells you everything you need to know about the carnivore diet. In this book, I'll show you why carnivore is one of a handful of proper diets for our species. There is a full starter guide that will get you through your first months and year on carnivore. I will walk you through the preparation phase and ensure you are set up for success long before day 1. There's an entire chapter on troubleshooting if you run into any issues. There are chapters covering all of the questions I'm asked every day on YouTube and another chapter that dispels common myths. Along the way, you'll find invaluable nuggets of information from long-term carnivores that can help you avoid some of the mistakes that my husband and I made in the beginning. And believe me, you are going to appreciate this knowledge. I wish I'd had this book when I started carnivore, because it would have saved me a lot of pain and suffering!

In addition to these chapters that cover the how-to of carnivore, there's an entire recipe section with over eighty recipes. They include a lot of the carnivore staples that you're going to be eating every day, like ribeyes and burgers, along with fully carnivore recipes that are a bit more complicated to make but super delicious for when you get bored, such as beef stroganoff and carnivore mac & cheese casserole. I also tell you which kitchen tools every carnivore should have and provide a meal plan, a grocery list, and so much more.

Whether you do carnivore for ninety days or one year, or you choose to stay carnivore long term, *Complete Carnivore* will be something you can refer to again and again.

After reading this book, I just know that you are going to feel fully confident in your ability to follow the carnivore diet and improve your metabolic health. Making the decision to change your life is one of the hardest steps in this entire process, so I commend you for your strength. Let's build on that momentum and get you started! First, let me give you a quick overview of carnivore before diving into preparing for your first day.

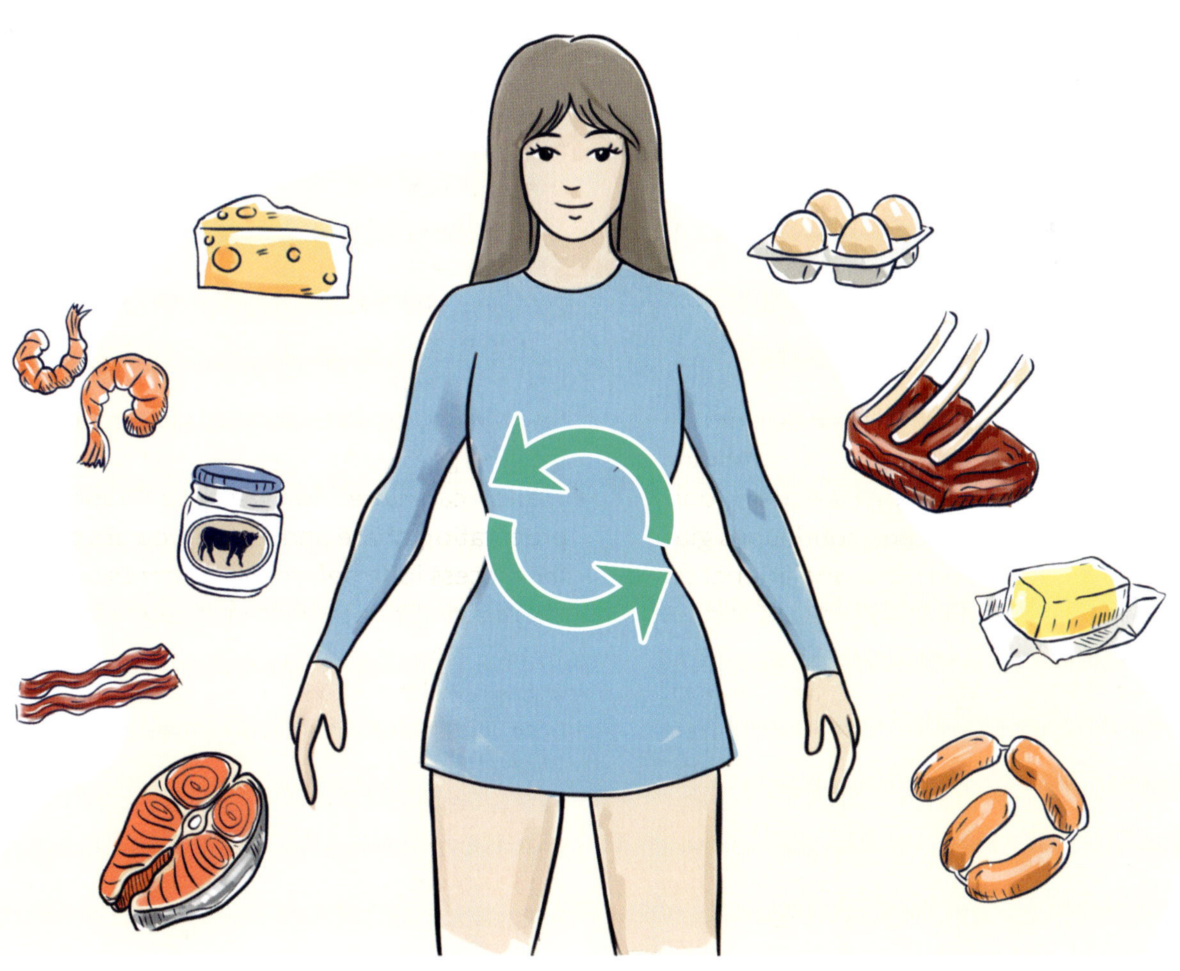

TESTIMONIALS

The carnivore diet has sparked so many amazing transformations. Here are just a few stories from members of my community to inspire you.

When my son was diagnosed with ADHD, our family faced the challenges many parents know all too well—emotional outbursts, trouble focusing, and constant worry. We tried multiple strategies, including counseling, occupational therapy, a school behavior plan, and even medication, but none of these interventions changed his symptoms. It felt like we were constantly battling, with little to no progress.

Then we discovered the carnivore diet, and everything changed.

I had already experienced significant health benefits from the carnivore diet myself, and after researching its potential for children with ADHD, I felt it could be worth trying for my son. With a focus on nutrient-dense, animal-based foods, we removed all processed foods, grains, and sugars from his diet. This was a big shift, but within weeks, the changes were undeniable.

The first improvement we noticed was his ability to organize complex tasks, like cleaning his room—something that had always been a struggle for him. Suddenly, he could break down the task into manageable steps and see it through without becoming overwhelmed. This was a huge breakthrough, as it showed he was gaining a new sense of focus and clarity.

In addition, his energy leveled out. Where once he swung between hyperactivity and exhaustion, he now had steady, balanced energy throughout the day. This balance was critical not just for his focus but also for managing his emotions. Prior to starting the carnivore diet, angry outbursts were frequent. He would often lash out in frustration, which made day-to-day life incredibly challenging. After switching to the carnivore diet, these outbursts became much less frequent, and when they did happen, he was more capable of calming himself down. The emotional regulation that came with the diet was life-changing.

Another unexpected benefit was the improvement in his physical health. He had suffered from digestive issues, but those disappeared entirely after the dietary switch. His sleep became more restful, his skin cleared up, and he started waking up each day feeling refreshed and ready.

Seeing my son heal from the inside out has been nothing short of miraculous. The carnivore diet didn't just improve his ADHD symptoms; it transformed his overall well-being.

—Cristie Kiehl

I am a 6-foot-tall sixty-one-year-old male. At my heaviest, I was 268 pounds and was eating a standard American diet and drinking A LOT of diet soda. I lived with sore knees, elbows, shoulders, hips, and lower back. I was diagnosed with high blood pressure and on two types of medication for it. I cut back on the size of my meals and soda and managed to lose 8 pounds and stalled out.

After researching many diets, I came across several YouTube videos pertaining to the carnivore way of eating, not so much a diet but eliminating all food except meat and meat products. I am a huge backyard BBQ person who cooks outdoors five or six days a week, and this sounded great to me. I found myself watching a lot of Jenny Mitich videos, and when I started carnivore I joined her carnivore group on Circle for great support and encouragement from others eating and living the same way.

I started eating carnivore on July 1, 2024. Within three days all the pain (inflammation) in my body disappeared. Within four weeks I noticed my blood pressure dropped to normal numbers, which it had never done, even on medication. Soon I stopped taking my medication and have not looked back. My blood pressure continues to stay in the 120s over 70s with a pulse in the high 50s.

Almost five months in, I continue to feel amazing, [with] lots of energy. I have lost 30 pounds, reducing my waist and chest by 5 inches and stomach by 7 inches. I am not at my goal yet, but I am certainly not going back. The bottom line is, carnivore removed my body pain, reduced my blood pressure, and gave me back the energy level I had twenty years ago. There have been zero negative results from this eating lifestyle.

—Curtis Rogers

I was 250 pounds, prediabetic, and possibly a little desperate. I started the carnivore diet in March 2023. The month prior I was sitting on the couch with my baby, and my last. I have ten children, five boys and five girls. With six of my pregnancies, I had gestational diabetes. For some, I was prescribed metformin. The dose would be low, like 0.05 grams, because I'd gotten rid of almost all carbs and only ate a large amount of vegetables and a little meat. (I now know that I should have eaten more protein.) Anyhow, I was sitting on my couch nursing my four-month-old and wanted to watch YouTube. One of the homesteaders I like to watch was sick with Lyme disease. He said he was going to start the carnivore diet. I immediately made fun of it! How's this guy supposed to poop? He's probably going to die of a heart attack! But because of that, I was recommended Dr. Ken Berry's channel. I watched almost all of his videos. I even took notes! I decided I was going to go carnivore.

My husband didn't think the carnivore diet was safe and thought it would be expensive. I told him it should be easy, and we'd just buy more butter and burger patties. I decided my start date would be March 3, the first Friday of Lent. We only eat fish, eggs, or cheese as proteins in Lent. I had ordered enough electrolytes to make it through the first month. I was ready. My first day was a little weird. I ate scrambled eggs with plenty of butter. I had my electrolytes and drank plenty of water. For dinner, I mixed egg, cheese, and salmon, pressed them into patties, and cooked them on the stove. Three days into carnivore I noticed my knees didn't hurt. I have had sore knees since I turned thirty. I used to skateboard as a youth, so I thought the knee thing was from an old injury. Then the best thing of all time happened! I woke up and my back didn't hurt. I thought my back hurt so bad because of all the babies I carried. Nope, it was inflammation! I lost 30 pounds in my first month. By September I lost 50 pounds. My brain has always been foggy, but on month six of carnivore my brain started to work better than it had before. I started back up my homesteading YouTube channel *(Boobie Goats)* because of carnivore and released a short in September 2023 about losing 50 pounds on a carnivore diet. Another YouTuber reached out to me and wanted to do an interview! I was so stoked. Old me would have been terrified to do an interview live on YouTube. I did the interview and told my story. I've told my story on a few other YouTube channels as well. The carnivore diet has made me so chill and relaxed.

On carnivore, I mainly eat beef, butter, bacon, and eggs. On occasion, I'll add cheese, chicken, and pork. I buy what's on sale or discounted. I have to make my diet sustainable. My children and husband are slowly transitioning to a meat-based diet. Now that my eyes are open, I have to be a food detective for my family. So far I have lost 82 pounds, and now losing weight doesn't matter. What matters is how good I feel and how much I want everyone to feel this great!

—Erin Dowdell

I was a relatively healthy kid growing up, but all that changed by the time I reach adulthood. I joined the United States Marine Corps on my 17th birthday and left home before I turned 18. While on active duty, my health began to decline, and none of the doctors could figure out what was happening to me and why. At twenty, I started to vomit every day. This affected my mental health because no one could tell me how to make it go away. I began to develop severe depression and anxiety. I was getting pumped full of prescriptions, began a battle with suicidal ideation, and had to figure out how to live with my health [problems] while also battling PTSD/MST. The doctors eventually removed my gallbladder thinking it was the source of all the vomiting, [but] they were wrong. By the time I got off active duty at twenty-one, I was told that I would be on a walker for the rest of my life because of a bilateral hip and knee injury from training, and the doctor told me I had the joints of an eighty-year-old. I began to have issues with debilitating migraines that added to the daily vomiting issues. My migraines were a beast: the left half of my face would swell, and I would lose vision in my left eye. All of this stress on my body started to cause my hair to fall out and become very thin.

With my first full-term pregnancy, I was diagnosed with insulin resistance, yet not a single doctor talked to me about diet because I was primarily eating the BRAT diet (bananas, rice, applesauce, toast) due to the vomiting. At twenty-six, I was involved in a car accident that changed my life drastically. I became bedridden with a spinal injury to my C3–C7 vertebrae with nerve damage. This caused me to lose all feeling and strength in my hands and arms. I lost most of my range of motion in my arms and shoulders and was told I had impact carpal tunnel. This caused severe constant pain and limited my mobility drastically. The doctors said I had to do a spinal surgery, two procedures two weeks apart, every six months for the rest of my life. My health continued to decline. I started to snore loudly, I began getting skin tags, my triglycerides went through the roof to 350+, and my skin was extremely dry and would crack and bleed. Then I noticed I was starting to struggle with shortness of breath and a racing heart. [When] I didn't think it could get any worse, my doctor told me I was on the verge of non-alcoholic fatty liver disease. He said my liver enzymes were too high; that's a red flag. Then he told me my weight (236 pounds) and the opioids I was taking were a contributing factor. At this point in my life, finding a way to keep living was all I was focused on.

In August 2022, I suffered the scariest moment of my life. I was home alone with my kids. It started with a migraine. Then everything went black in my left eye. After that I realized I couldn't speak; I couldn't move my left side at all. Luckily, I managed to move my right hand just enough to text a friend for help. At thirty-three years old, I had suffered a mild stroke.

By July 2024, I felt like my whole world had come crashing down around me. The doctor had more bad news. She said my insides looked ten years older than they should, and I might have celiac disease. So, I had even more testing. The blood test came back negative, but the other came back positive. I then had to have surgery to remove a celiac cyst in my mouth that required a bone graft and was affecting three teeth. In this process I got diagnosed with two MTHFR gene mutations as well.

At this point I was following everything the doctors were saying, but I was so tired of living in constant sickness and pain. My husband's best friend happened to mention the carnivore diet, [and] it sounded crazy to me. When my husband asked me to try it, I went off the deep end, repeating everything we have been taught our whole lives, all the propaganda we are programmed to believe. After a lot of carnivore research and anecdotal evidence, he convinced me to take the dive and do our own experiment because "what's the harm in trying it for thirty days?" Now, I have my life back. After a few weeks my vomiting stopped after fifteen years, [and] no more snoring. Slowly my depression and other mental health issues started to subside. Finally, after thirty-six spinal surgeries, I don't have to do them anymore, and the neuropathy in my hands and arms has healed. Carnivore saved my life and has given me the quality of life everyone deserves.

—Erin Fisher

My journey into carnivore didn't happen out of a massive need like so many I hear about online. I'm pretty much an average sixty-year-old woman, retired after thirty-five years of teaching. I don't have a huge amount of stress in my life. My health, I thought, was on track, but still I was curious about all of the positive things I was hearing about the carnivore way of eating. Little did I know the massive difference I was about to experience!

I was crossing the country in a van my husband and I designed and built. With lots of time on my hands, I happened upon a few podcasts promoting this lifestyle. One podcast led to a couple dozen more featuring many doctors and people that swear it changed their lives. Since I was traveling alone, I had no one to cook for or answer to, so I said, what the heck, let's give this a try.

Prior to this experiment I was basically a vegan eating fairly clean. I limited my sugar to fruits and consumed very few processed carbs. I ate lots of vegetables and took pre- and probiotics every day to keep my gut regulated. I think that's why my switch to basically beef, salt, a few eggs, and water for the first month was an easy slide. I had no keto flu symptoms, no digestive distress, no major cravings. It was pretty smooth sailing.

The things that did change included not being hungry all the time! I was a snacker prior to this. I ate carrots and hummus, cut-up fruit, smoothies, and so on. It was like I could never get filled. Within a few days of eating only beef, salt, and butter I was forgetting to eat! I settled into two meals a day for several weeks while crossing the country. One morning I woke up and realized how different my gut issues were. No longer was I swinging without warning from light diarrhea to constipation. I had become "regular" in a week! The next thing I noticed was that I was sleeping so much better! It was a deep, dreamless sleep that I slipped into so quickly, and when I woke, I was totally awake and ready to go. My energy bloomed, my hikes became longer, and then my knees began to feel so much less cranky!

Coming back home after five weeks on the road was a bit of a challenge because there were people to face. This food style is not understood in general; after all we have been taught the "food pyramid" and "limit red meat, salt, and fat" all of our lives, so the fact that I was not eating the standard American diet that everyone else was presented a concern—for them! It wasn't until I had blood work that they took a breath. My numbers looked better than they ever had. One interesting thing is that my cholesterol level has dropped!

Six months [later] I continue to walk/hike daily, lift weights at least four days a week, and foster my mental health. I have added a small amount of dairy without much effect, and I eat several different meats now. My weight was never a big driver for any of this; however, I slowly dropped about 15 pounds without losing my treasured muscle. I have lost much of that post-menopausal belly fat, and pants I thought I'd never get back into are now a bit large on me. I started with around 38% body fat. I dropped to 27.7%. My goal is to be just under 25% and see how I feel. I can work to adjust it up or down from there.

Here's the part I really wanted to share. I had told my hubby that I wanted to celebrate breaking the 30 mark on % body fat. I thought we could go out to a local wings restaurant. Lots of good carnivore stuff to eat there. This going out to eat thing is something we don't do very often for two reasons: one, it's gotten ridiculously expensive, and two, I can eat better food at home. Anyway we went and enjoyed twenty traditional wings between us with dipping sauces on the side for him and a bacon double cheeseburger without the bun and such. The burger was excellent!

I felt fine leaving the restaurant. It was nice to be out on a date night. [But] the next morning, my joints hurt so badly. My knees were so cranky, and the pain in my fingers was excruciating! Keep in mind I had changed nothing else. If I was not so aware of my body at this point, I would've had no idea the connection. It took me three days to get the seed oils those wings were fried in out of my system. It affected my sleep with disturbing dreams and nasty calf pain off!

I think so many people walk around in so much pain, mental fog, high blood pressure, diabetes, depression, anxiety, and have no idea the root cause of so much of it. They think they are getting older and it's just how it is. Those are just physical signs. That's not blood work showing what's really happening inside the body.

The reason I agreed to write about my carnivore journey is I just want to shout it from the rooftops! You don't have to hurt so badly all the time. You can become less dependent on big pharma. You can choose a very different path that will allow you to get back in touch with your body's natural healing abilities. You don't have to live in their fog! It all comes down to choice!

—Jo Hagerty

I am fifty-five years old and have been following carnivore for seven months. I prefer to refer to it as a lifestyle rather than a diet, as I have previously attempted various diets for weight loss, only to regain the weight once the diet ended. By calling it a lifestyle, I emphasize that this is my new way of living, not just a temporary fad.

Regrettably, I am unable to share before-and-after photographs, as I did not consider taking them when I commenced this journey. I was not pleased with my appearance and was concerned about the need to increase my pants size and the potential for developing obesity, high cholesterol, and diabetes. For the past four years, my medical professionals have expressed concerns about my cholesterol levels, and my blood sugar levels have placed me at risk of developing prediabetes.

Three years ago, my mother passed away, and this year, my father passed away. These events served as a wakeup call for me. On March 12, I weighed 230.8 pounds and am 5-foot-10. The carnivore lifestyle appealed to me because I genuinely enjoy consuming beef, pork, and lamb. While I am able to eat two or three meals a day on this diet, I wondered if I could achieve satiety and maintain a healthy weight.

Fast-forward seven months, and I can affirm that the answer is a resounding "yes." While I have indulged in two cheat days which made me feel ill, [overall] I have experienced significant positive changes. My waist size has decreased from a 38 to a 33, and I have had to replace all of my clothing. I have also lost 39.8 pounds. This has been a transformative experience, and I am committed to continuing this lifestyle for the long term.

Adopting the carnivore lifestyle has significantly improved my overall health. I have undergone two blood tests, and after my blood test in August, my doctor reported positive improvements. I am no longer prediabetic and believe that continuing this lifestyle, as it appears to be beneficial for my body, is the appropriate course of action.

—Jonathan Tripp

I started my carnivore journey on January 4, 2024. I weighed 149.6 pounds. Since I was already fat adapted from experimenting with keto and intermittent fasting, I went all in (not recommended for first-time participants). I was strict carnivore eating nothing but beef, bacon, butter, and eggs. I was not hungry at all, and some days I effortlessly ate only one meal. By the end of the month, I was down to about 138. Then I got the flu and the only thing that tasted good was fruit. For the next two weeks I gained back a bunch of weight (think high blood sugar), but as soon as I recovered, I returned to the carnivore diet. By mid-March I was down to about 135.

Not long ago, my son asked me about a particular supplement to help him lose weight. I told him that all those "super supplements" don't work. It has to be a lifestyle change, and the best thing he could do was the carnivore diet. Taking after his dad, he went all in. It was a bit uncomfortable for him at first as he had been eating the standard American diet, but he dropped from 152 to 142 in less than a month. He was amazed that his dad was right.

—Steve Gould

I've been a carnivore for five years. Prior to that I did low carb for a little over two years and found many benefits. I got off my cholesterol and blood pressure meds. I also got off my CPAP machine. [But] I still had many binges and joint pain.

I heard about carnivore from Dr. Ken Berry and Kelly Hogan, and I jumped in. The ankle pain I'd had for a few weeks was gone in three days! I sleep so much better without tossing and turning all night in pain. Of course, the 60 pounds that I have lost since low carb and carnivore has been awesome.

At age sixty-five I go to the gym, kayak, bike, hike, snowshoe, play pickleball. and am active with my grandkids. I'm not going back to the standard American diet!

—Karen Miles

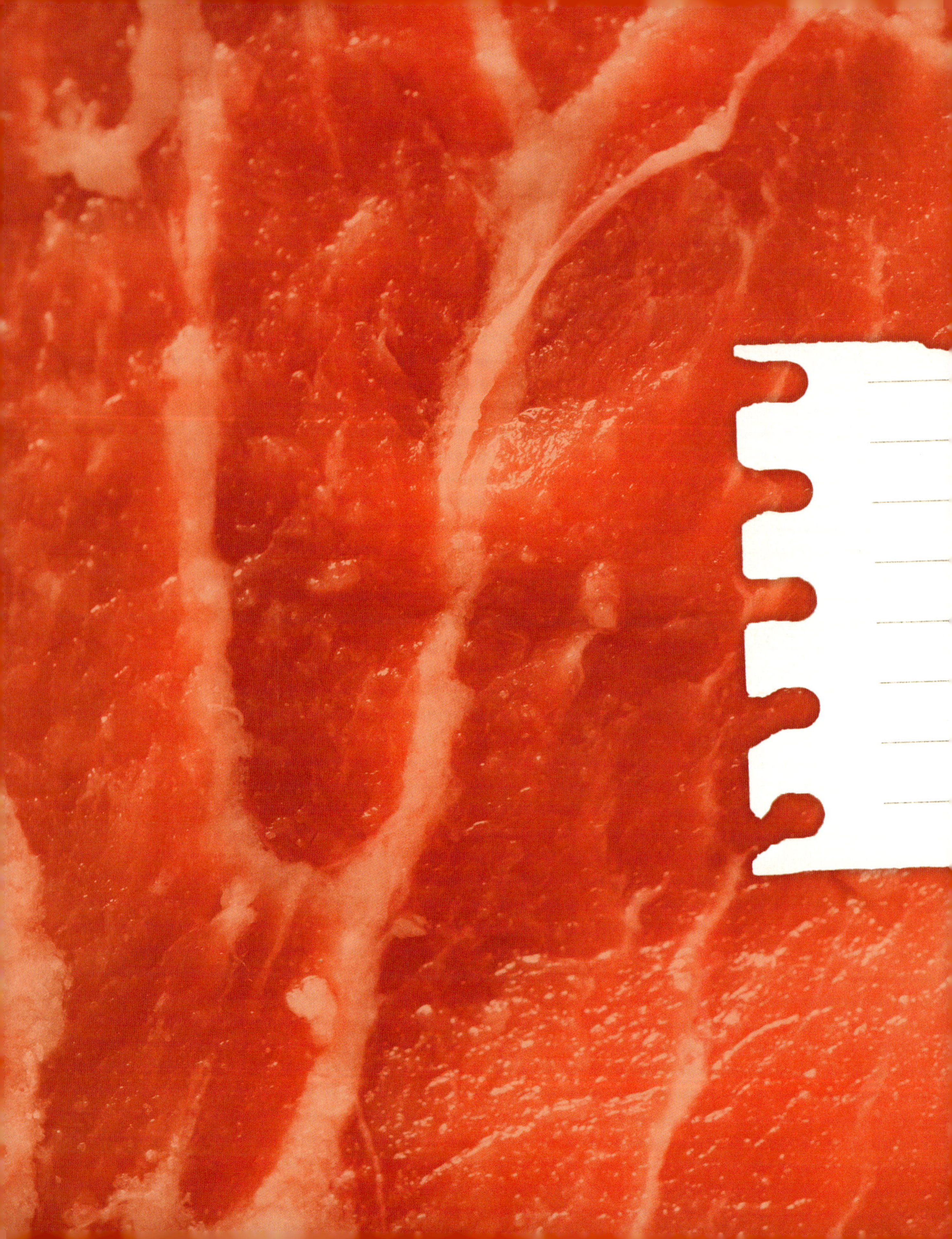

PART 1

A COMPREHENSIVE GUIDE TO THE CARNIVORE DIET

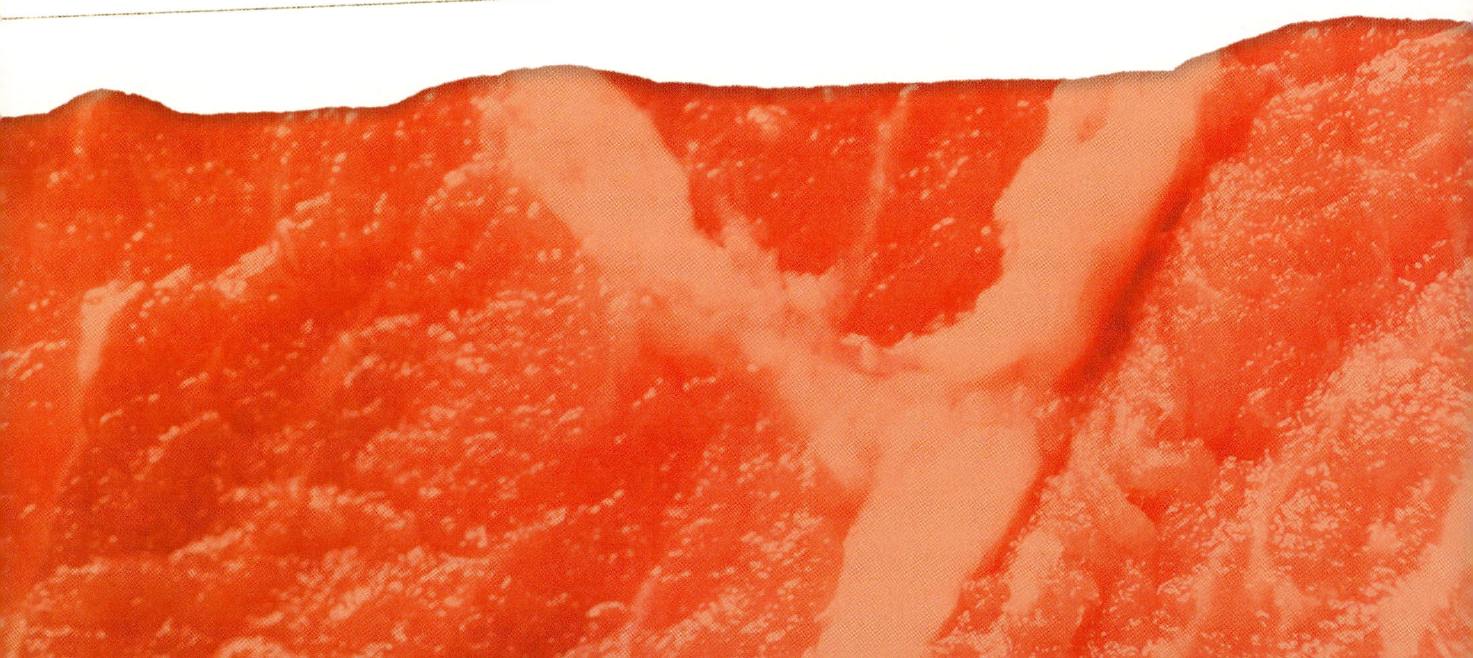

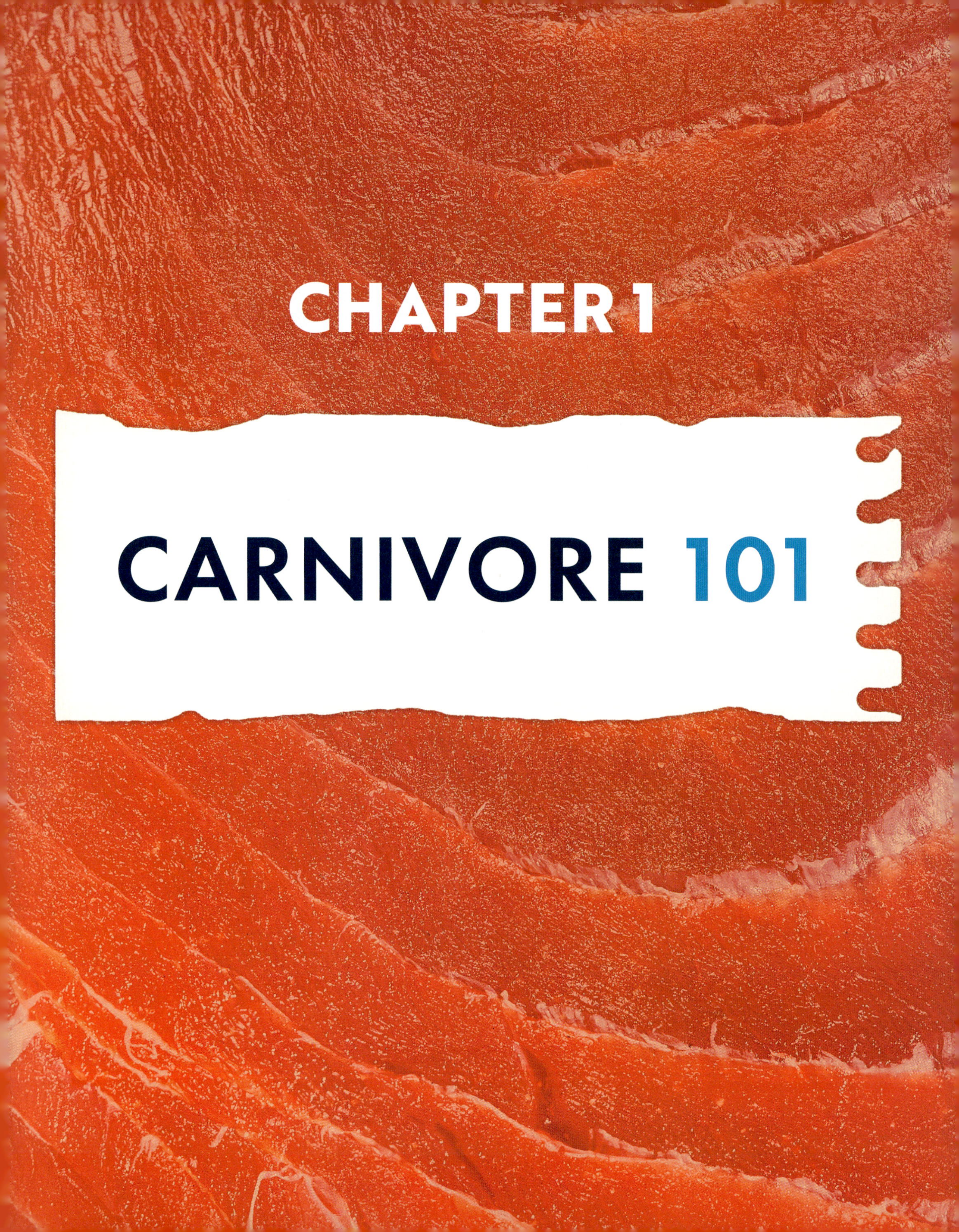

CHAPTER 1

CARNIVORE 101

The carnivore diet is a way of eating that focuses on meat and animal products as the sole sources of sustenance. It is considered a ketogenic diet. A ketogenic diet is a high-fat, very low-carbohydrate eating plan that shifts the body into a state of ketosis, where it burns fat for fuel instead of carbs. Carnivore is typically the lowest-carbohydrate ketogenic diet you can do. Some people consume zero carbohydrates in their version of carnivore. (You'll read about the different versions in chapter 2.)

When building any kind of diet, you consume some mix of three macronutrients: carbohydrates, protein, and fat. These macronutrients provide your body with the fuel and building blocks it needs so that it can function in a metabolically healthy way.

Carbohydrates are broken down into glucose in the body, which raises blood sugar levels. While humans *can* consume carbohydrates, carbs are not *required* for life. You will not die if you don't eat carbs. Your body can manufacture all of the glucose it needs. That leaves us with the other two macronutrients: protein and fat. You could die if you didn't eat protein or fat for a long enough period. Carnivores meet their protein and fat needs using animal sources and exclude most carbohydrates.

But why choose animal proteins and fats over plant-based proteins and fats? Why cut plants or carbohydrates from your diet?

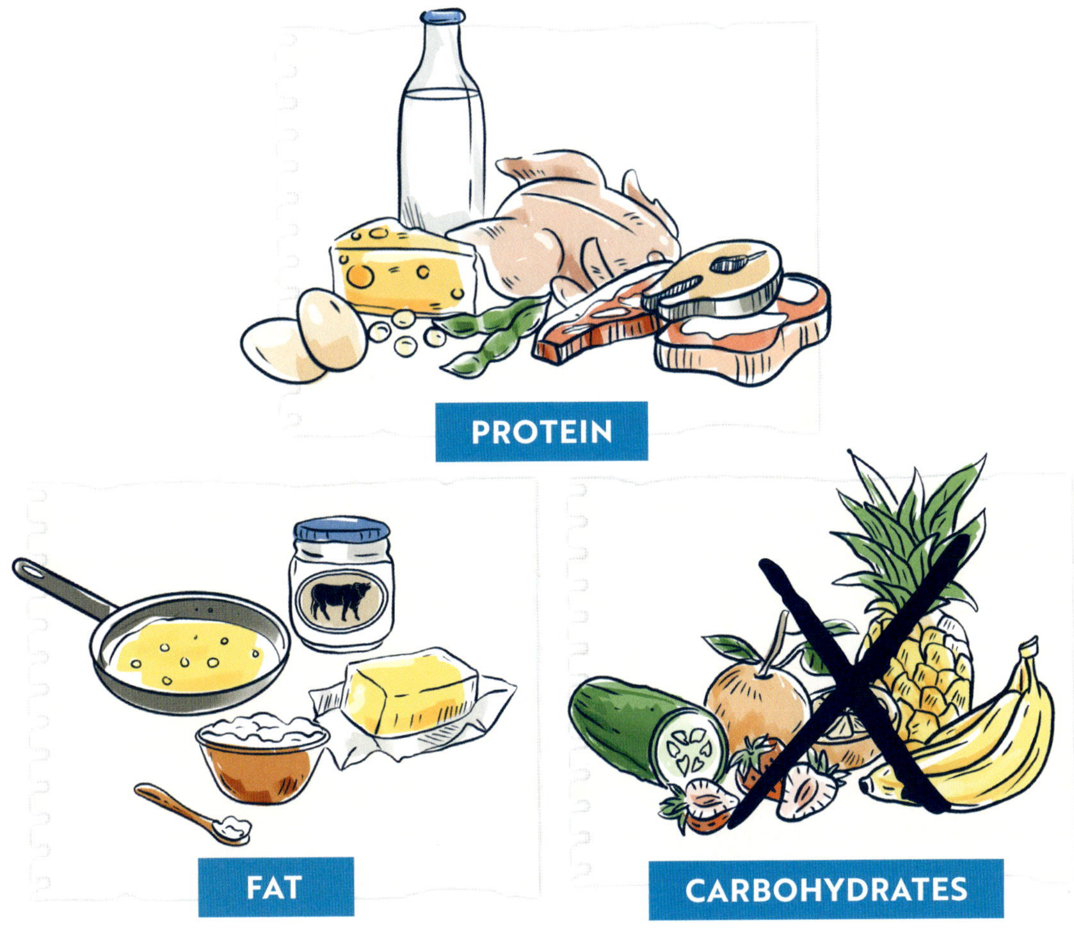

WHY CARNIVORE WORKS

Starting with protein, it boils down to **bioavailability**. Proteins sourced from animals are broken down more efficiently by the body and are absorbed better than plant-based proteins. This is partly due to their highly digestible nature. Proteins are broken down into amino acids, of which there are twenty. Nine are considered essential amino acids because they need to be gotten from food; your body is unable to manufacture them itself.

Animal proteins are *complete proteins*, which means they contain all nine essential amino acids that are the building blocks of your muscles, bones, and internal organs. Most plant proteins are incomplete, meaning they do not contain all nine essential amino acids. Even if they do contain all nine, as is the case with soybeans, those amino acids are not as bioavailable as the ones in meat. Your body simply cannot utilize them as easily, if at all.

The twenty amino acids that comprise proteins are alanine, arginine, asparagine, aspartic acid, cysteine, glutamic acid, glutamine, glycine, histidine, isoleucine, leucine, lysine, methionine, phenylalanine, proline, serine, threonine, tryptophan, tyrosine, and valine.

Among these twenty amino acids, nine are essential: phenylalanine, valine, tryptophan, threonine, isoleucine, methionine, histidine, leucine, and lysine.

Amino Acids

NONESSENTIAL	ESSENTIAL
ALANINE	PHENYLALANINE
ARGININE	VALINE
ASPARAGINE	TRYPTOPHAN
ASPARTIC ACID	THREONINE
CYSTEINE	ISOLEUCINE
GLUTAMIC ACID	METHIONINE
GLUTAMINE	HISTIDINE
GLYCINE	LEUCINE
PROLINE	LYSINE
SERINE	
TYROSINE	

Animal fats are also highly bioavailable and are the perfect fuel source for the human body. Fats are broken down into glycerol and fatty acids, which in turn are broken down into *ketone bodies*, a highly efficient fuel.[1] (I will talk a lot more about ketones later in the book.) Fat also helps you synthesize essential hormones such as estrogen, testosterone, and thyroid hormone and aids in the formation of fat-soluble vitamins such as A, D, E, and K. Animal fats are anti-inflammatory, and our bodies are perfectly adapted to use them.

While there are a lot of plant fats out there, most of them do not exist in nature; they are created in factories using lots of chemicals, bleaching, high pressure, and heat. Specifically, vegetable seed oils are basically industrial lubricants that were repurposed into food products so that the corporations producing them could make more money. If you ever saw the way these oils are produced, you would not consume them.[2] They are highly inflammatory to the human body.[3]

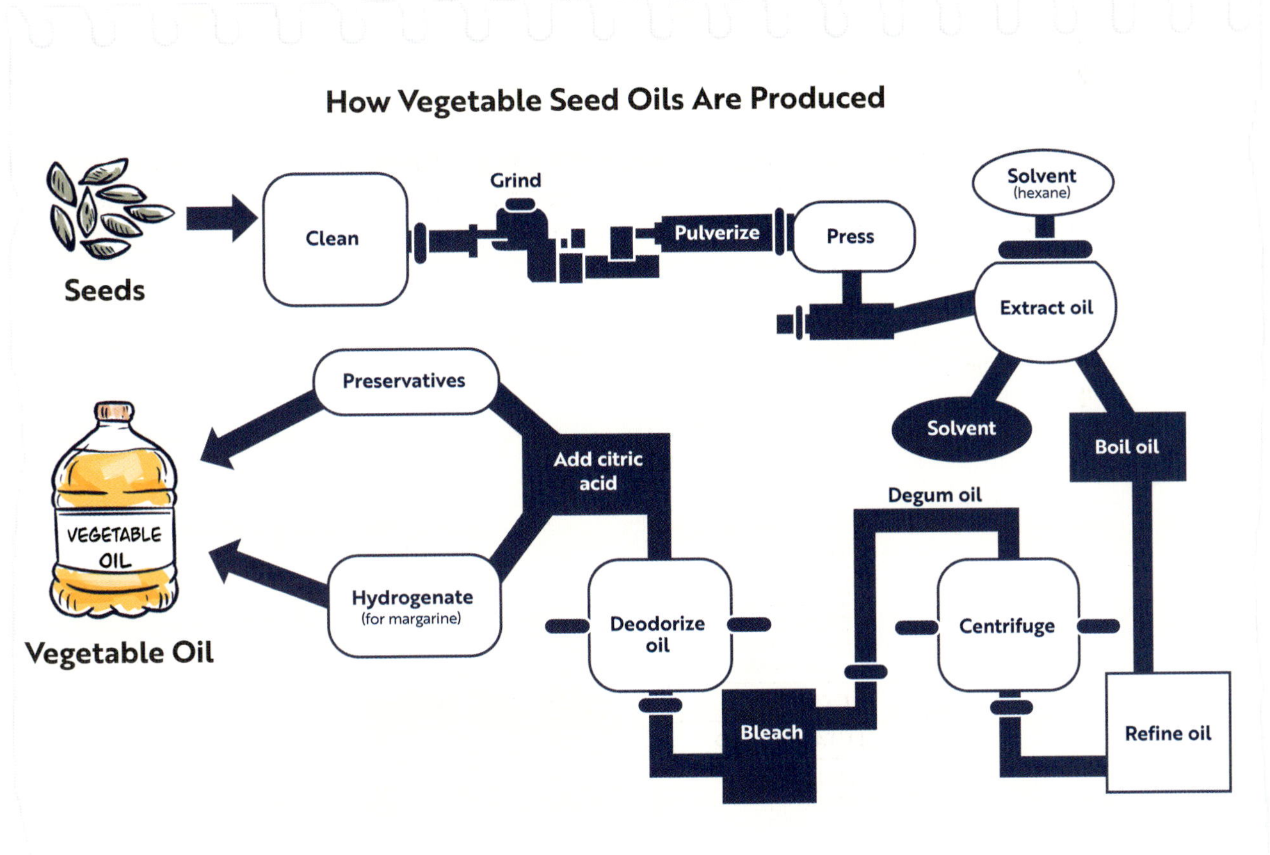

---

[1] Caleb B. Cantrell and Shamim S. Mohiuddin, "Biochemistry, ketone metabolism," In: StatPearls, https://www.ncbi.nlm.nih.gov/books/NBK554523/.

[2] Catherine Shanahan, *Dark Calories: How Vegetable Oils Destroy Our Health and How We Can Get It Back* (New York: Hachette Books, 2024): 9–12.

[3] Shanahan, *Dark Calories*: 12–27.

But bioavailability of nutrients isn't the only reason to exclude plants from your diet. Another great reason is the **phytochemicals**, or plant toxins, that many plants contain. Did you know that plants do not want to be eaten? They can't run away like animals, so they protect themselves by engaging in chemical warfare! Lectins, oxalates, tannins, and other natural phytochemicals are found in many of the plants we eat, sometimes at very high levels. That green smoothie made with spinach is causing more damage than you might think, including digestive distress, inflammation, skin conditions, brain fog or mood problems, kidney issues, gout, and more.[4]

When you consume plant material, you are dealing with not only the natural phytotoxins but also the massive amounts of **pesticides** that are used to grow conventional produce. According to the Environmental Protection Agency, 280 million pounds of glyphosate are applied to an average of 298 million acres of crop land annually in the United States.[5] Glyphosate (also known by its brand name, Roundup) has been linked to neurological disorders,[6] gastrointestinal issues,[7] liver inflammation,[8] and respiratory effects,[9] and its residue is present on a large proportion of our conventional produce supply. Organic fruits and vegetables aren't completely pesticide free, either. Though not sprayed with the same pesticides as their conventionally grown counterparts, plenty of organic produce is treated with pesticides that utilize some of those same phytotoxins. Also, organic farms can be affected by pesticide drift from nearby conventional farms.[10] Organic farmers cannot control the wind.

Years of tillage-based agriculture and monoculture have decimated our soil and stripped it of nutrients.[11] Monoculture is the agricultural practice of growing a single crop or plant species over a large area. It can lead to reduced biodiversity and increased vulnerability to pests and disease. Because of **declining soil health**, the produce we consume today is not as nutrient dense as produce used to be. If the soil in which a plant is grown is depleted of nutrients, the plant itself cannot contain those nutrients.

---

[4] Sally K. Norton, *Toxic Superfoods: How Oxalate Overload Is Making You Sick—and How to Get Better* (New York: Rodale Books, 2023): 9–10.

[5] United States Environmental Protection Agency, https://www.epa.gov/sites/default/files/2019-04/documents/glyphosate-response-comments-usage-benefits-final.pdf.

[6] Carmen Costas-Ferreira et al., "Toxic effects of glyphosate on the nervous system: A systematic review." *International Journal of Molecular Sciences* 23, no. 9 (2022): 4605.

[7] Pere Puigbò et al., "Does glyphosate affect the human microbiota?" *Life* (Basel, Switzerland) 12, no. 5 (2022): 707.

[8] Brenda Eskenazi et al., "Association of lifetime exposure to glyphosate and aminomethylphosphonic acid (AMPA) with liver inflammation and metabolic syndrome at young adulthood: Findings from the CHAMACOS study," *Environmental Health Perspectives* 131, no. 3 (2023): 37001.

[9] "Glyphosate—ToxFAQs" https://www.atsdr.cdc.gov/toxfaqs/tfacts214.pdf.

[10] Joanna Ory, "Avoiding pesticide drift impacts on organic farms." Organic Farming Research Association, 2017, https://ofrf.org/wp-content/uploads/2019/09/OFRF.Pesticide.Drift_.pdf.

[11] Rolf Derpsch et al., "Nature's laws of declining soil productivity and conservation agriculture," *Soil Security* 14 (2024): 100127.

Good vs. Compacted Soil

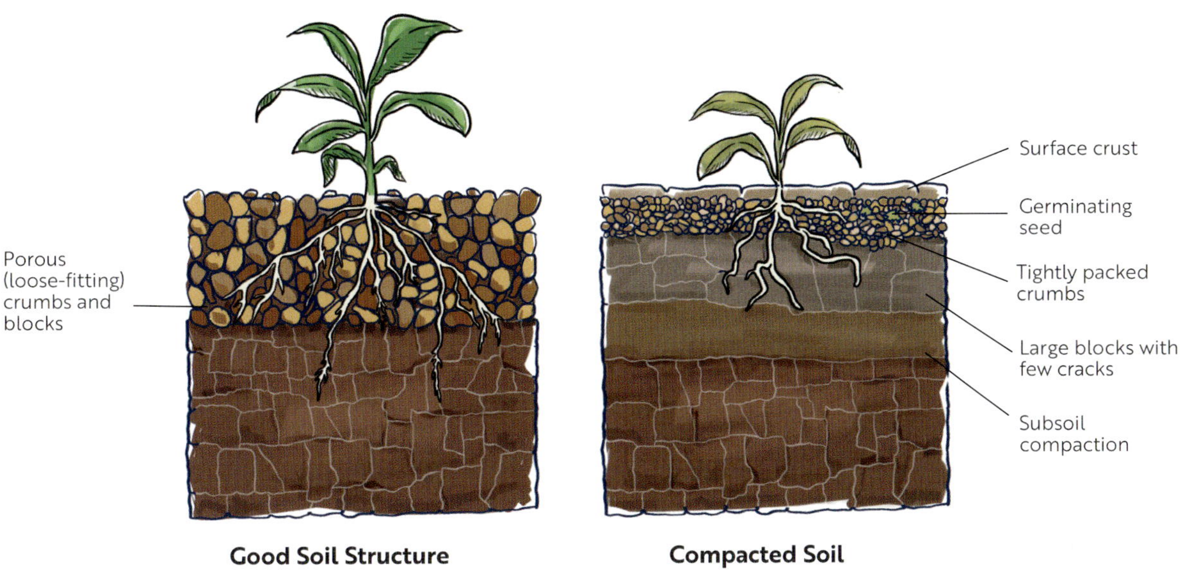

Healthy Soil Matrix

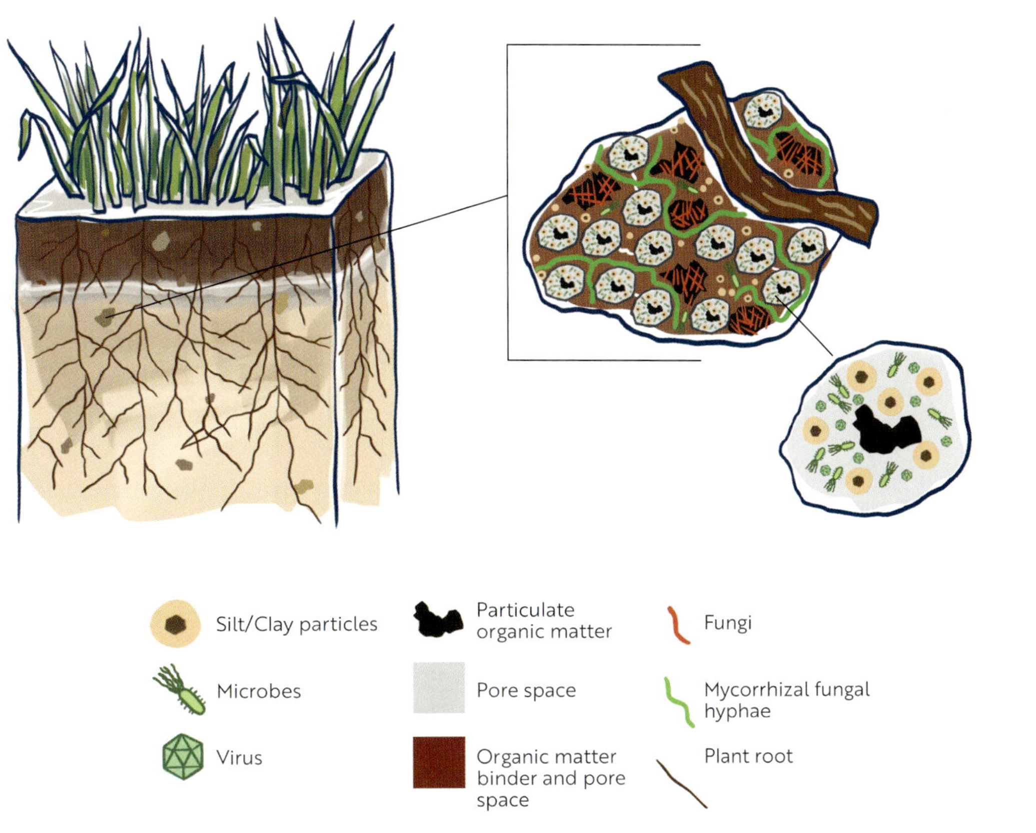

You may worry that once you get rid of all plant foods, you won't be left with much in the way of vitamins and minerals. We have been indoctrinated to think that vitamins and minerals come from the plants we eat, but the truth is that most of them come from the meat we consume. Meat and other animal products are the best sources of protein and fat while being the most nutrient-dense foods on the planet.

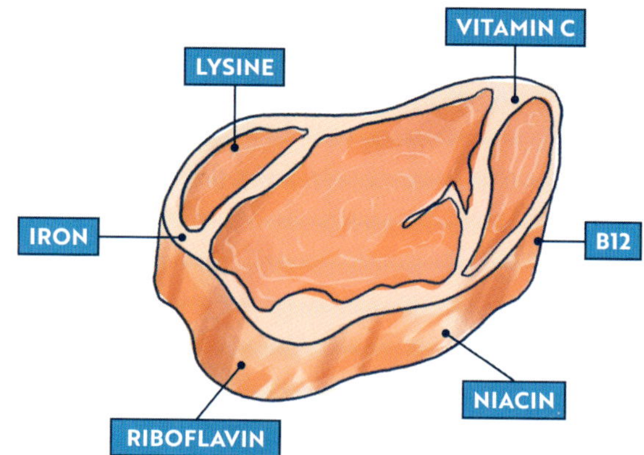

Another benefit of excluding plants is getting rid of the sugar in your diet. A lot of people don't realize that plants = carbs = sugar. Our bloodstreams only circulate the equivalent of 1 teaspoon of sugar in the form of glucose at a time.[12] It doesn't take much plant material to raise your blood sugar to dysfunctional levels. One of the cornerstones of metabolic dysfunction is chronically elevated blood glucose. We are simply not meant to consume sugar all the time, even in modest amounts. Your body manufactures all of the glucose it needs.

While avoiding plant foods can improve your blood glucose levels drastically, the carbs and sugar in some lettuce or a strawberry aren't what get most people to a state of metabolic disorder. The main culprit is ultra-processed foods, which are filled with carbohydrates, added sugars, seed oils, shelf stabilizers, and other chemicals. **Ultra-processed foods are not real food**, even though they may look like it. They are designed to be addictive and never fully satisfying, leading to cravings for more. They lack the essential nutrients humans require for optimal health and cause harm over time. If you are consuming a diet full of ultra-processed foods, it is entirely possible to be malnourished despite being overweight or obese. The biggest benefit of the carnivore diet is its lack of ultra-processed foods. Ultra-processed foods have no place in this way of eating. ("Ultra-processed" and "processed" are different things, and I will touch on that distinction later in the book.)

Simply put, the carnivore diet is a human species–appropriate way of eating that allows us to regain and maintain our metabolic health and enjoy a higher quality of life due to the nutrient bioavailability of meat and animal products along with the lack of phytotoxins, pesticides, added sugars, and ultra-processed food products. As leading carnivore advocate Dr. Ken Berry says on his YouTube channel, carnivore is the Proper Human Diet.

Why Carnivore Works

- Bioavailability of nutrients
- Eliminates plant toxins
- Eliminates pesticides
- Eliminates added sugar
- Eliminates ultra-processed foods
- Meat is the most nutrient-dense food on the planet
- Evolutionarily appropriate for humans

---

[12] World Health Organization, "Mean fasting blood glucose," https://www.who.int/data/gho/indicator-metadata-registry/imr-details/2380, accessed April 8, 2025.

ANCESTRAL ORIGINS OF CARNIVORE

Let's briefly return to the ancestral origins of a meat-based diet. According to an abundance of anthropological data, human diets have been primarily meat based since our ancestors began migrating from the trees to bipedalism around 2.6 million years ago.

Some of the strongest evidence that early humans ate meat comes from marks found on animal bones—cuts from sharp tools and dents from breaking bones open to get the marrow inside.[13] Fossils from early human relatives like *Australopithecus* and *Paranthropus* show signs of meat-eating as far back as 2 million years ago in places like Kanjera, Kenya.[14] Scientists can also study chemical markers in ancient bones to learn about diets; these tests show that Neanderthals ate mostly land animals, while some early modern humans also ate a lot of seafood.[15]

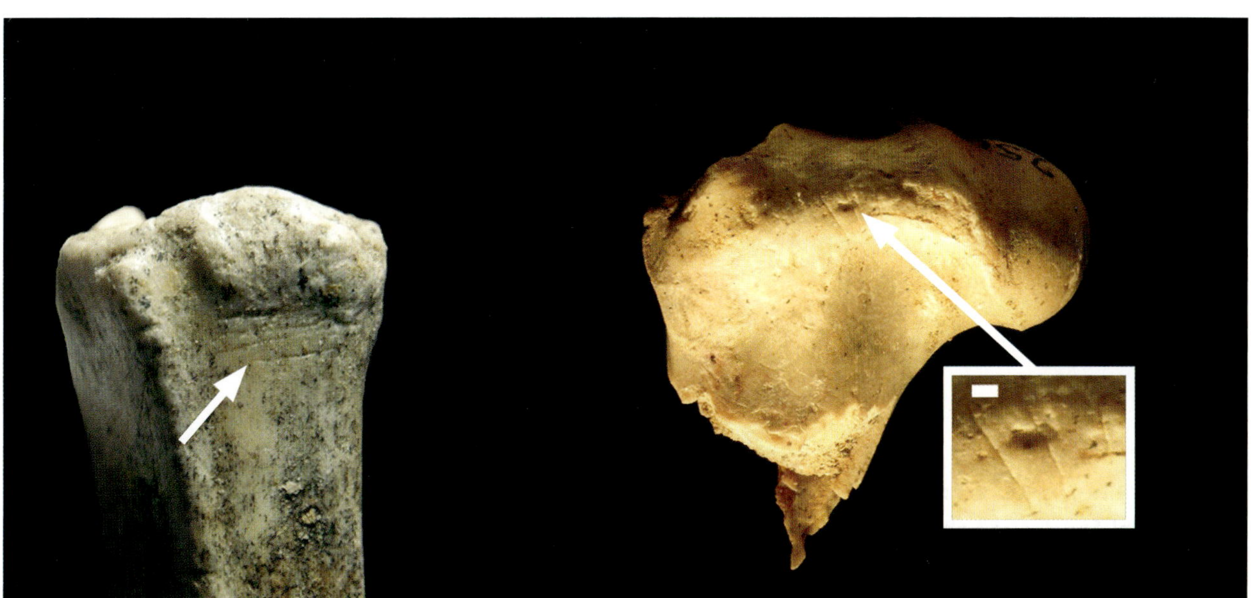

Kanjera Bone A by Joseph V. Ferraro, Thomas W. Plummer, Briana L. Pobiner, James S. Oliver, Laura C. Bishop, David R. Braun, Peter W. Ditchfield, John W. Seaman III, Katie M. Binetti, John W. Seaman Jr., Fritz Hertel, and Richard Potts, licensed under CC BY 4.0, via Wikimedia Commons.

Kanjera Bone D by Joseph V. Ferraro, Thomas W. Plummer, Briana L. Pobiner, James S. Oliver, Laura C. Bishop, David R. Braun, Peter W. Ditchfield, John W. Seaman III, Katie M. Binetti, John W. Seaman Jr, Fritz Hertel, and Richard Potts, licensed under CC BY 4.0, via Wikimedia Commons.

---

[13] Briana Pobiner, "Evidence of meat-eating by early humans," *Nature Education Knowledge* 4, no. 6 (2013): 1.

[14] Joseph V. Ferraro et al., "Earliest archaeological evidence of persistent hominin carnivory," *PLOS One* 8, no. 4 (2013): e62174.

[15] Michael P. Richards and Erik Trinkaus, "Isotopic evidence for the diets of European Neanderthals and early humans," *PNAS* 106, no. 38 (2009): 16034–16039.

We also see the importance of animals as a main food source in the art that these ancient peoples created. They weren't making cave paintings about salad; they were memorializing hunting scenes. At the famous Lascaux cave in France, paintings and engravings of bison, deer, aurochs, ibex, and horses decorate the chambers.[16] Some of the walls are sixteen feet high, and the highest points must have required some sort of scaffolding to reach. It has been hypothesized that there may have been a shamanistic purpose to these paintings, or perhaps the artists were commemorating hunts or even using the paintings to teach younger members of the tribe how to hunt effectively.

A recent study looked at some peculiar marks that appear in a lot of these cave paintings. These sequences of dots, lines, and Y-shapes seem to indicate when a particular animal would be in mating or birthing season. This would have been important information to the hunters, as it is much easier to harvest an animal from a herd than a solitary animal.[17]

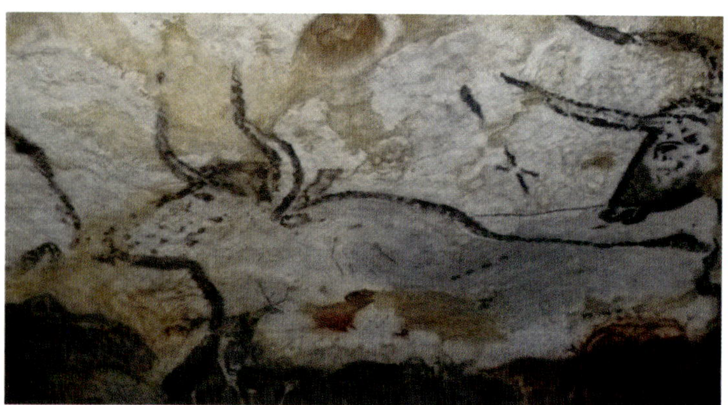

Interior of the Lascaux cave (Lascaux 004.jpg) by JoJan, licensed under CC BY 4.0, via Wikimedia Commons.

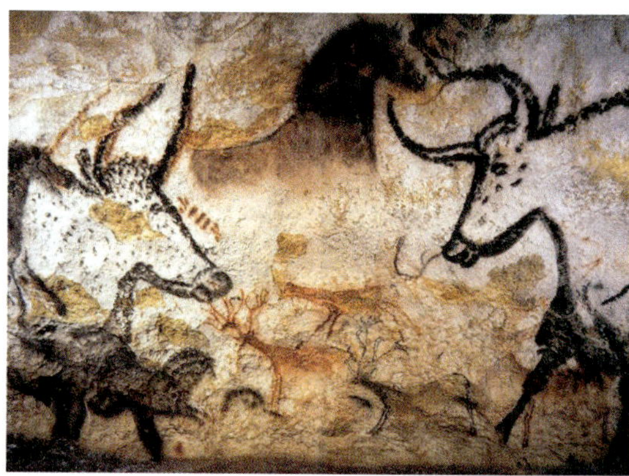

Lascaux painting by EU, licensed under CC BY 3.0, via Wikimedia Commons.

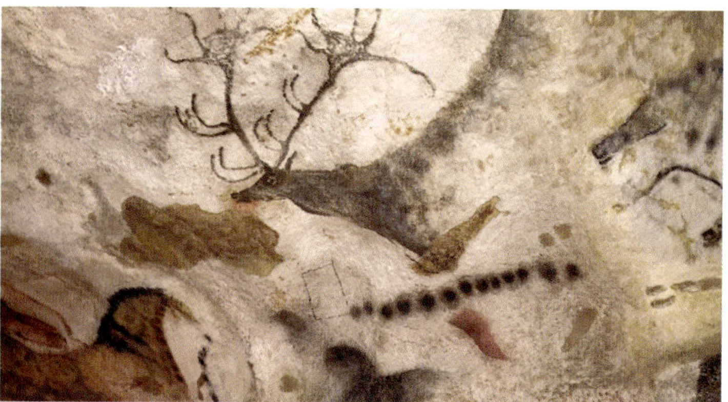

Élan aux bois 2.jpg by Codex, licensed under CC BY 4.0, via Wikimedia Commons.

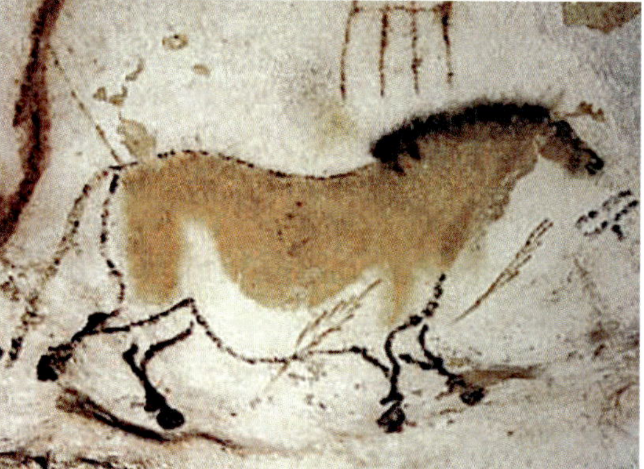

Höhle von Lascaux, public domain, via Wikimedia Commons.

[16] Laura Ann Tedesco. "Lascaux (ca. 15,000 B.C.)." The Met, October 1, 2000. https://www.metmuseum.org/toah/hd/lasc/hd_lasc.htm.
[17] Bennett Bacon et al., "An upper Palaeolithic proto-writing system and phenological calendar," *Cambridge Archaeological Journal* 33, no. 3 (2023): 371–89.

Another possible piece of evidence of humans' insatiable desire for meat and animal fats is the extinction of the megafauna of the Ice Age: woolly mammoths, mastodons, giant sloths, cave bears, and saber-toothed tigers.[18] A leading theory is that these species were hunted to extinction, though other theories include rapid climate change or a catastrophic comet impact.[19] It may even have been a mix of these causes. But evidence has been found that these animals were often on the menu for the people who coexisted with them.

The layout and function of the human digestive system also suggest a mostly meat-based past. According to a study published in *Current Anthropology*, over millions of years, the human digestive system changed from being better at digesting plants to being better at digesting meat, and today we have very acidic stomachs to help break down animal foods.[20] Humans have highly acidic stomach acid with a pH of 1.5 to 2.0.[21] This level of acidity is similar to that of other carnivores and scavengers and is helpful for digesting meat and animal fats. Another noteworthy anatomical feature of the human digestive system is our small cecum, which is a pouchlike structure at the beginning of the large intestine. In herbivores, the cecum is much larger to allow for the fermentation of cellulose or plant materials, among other things.[22] Humans have evolved to no longer need this large fermentation chamber because our species moved away from plant-based diets millions of years ago.

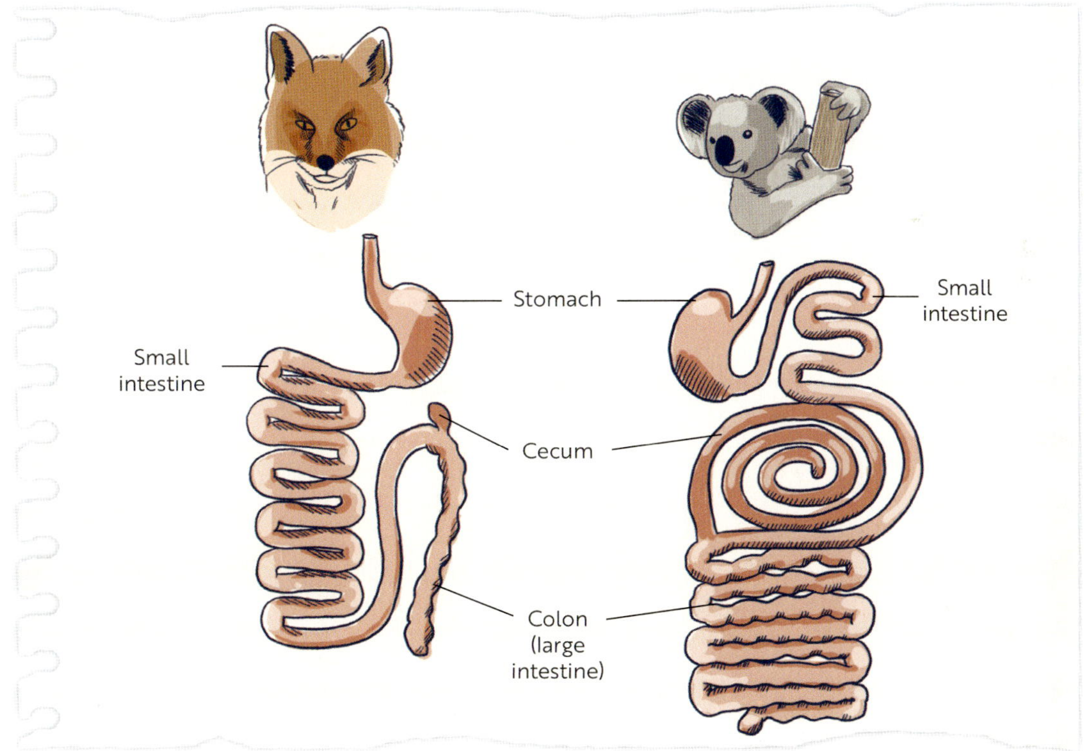

[18] Leoma Williams, "10 Ice Age animals: Meet the extraordinary prehistoric beasts that survived when the world was frozen," *Discover Wildlife*, March 3, 2025.

[19] Christopher R. Moore, "Forensic evidence suggests Paleo-Americans hunted mastodons, mammoths and other megafauna in eastern North America 13,000 years ago," *The Conversation*, University of South Carolina, June 14, 2023, https://sc.edu/uofsc/posts/2023/06/hunting_mammoth.php.

[20] Leslie C. Aiello and Peter Wheeler, "The expensive-tissue hypothesis: The brain and the digestive system in human and primate evolution," *Current Anthropology* 36, no. 2 (1995): 199–221.

[21] DeAnna E. Beasley et al., "The evolution of stomach acidity and its relevance to the human microbiome," *PLOS One* 10, no. 7 (2015): e0134116.

[22] "Cecum," *Science Direct*, https://www.sciencedirect.com/topics/agricultural-and-biological-sciences/cecum.

Human Digestive System

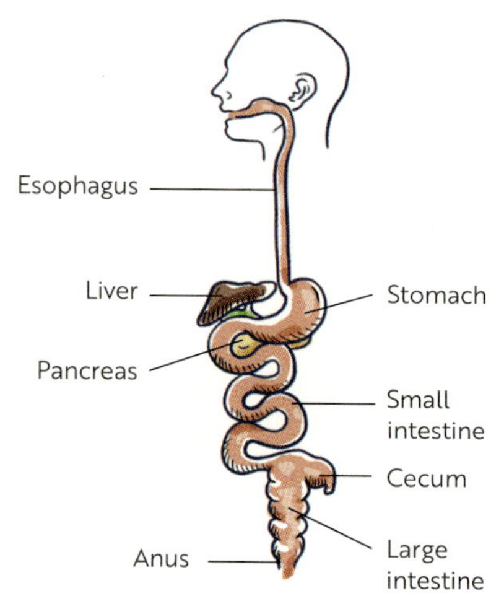

Rabbit Digestive System

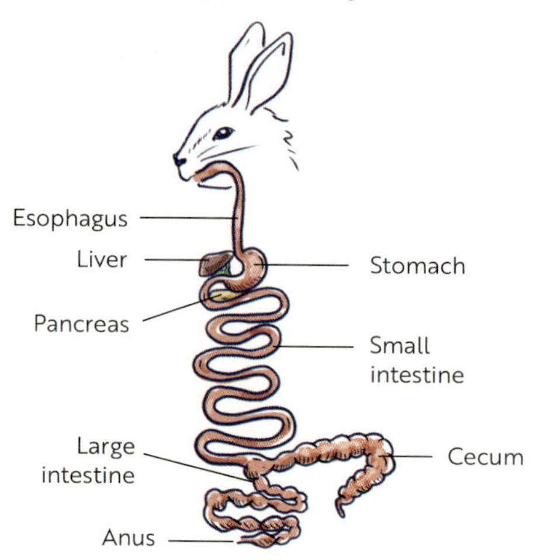

Non-ruminant Herbivore

Simple stomach, large cecum

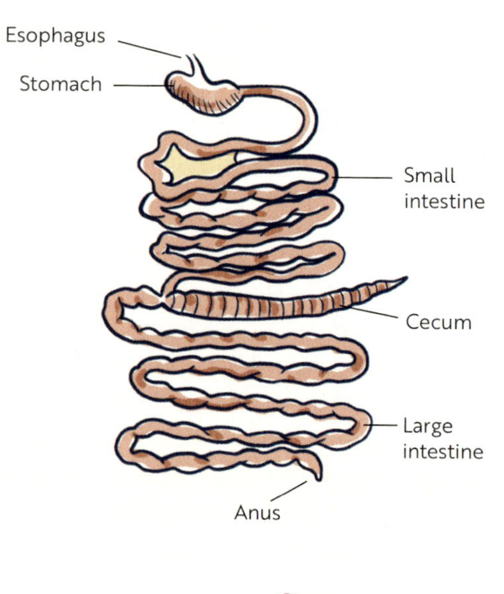

Ruminant Herbivore

Four-chambered stomach with large rumen; long small and large intestines

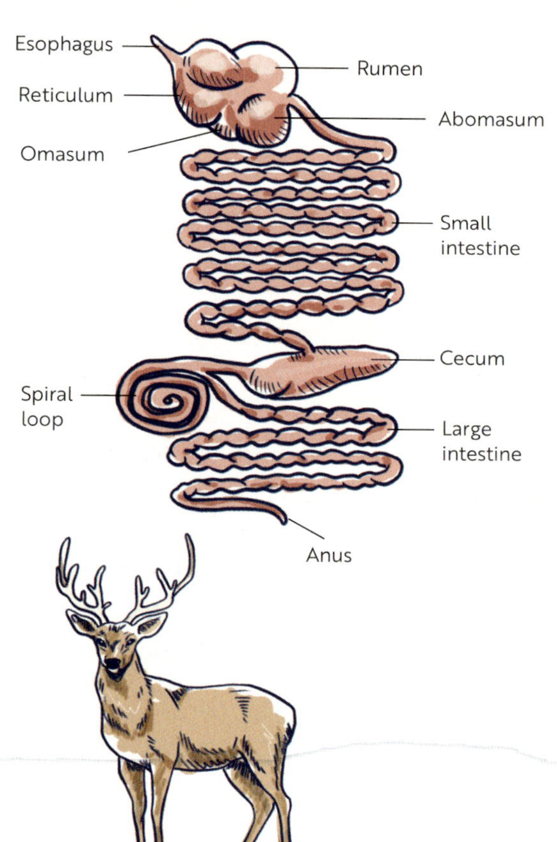

There are more modern examples of meat-based diets, too. We have in-depth knowledge of the Inuit because of an anthropologist named Vilhjalmur Stefansson. Starting in 1906, he spent twelve years on and off living with them and eating like them. The Inuit ate plants only if there was a famine or, for inland tribes, when certain berries were ripe in the springtime. The main sources of food for the Inuit were caribou, fish, eggs, seals, rabbits, moose, beavers, mountain sheep, polar bears, and whales. They favored fattier cuts of meat as well as bone marrow from specific areas of the animal. The lean meats and most of the organs were fed to the dogs.[23]

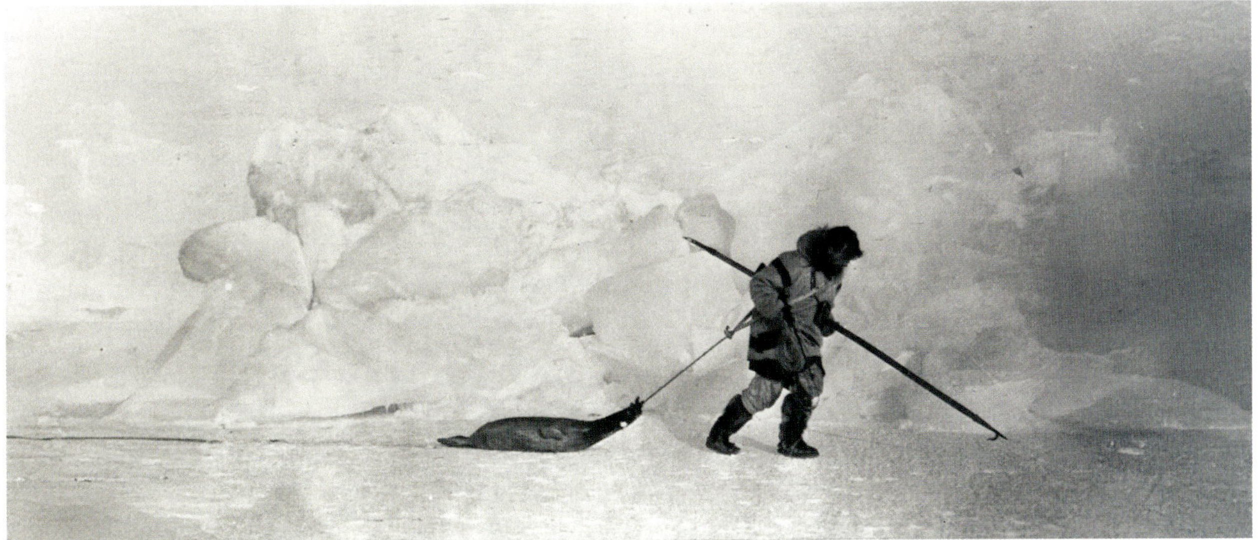

Adapted from *"Vilhjalmur Stefansson pulling a dead seal near Martin Point"* by George H. Wilkins, licensed under CC BY-SA 4.0, via Wikimedia Commons.

Another recent example of meat-based diet adherents are the Maasai. This East African tribe traditionally lived on meat, blood, milk, fat, honey, and tree bark.[24] The measures of a tribesman's wealth were the numbers of cattle and children he had. The Maasai are significantly taller than the worldwide average and do not suffer from chronic diseases when eating their traditional diet. Interestingly, when the Maasai transitioned to more carb-heavy, processed-food diets, their metabolic health declined, and they experienced increases in BMI and diabetes.[25]

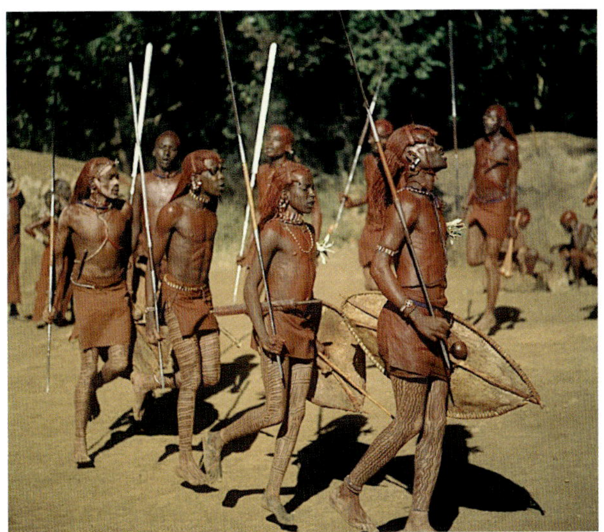

Original image by H. W. van Rinsum. Uploaded by Mark Cartwright, published on 18 November 2019. CC BY-SA 4.0, via worldhistory.org.

[23] Vilhjalmur Stefansson, *Not by Bread Alone* (Brattleboro, Vermont: Echo Point Books & Media, 2017): 15–39.

[24] "Maasai Tribe," https://www.masaimara.travel/maasai-tribe-facts.php.

[25] Mariel Pressler et al., "Dietary transitions and health outcomes in four populations—Systematic review," *Frontiers in Nutrition* 9 (2022): 748305.

These are just a few examples of our carnivorous roots. Humans relied on meat and animal products for the bulk of their calories until the advent of agriculture. It's no coincidence that once grains became the foundation of human diets, people became shorter in stature[26] and chronic disease started to take hold.[27]

I would like you to consider a few other things before we move on to the therapeutic uses of an animal-based diet. First, when our ancestors consumed plants, it was only when they were in season. Ancient peoples didn't have refrigerators or grocery stores. So, when berries were ripe, people gorged on them for a couple of weeks and then did not eat them again until the following year. Similarly, honey was consumed only when a hive was discovered. It took quite a bit of effort and time to get the bees to surrender their hive, with the risk of injury and death. Ancient people didn't eat honey every day. Again, they would find a hive on occasion, partake of the honey, and that was the end of it.

Second, the fruits and vegetables that exist today are different from what our ancient or even more recent ancestors would have consumed. We have hybridized and grafted our way to monster-sized fruits and vegetables that are hyper-palatable. For example, wild bananas are full of seeds and nowhere near as sweet as the bananas you and I would recognize. Watermelons used to have a lot more rind and many more seeds. Wild strawberries are small and bitter.

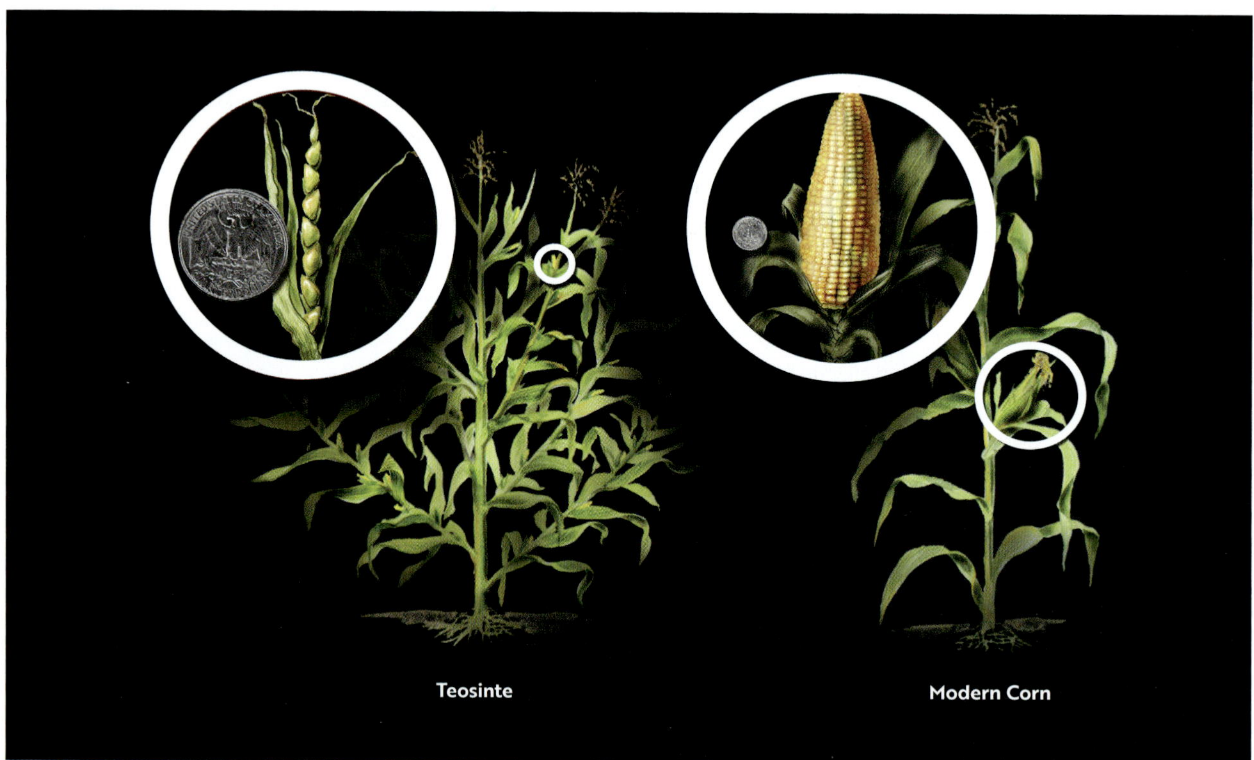

Teosinte and Modern Corn Comparison by the National Science Foundation, public domain, via Wikimedia Commons.

---

[26] Stephanie Marciniak et al., "An integrative skeletal and paleogenomic analysis of stature variation suggests relatively reduced health for early European farmers," PNAS 119, no. 15 (2022): e2106743119.

[27] Valerie Ross, "Early farmers were sicker and shorter than their forager ancestors," *Discover*, June 17, 2011.

Third, you can peruse cookbooks from the past few hundred years to see what people were preparing. Most of the surviving cookbooks from the 1500s to the 1800s focus on meat-heavy dishes, with vegetables as garnishes or sides or used in stews.[28] Roasted veal, a baked venison tart, and a shoulder of mutton were not out of the ordinary.[29] Why? Because meat has always been considered the most important part of a meal, and because it is always available, regardless of the season.

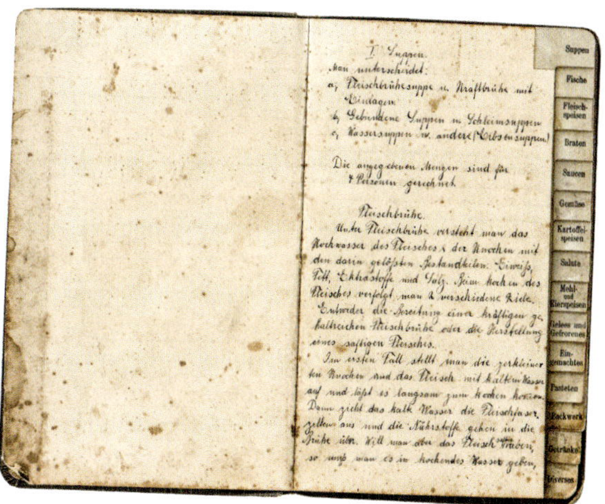

HOW ANIMAL-BASED DIETS HAVE BEEN USED IN MEDICINE

The innate healing abilities of animal-based diets were well known in the not-so-distant past. They were the sole treatment for type 2 diabetes before insulin was discovered. The first doctor on record to bring a case of diabetes under control using an "animal diet" was Dr. John Rollo in 1796. This mostly animal-based, ultra-low-carb diet restored the health of his patient, Captain Meredith, in the span of a few months. Various animal-based diets remained the standard of care for the next 125 years, until the advent of insulin therapy.[30] After insulin, animal-based diets fell out of favor because doctors assumed people wanted to have more variety in what they ate.

As carnivore has been gaining in popularity, many people have put their type 2 diabetes into remission by using it.[31] Those with type 1 diabetes can restore normal blood glucose and A1c levels and reduce the amount of insulin they need to take by using an ultra-low-carb diet like carnivore.[32] We are rediscovering the knowledge that removing dietary

[28] *A Proper Newe Booke of Cokeyre*, Catherine F. Frere, ed., https://www.uni-giessen.de/de/fbz/fb05/germanistik/absprache/sprachverwendung/gloning/tx/bookecok.htm.

[29] *A Book of Cookrye*, https://jducoeur.org/Cookbook/Cookrye.html.

[30] Gary Taubes, *Rethinking Diabetes* (New York: Vintage Books, 2024): 34.

[31] Amy L. McKenzie et al., "5-year effects of a novel continuous remote care model with carbohydrate-restricted nutrition therapy including nutritional ketosis in type 2 diabetes: an extension study," *Diabetes Research and Clinical Practice* 217 (2024):111898.

[32] Belinda S. Lennerz et al., "Management of type 1 diabetes with a very low-carbohydrate diet," *Pediatrics* 141, no. 6 (2018): e20173349.

carbohydrates can normalize blood sugar. While the American Diabetes Association suggests reducing carbs, their guidelines may not go far enough to achieve optimal blood sugar control. With an ultra-low-carb diet like carnivore, we could make type 2 diabetes a disease of the past.

Another condition that responds well to an ultra-low-carb diet is epilepsy. As early as 500 BCE, fasting was listed as an effective treatment for epilepsy. But in 1921, it was observed that just lowering carbohydrate intake to almost nothing leads to similar effects. The protocol was 1 gram of protein per kilogram of body weight, a maximum of 10 to 15 grams of carbohydrates, and the rest of daily calories from fat. Dr. Russell Morse Wilder of Mayo Clinic coined the term "ketogenic diet" because this ultra-low-carb diet leads to the production of ketone bodies.[33] Carnivore is the lowest-carb version of a ketogenic diet and continues to be used as a medical intervention for epilepsy.

Another key use of an ultra-low-carb diet, be it keto or carnivore, is in the management of cancer. Cancer is simply the body's own abnormal cells multiplying uncontrollably, and cancer cells *love* glucose. It is their primary fuel source. Lowering or eliminating dietary carbohydrates creates a hostile environment for cancer cells. There isn't an abundance of glucose for them to feed on. While I cannot say that carnivore can cure cancer, I can say that it can help the body deal with cancer treatment and perhaps minimize tumor progression.[34] Many oncologists in the low-carb space are using therapeutic ketogenic diets to help their patients manage the condition and heal during cancer treatment.

Therapeutic ketogenic diets are also showing great promise in the treatment and remission of mental health issues such as anxiety, depression, bipolar 1 and 2, schizophrenia, and eating disorders. Over the past several years, the Baszucki Group has been funding research in this area after David and Jan Ellison Baszucki's son experienced complete remission of his bipolar disorder after going on a therapeutic ketogenic diet. One of their primary objectives "is to transform mental health outcomes, beginning with bipolar disorder, by supporting initiatives at the intersection of metabolism, psychiatry and neuroscience."[35]

Perhaps the reason we are experiencing an abundance of these chronic conditions is because so many people have strayed from our original species-appropriate diet, and their bodies are rebelling. That is just speculation, but it is an interesting thought experiment. Our ancient ancestors had shorter life spans for sure, but that was mostly due to high infant mortality rates, acute infections and illnesses, accidents, and injuries. They were not dying from chronic disease like people do today. Without infections, would our animal-based ancestors have lived longer than us? Would they have had better health in their elder years? We can only guess, but I think that they would have.

---

[33] James W. Wheless, "History of the ketogenic diet," *Epilepsia* 49, s8 (2008): 3–5.
[34] Bryan G. Allen et al., "Ketogenic diets as an adjuvant cancer therapy: History and potential mechanism," *Redox Biology* 2 (2014): 963–70.
[35] https://baszuckigroup.com/metabolic-psychiatry-scholar-award/, accessed August 29, 2025.

THE BENEFITS OF CARNIVORE

Let's dive into some of the benefits of following a carnivore lifestyle. If it didn't work, it would've faded from popularity quickly. You may have heard about some of the advantages on social media or from a friend. I've had the opportunity to talk with thousands of people every month on YouTube, and here are some of the positive changes that they have reported:

Metabolic health improvements:

- Weight loss, sometimes profound
- Complete remission of type 2 diabetes, with blood sugar levels returning to normal
- Reduced insulin requirements for managing type 1 diabetes, with normal glucose and A1c levels
- Much tighter variability in blood glucose levels, with lower average glucose overall
- Reduction or elimination of inflammation
- Reduction or elimination of chronic pain
- Resolution of digestive issues
- Improvements in or resolution of mental health conditions
- Normalized menstrual cycles, reduction or elimination of menstrual cramping and PMS symptoms
- Return of fertility and the ability to have a healthy, full-term pregnancy
- Normalized blood pressure
- Resolution of or reduction in symptoms of autoimmune conditions

Unexpected changes:

- Reduction in excess skin after weight loss
- Not hungry all the time, never "hangry"
- Lower grocery bills
- Virtually zero food waste
- Reduction or elimination of the need for medications
- Better overall health leading to lower healthcare costs
- Faster healing after sickness or surgery
- No longer rolling or spraining ankles
- Cleared, glowing skin
- Virtually zero gas or bloating
- Disappearance of skin tags
- Stronger hair and nails
- Increased energy
- Muscle gains
- Improvements in oral health (gums no longer bleeding, no more bad breath, etc.)
- Better and more sound sleep
- Improvements or reductions in cellulite

These are just some of the many benefits of following a carnivore lifestyle. What improvements or changes will you see when you adopt this way of life? Only time will tell, but it is an exciting prospect!

WHY CHOOSE CARNIVORE OVER OTHER DIETS?

There are several reasons why you would choose carnivore over other dietary lifestyles. First, if you have tried keto, Paleo, primal, whole food, Mediterranean, or some other approach but saw only marginal improvements in your health, perhaps carnivore is the natural next step. Some people need to cut out plant foods completely to restore metabolic health and see the benefits they are looking for.

Next, if you can't seem to break your sugar/carb addiction, you would probably benefit from going carnivore. Trying to overcome a sugar addiction while still consuming carbs is like trying to heal from alcoholism by drinking alcohol. Cut the cord by omitting carbs completely, and you are likely to see your sugar addiction fade within a few months.

If you are metabolically unhealthy (that is, if you have high blood sugar, high blood pressure, autoimmune issues, etc., and/or if you are overweight or obese), it is in your best interest to get things under control as soon as possible. Tomorrow is not promised, and the sooner you restore your metabolic health, the more likely you are to avoid permanent damage from a chronic health condition. It's never too late to get started, but the sooner, the better.

If you have tried and failed at everything else, carnivore could be what you need to reset your system and heal your relationship with food. Before taking more drastic steps such as bariatric surgery or using a prescription weight-loss drug, give carnivore a shot! You can get many of the same benefits without the negative side effects that are so common with those interventions.

Another great reason to choose carnivore is as a fun experiment. Carnivore is gaining in popularity, and maybe you want to see if it will work for you! The only way to know is to give it a fair shot. There are many people out there who are looking to lose a bit of weight and feel better, and carnivore is a great way to achieve those goals.

WHO DOES CARNIVORE WORK FOR?

Carnivore is appropriate for all ages, genders, races, and ethnicities. Children benefit from the extremely high nutrient density of meat, which nourishes their bodies and brains. It is not abnormal for meat-based kids to be taller than their peers, along with meeting developmental milestones much quicker. My twin toddlers tower over other kids their age and started reading at two and a half years old. There are many peer-reviewed studies showing that meat is a necessary food for children and should make up a large portion of their diet.[36]

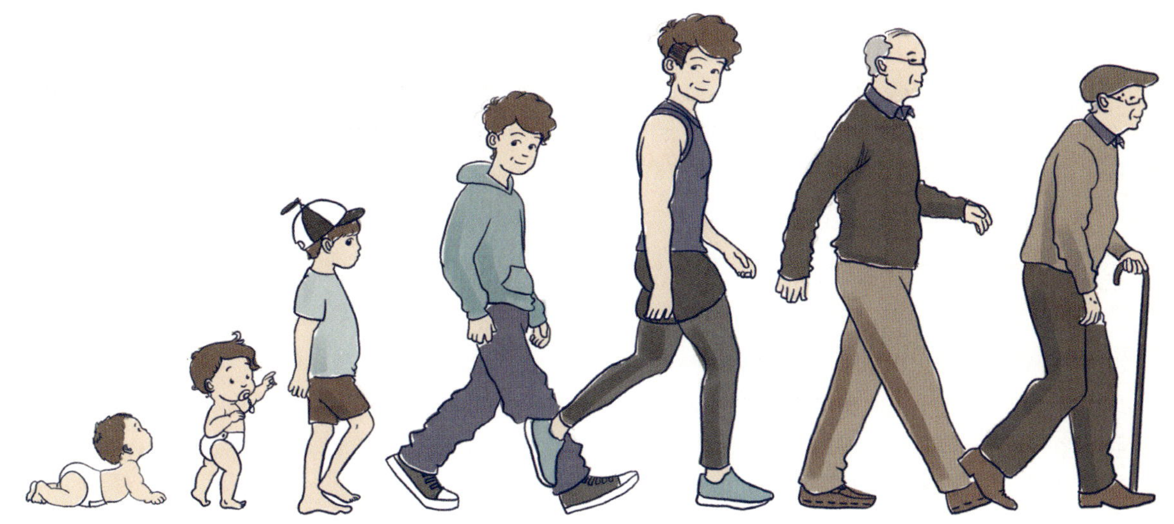

CARNIVORE IS APPROPRIATE FOR EVERY STAGE OF LIFE!

[36] Michael Hopkin, "Meat diet boosts kids' growth," *Nature* (2005): published online.

[37] Victoria C. Wilk et al., "Early Life beef consumption patterns are related to cognitive outcomes at 1–5 years of age: An exploratory study," *Nutrients* 14, no. 21 (2022): 4497.

[38] Keli M. Hawthorne et al., "Meat helps make every bite count," *Nutrition Today* 57, vol. 1 (2022): 8–13.

Once children hit puberty, animal fats and proteins can help them develop into healthy adults with healthy reproductive systems.[39] Stable blood glucose levels from eating a low-carb, ketogenic diet can help stave off behavioral problems[40] as well as the many mental health issues[41] that affect today's youth.

As you hit your prime reproductive years, feeding your body a carnivore diet can help you stay healthy, fit, active, and fertile.[42] But it doesn't stop there. Once you reach middle age, carnivore eating can help you avoid those aches and pains that everybody seems to complain about, along with healing from and/or preventing metabolic health dysfunction that can lead to chronic disease. And if you are in your golden years, carnivore can help you enjoy a higher quality of life, enabling you to do all of the things you have on your bucket list for after retirement.

Carnivore athletes benefit from increased power, stamina, and strength. They enjoy faster recovery from an intense workout or match, along with better healing if they get injured. While there is an adaptation period for athletes going from carb-heavy to virtually carb-free diets, it is typically short (two to three weeks for most) and can be done during the off-season to minimize the impact.

Carnivore can truly work for anyone, simply because it is the way humans evolved to eat. It is literally written into our DNA.

---

[39] Dr. Elizabeth Bright, *Good Fat Is Good for Girls* (Zenabright Press: 2024).

[40] Patricia Murphy and W. M. Burnham, "The ketogenic diet causes a reversible decrease in activity level in Long-Evans rats," *Experimental Neurology* 201, no. 1 (2006): 84–89.

[41] Tracy S. Gertler and Robyn Blackford, "Bringing nutritional ketosis to the table as an option for healing the pediatric brain," *Frontiers in Nutrition* 11 (2024).

[42] Liam McAuliffe, "Carnivore diet for fertility: how and why it works," DoctorKiltz.com, December 11, 2023.

IF YOU HAVE RESERVATIONS ABOUT GOING CARNIVORE

Some people may be hesitant to try carnivore because of their unique circumstances. Let's go over some of those reservations now.

PEOPLE WHO HAVE SEVERE HISTAMINE REACTIONS TO MEAT

In my years of coaching, I've seen many people react strongly to certain meats and cheeses, though pinpointing the cause isn't always simple. Often, histamine reactions stem from leaky gut, so addressing gut health is essential. In the meantime, avoiding processed meats and aged cheeses can help, and freezing fresh meat right away keeps histamine levels lower. Some highly sensitive individuals do better avoiding single-stomach animals like pork and chicken, focusing instead on ruminants such as beef, lamb, venison, and elk. Beginning with the strictest version of carnivore while your gut heals is often the best approach. Keep in mind that histamine issues can also be triggered by external factors like mold or parasites, so testing for these may be necessary if symptoms persist.

PEOPLE WITH KIDNEY DISEASE

A lot of people assume that meat or protein is bad for the kidneys. This couldn't be further from the truth. What is harmful to the kidneys is "overnutrition leading to hyperglycemia, insulin resistance and diabetes mellitus."[43] Overnutrition just means eating too many sugar-containing foods or excess carbohydrates. It is a common misconception that carnivore is a high-protein diet. It is typically a high-fat, moderate-protein diet, and "dietary analysis of very low carbohydrate studies usually reports daily protein intake ranging from 0.6 g/kg to 1.4 g/kg, which is similar to that in the standard American diet and below the high protein threshold (≥2.0 g/kg) believed to be of concern."[44] These amounts of protein are more than doable on carnivore.

Many conventional doctors see chronic kidney disease (CKD) as an incurable condition, but when using a therapeutic ketogenic diet, kidney function might improve.[45] Among the best things a person with CKD can do are to clear their diet of ultra-processed foods, seed oils, and sugar and then focus on a therapeutic ketogenic diet. I recommend finding a low-carb-friendly healthcare practitioner to guide you through the process, though, as each case is unique.

---

[43] Thomas Weimbs et al., "Ketogenic metabolic therapy for chronic kidney disease—the pro part," *Clinical Kidney Journal* 17, no. 1 (2024): sfad273.
[44] Marta Cuenca-Sánchez et al., "Controversies surrounding high-protein diet intake: Satiating effect and kidney and bone health," *Advances in Nutrition* 6, no. 3 (2015): 260–266.
[45] Shaminie J. Athinarayanan et al., "The case for a ketogenic diet in the management of kidney disease," *BMJ Open Diabetes Research and Care* 12, no. 2 (2024): e004101.

PEOPLE WITH CANCER

Earlier in this chapter, I briefly mentioned therapeutic ketogenic diets and their use in cancer treatment. If you are facing a cancer diagnosis, I know this is a scary time for you. It can feel like everything is out of your control, but one thing you do have control over is what you eat. While I cannot say that therapeutic ketogenic diets can cure your cancer, clearing your diet of glucose, cancer's main fuel source, could be helpful. I recommend working with a low-carb practitioner who knows how to get you into the proper level of therapeutic ketosis when dealing with a cancer diagnosis. A great place to start your search is the Society of Metabolic Health Practitioners' provider directory at thesmhp.org/directory. Carnivore can be a therapeutic ketogenic diet, and many people with cancer have used it in tandem with their medical treatment to improve healing and possibly slow tumor progression.[46]

PEOPLE WITH HIGH CHOLESTEROL

Contrary to popular belief, the carnivore diet doesn't typically raise LDL cholesterol. Most people see reductions in their triglycerides and increases in their HDL cholesterol, while LDL tends to stay the same or even decline. For a small subset of the population, a ketogenic diet can cause LDL cholesterol levels to skyrocket, while triglycerides are very low and HDL is very high. These people are called lean mass hyper responders (LMHR), and they are unique in that they are typically lean and athletic, and all of their other biomarkers are excellent.

Dave Feldman is the person who discovered this phenomenon and coined the term LMHR based on his early observation that people tended to be lean and fit. He and a team of researchers are trying to determine if the elevated LDL-C levels seen in LMHRs are leading to increased plaque buildup in their coronary arteries. This research is ongoing, and you can learn more in several ways. First, you

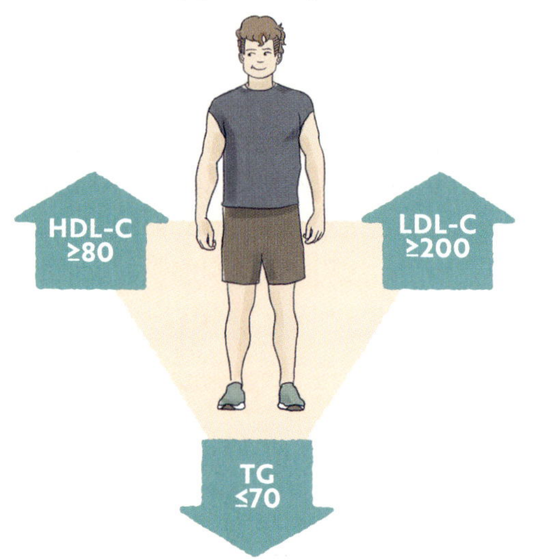

Typically in leaner people, all other biomarkers are excellent, including glucose, inflammation, and visceral fat levels.

[46] Daniela D. Weber et al., "Ketogenic diet in cancer therapy," *Aging* 10, no. 2 (2018): 164–165.

can head to the Citizen Science Foundation's website (citizensciencefoundation.org) to get updates on this important research and donate to the next study. Second, you can follow Feldman and his frequent collaborators Nick Norwitz and Adrian Soto-Mota on YouTube and Instagram; they are constantly releasing excellent content in this area. Finally, you can head to conferences such as the Collaborative Science Conference (cosci.org), the Symposium for Metabolic Health (lowcarbusa.org/events), and Low Carb Down Under (lowcarb-downunder.com.au) to learn more about how ketogenic diets are being used in clinical practice and the exciting research being conducted in this field.

When people come to carnivore, this question about its effects on blood cholesterol ranks in the top five most frequently asked, so I will be discussing this topic a few more times throughout this book. In chapter 7, I dive into why cholesterol has been demonized for the past sixty to seventy years. In chapter 8, I touch on some goals you should aspire to in your standard lipid panel and where you can get a CAC scan.

PEOPLE WHO CAN'T STAND THE THOUGHT OF EATING AN ANIMAL

If you have been vegan or vegetarian for a long time, the thought of eating an animal may be daunting. Unfortunately, long-term veganism/vegetarianism can cause serious health problems[47] and vitamin deficiencies,[48] so finding a way to incorporate animal foods in some way is strongly encouraged. An excellent book that could help you reframe the consumption of animals as something positive is *The Vegetarian Myth* by Lierre Keith. Written by a former vegetarian who wrestled with a lot of these existential questions, this great read helped me consider the ethical dilemma that many vegans and vegetarians have in a new way. It and several other excellent books are listed in Appendix B.

If you still can't wrap your mind around eating meat, at least begin to incorporate eggs and/or dairy products so that you can get some essential nutrients, and be sure to take high-quality supplements, including B12 and iron. It is possible to do a therapeutic ketogenic diet while consuming a mostly vegetarian diet that includes eggs, fish, and/or chicken. I also know of a few people who are doing a vegan therapeutic ketogenic diet. But carnivore is not an option if you can't overcome this hurdle.

---

[47] Vicente J. Clemente-Suárez et al., "Impact of vegan and vegetarian diets on neurological health: a critical review," *Nutrients* 17, no. 5 (2025): 884.
[48] Dimitra R. Bakaloudi et al., "Intake and inadequacy of the vegan diet. A systematic review of the evidence," *Clinical Nutrition* 40, no. 5 (2021): 3503–3521.

PEOPLE WHO HATE EATING MEAT

If you dislike the taste or texture of meat, it may be difficult for you to do the carnivore diet. Sometimes this is a psychological issue that can be overcome with therapy, but for certain people it is an insurmountable obstacle. If you are only averse to certain meats, then you can do carnivore! The great thing about this dietary lifestyle is that you can customize it to your tastes and budget. If you hate beef, for example, you don't have to eat it. And perhaps with time, you will come to love meats that you used to find unappealing.

PEOPLE OBSERVING RELIGIOUS RESTRICTIONS

There are many people who cannot eat meat from certain species, such as pork or beef, due to religious restrictions. You can still have a diverse and nutrient-dense carnivore diet even while heeding those restrictions. There is a comprehensive grocery list on pages 73–74, and you are free to exclude anything you are not allowed to consume. When you head to the recipe section of this book, you can substitute any restricted meats with meat you can eat.

PEOPLE WITH A LIMITED BUDGET

Budget is a real hurdle for a lot of people. Food prices can be astronomically high. Thankfully, there are ways to save money on carnivore. I have an entire section in this book that gives you money-saving tips; turn to page 79. I also have videos on my YouTube channel showing how I successfully fed one person for one month on $100 and fed a family of four for one month on $300. (I did an updated $100 budget video in June 2025, and I was still able to feed one person for a month on $100!) It is entirely possible to do carnivore on a tight budget.

You have now completed your crash course on the carnivore diet! Are you ready to get started? In the next chapter, I've laid out an in-depth guide for you that walks you through the entire process, from preparation to the first ninety days and beyond. Turn the page to get started!

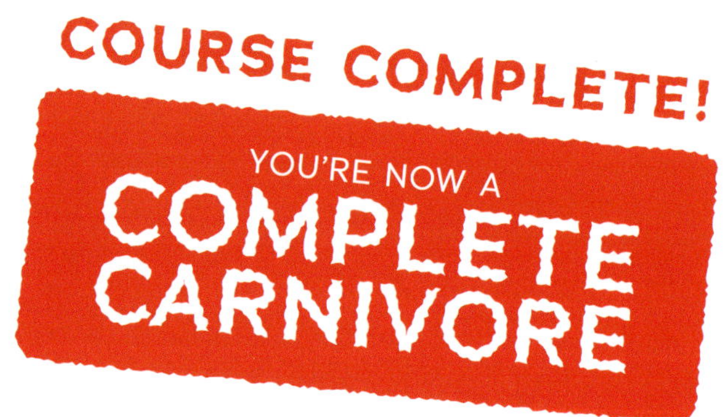

CHAPTER 2

IN-DEPTH GUIDE

Half the battle in making a lifestyle shift is making the decision to change. Now that you have made up your mind to try the carnivore diet, it's time to get started. But there are a few things to take care of before you eat your first carnivore meal. By laying the groundwork, you will increase your likelihood of success and avoid some of the pitfalls and mistakes that I and so many other carnivores made in the beginning. You are lucky in a way; you are reaping the benefits of other people's years of experience, troubleshooting, and tweaking.

My goal with this chapter and the next is to give you everything you need to prep for the first days of carnivore, get through the first few months, and, if you decide to go longer, the first year and beyond. This in-depth guide is laid out in chronological order, beginning with defining your Whys and choosing a version of the carnivore diet.

It's not required, but I find that writing things down on paper can be incredibly helpful. The physical act of writing reinforces your commitment to change, and seeing your goals and plans in your own handwriting serves as a powerful reminder of the path you've chosen.

To help you prepare for this lifestyle shift, I've built you a "Prepping for Day 1 Worksheet" that you can print out (find it at JennyMitich.com). Or, if you prefer, you can write directly on the worksheet in this book and work your way through the activities so that you are fully prepared to start the carnivore diet. You can also write everything out on a blank sheet of paper or in a journal or notebook. The activities include defining your Whys, figuring out which version of carnivore to start with, cleaning out your pantry, and so much more. And don't worry, most of these preparatory tasks are short and sweet. I don't want you to feel bogged down with complicated homework. But please be sure to complete the worksheet. It will help you be successful down the road.

Then pick a date to take the plunge with carnivore! I will talk about timing and other factors here in a little bit, but in general, you need to give carnivore at least thirty days to let your body adjust to a new fuel source, with most carnivore experts recommending a *minimum* of ninety days. That amount of time may seem intimidating right now, but don't worry. Focus on making it through the first thirty days first, and then you can think about committing to another thirty. No need to overwhelm yourself right now.

REMEMBER:

Health is highly individualized. You must figure out what works for you.

COMPLETE CARNIVORE PREPPING FOR DAY 1 — WORKSHEET

Which version of carnivore are you starting with? ______________________

What are your Whys?

____

____

____

____

____

____

Are you going cold turkey or easing in?

◯ Cold turkey ◯ Easing in

Any other special considerations you need to keep in mind?

____

____

Visioning:

Close your eyes and envision a future where you have reached your goals. What does that look like? Write about it here:

____

____

____

Positive affirmations:

____

____

____

____

____

____

____

____

What are your goals?

____

____

____

____

____

____

____

____

Pick 1-3 pieces of clothing that don't fit you well right now; you are going to try these on in a month. Which clothing items did you pick?

1. ______________________
2. ______________________
3. ______________________

Put these clothes somewhere you can find them easily, or hang them on a hanger and put them somewhere prominent in your home to motivate you.

In addition, take measurements of your chest, waist, hips, thigh, and upper arm and record them here.

____

____

____

____

____

How are you feeling physically? How are you feeling mentally/emotionally?

____

____

____

____

____

***(Fill out after 30 days on carnivore)* How are you feeling physically? How are you feeling mentally/emotionally?**

____

____

____

____

Checklist:

- ◯ Purchase or make some electrolytes *before* starting.
- ◯ Clear your fridge, shelves, and pantry of non-carnivore foods.
- ◯ If you need a meal plan, print it out and use it to make your grocery list (you can also use the blank meal plan template and make your own).
- ◯ Go grocery shopping.
- ◯ Meal prep at least a few items so you have carnivore food on hand.

You are now ready for Day 1! Pick a day on the calendar to get started and write it here: ☐

WHAT ARE YOUR WHYS?

When you are trying to do a complete lifestyle shift, it helps to have clearly defined reasons for making the change. These are called "Whys," and they will help you define your goals and keep you on track when you encounter difficulties.

A Why can be as simple as:

- "I want to see my child get married someday."
- "I want to age gracefully."
- "I don't want to die at a young age from a chronic condition."

Or it can be something specific, such as:

- "I want to feel my best for my thirtieth wedding anniversary."
- "I want to climb Mount Everest next year."
- "I want to recover fully after a severe injury."

It can be related to your metabolic health:

- "I want to heal from type 2 diabetes."
- "I need to lower my inflammation levels."
- "I want to be free from having to run to the bathroom unexpectedly."

For many people, weight loss is a huge Why. But try to tie the Why to more than just a number on the scale. For instance:

- "I want to lose weight so that my joints don't ache and I am able to go hiking again."
- "I want to lose weight to lower my blood pressure and glucose levels."
- "I want to lose that last 30 pounds so that I can look my best and feel confident again."

I don't recommend getting your heart set on a particular weight, because the scale is the worst measurement tool we have in our arsenal. Also, sometimes our idea of what we *should* weigh and what our body *wants* us to weigh diverge a bit, and I don't want you to get discouraged if you are unable to hit that number on the scale. I will talk about better and more accurate measurement tools in a bit.

Once you have figured out your Whys, write them down on your prepping worksheet and keep them somewhere you can see them every day. I like using sticky notes, writing them on the dry erase board in my office, or typing them out and printing them to put on the fridge. The key is to have them front and center.

Be sure to write down at least one to three Whys. You are going to use them to determine which version of the carnivore diet you will start with and to formulate your goals. Your Whys will also come in handy if you run into difficulty during your time on carnivore. Sometimes it helps to remember why you are doing this "crazy" diet in the first place.

If one or several of your Whys are related to metabolic health conditions, be sure to refer to the index at the back of this book to find all of the mentions of your condition.

WHICH VERSION OF CARNIVORE SHOULD YOU START WITH?

You may have thought that carnivore was as simple as eating meat and drinking water, but like everything in life, it's a bit more complicated than that. There are several versions of the carnivore diet, along with many carnivore lookalikes that I do not consider to be technically carnivore.

THE DIFFERENT VERSIONS OF CARNIVORE

Let's go over the variations quickly, from most to least strict, and then talk about who would benefit from each level of strictness:

- **Beef, salt, and water:** Known as the lion diet, this is the strictest version of carnivore. Some carnivore experts include other ruminants (animals with chambered or "four" stomachs) in this version of the diet. But, at its strictest, lion is only beef, salt, and water. You cook with beef fat or tallow.
- **Only ruminant animals:** This next level of strictness includes all ruminants: cows, sheep, lambs, goats, elk, moose, deer, etc. Any fats from those animals can be used for cooking.
- **All meat and all seafood:** This level of strictness is middle of the road and still does not include products produced by animals, only the meat from those animals.
- **All meat, all seafood, eggs, and butter:** This is the version of carnivore that I follow most of the time.
- **All meat, seafood, eggs, butter, and high-fat dairy:** This is the least strict version of carnivore. Some experts consider it to be more keto than carnivore because of the dairy.

Finally, there are a couple of "carnivore lookalikes":

- **Meat and fruit:** Proponents of the meat and fruit diet eat lots of meat and organs along with lots of fruit, a handful of low-phytotoxin vegetables (more on phytotoxins later), and some dairy. While it's a whole-food diet, it's also very high in sugar. I do not recommend starting with the meat and fruit diet if you have metabolic health issues or if you are addicted to sugar. The sugar in the fruit can keep that addiction alive, and you want to put the kibosh on it.
- **Atkins diet:** While Atkins is like carnivore, it has some distinct differences. Atkins is a low-carbohydrate diet that has four phases: induction, balancing, fine-tuning, and maintenance. It allows for a broader range of food, including fruits, vegetables, grains, legumes, nuts, seeds, and dairy. Including these plant materials can be problematic for some people. Carnivore excludes plant materials and focuses solely on meat and animal products.

As far as seasonings go, salt is included at all levels of strictness. I think it's fine to include some spices and seasonings if you are not sensitive to them, such as garlic powder, onion powder, and smoked paprika, although I advise people at the stricter levels to avoid them for at least the first ninety days. I will dive more into who may be able to use seasonings and who should probably avoid them later in this chapter.

CHOOSING A VERSION OF CARNIVORE

It's time to pick which version of carnivore you should start with. You can always shift versions down the road, but it's nice to have a starting point. Keep your Whys close by because they will aid you in your decision.

STRICTEST (LION DIET OR ONLY RUMINANTS)

If your Why is related to:

- Severe autoimmune issues such as rheumatoid arthritis
- Severe allergies or reactions you can't seem to pin down
- Severe digestive issues such as Crohn's or IBS
- **AND/OR** is affecting the quality of your life so severely that it is all you can focus on...

then you would likely benefit from a stricter version of carnivore, at least in the beginning.

You may have heard of Mikhaila Peterson, the daughter of media commentator Jordan Peterson. She had severe childhood rheumatoid arthritis and had to eliminate everything except for beef, salt, and water from her diet to find relief from her symptoms. Eating only beef is the original elimination diet. It can cut through the noise and allow your body to begin to heal from extreme inflammation. Yes, it does seem a bit radical on the surface, but in the end, thirty to ninety days of lion is a drop in the bucket when compared to the symptoms and low quality of life you may have been experiencing. The human body wants to be healthy. You likely won't have to do lion forever. Once the healing is done, you can slowly reintroduce foods and see if you have a reaction to them (I touch on the reintroduction process on page 100).

After five-plus years on carnivore, Peterson diversified her diet a bit and now consumes both beef and lamb. That is how she has determined she can stay symptom free and have a high quality of life, so she sticks with a very strict version of carnivore.

If eating only beef or ruminants seems overly restrictive to you, you can start with a less restrictive version of carnivore. If, after ninety days, you are not feeling much better, you can always go stricter and see what happens.

MODERATELY STRICT (MEAT & SEAFOOD OR MEAT, SEAFOOD, EGGS & BUTTER)

If your Why is related to:

- A chronic disease or ailment such as high blood pressure or type 2 diabetes
- Chronic acne or other skin issues
- Mental health issues such as depression, anxiety, bipolar disorder, or schizophrenia
- **AND/OR** is affecting the quality of your life, but you can still do a lot of the things you want to do...

then you can start with a moderately strict version of carnivore. I recommend all meat, all seafood, eggs, and butter. You may be able to include some spices other than salt.

I don't include dairy for this group because for most people, dairy is inflammatory and they don't even realize it. Also, dairy is easy to overeat, and many who would otherwise have success on carnivore may not if they continue eating a lot of dairy.

Butter vs. Dairy: When I say dairy, I am not talking about butter or ghee. I am referring to liquid dairy and cheeses. Butter and ghee have most if not all of the lactose and milk proteins removed from them, so for most people, they don't have the same effect as other dairy products.

After ninety days at a moderate level of strictness, you can experiment with adding a little dairy if you want to. But you may find that it bogs you down, makes depression and anxiety symptoms return, and/or slows your weight loss. Indigestion and bloating are common symptoms of dairy intolerance. You may not think you are intolerant to dairy, but try cutting it for ninety days and then reintroducing it one item at a time. You may be surprised that your daily upset stomach or gas disappears when you are dairy free and returns with a vengeance the minute you eat some cheese or add some heavy cream to a recipe.

Special Resources if your Why is mental health related:

If you are coming to carnivore because of mental health issues, I strongly suggest reading the book *Change Your Diet, Change Your Mind* by Dr. Georgia Ede. This amazing book talks about the effects of a ketogenic diet on mental health, and I think it will be helpful for you in navigating your unique situation.

Another excellent book on this topic is *Brain Energy* by Dr. Christopher Palmer. In it, Palmer argues that mental disorders are metabolic brain conditions rooted in mitochondrial dysfunction. He explains how improving metabolic health—especially through diet—can significantly improve psychiatric symptoms.

Yet another great resource for learning more about how to use ketogenic diets in the treatment of mental health conditions is the YouTube channel *Metabolic Mind*. This channel has a research focus and will be invaluable to you in navigating your mental health condition.

LEAST STRICT (MEAT, SEAFOOD, EGGS, BUTTER & DAIRY)

If your Why is related to:

- Weight loss
- Improving your energy levels or overall metabolic health
- Other general health improvements
- **OR** is not significantly affecting your quality of life, but improvements would be great...

then I think you can start with whatever level of strictness you want to. I recommend all meat, all seafood, eggs, and butter, and you could probably throw in a little bit of dairy, too. You could also use some spices in addition to salt.

But if you do carnivore at the least strict level for a few months and you're not feeling great, not losing weight, or otherwise not making progress toward your Why, consider going to a stricter version. Chapter 5 discusses troubleshooting the carnivore diet.

While nutrition can help with a lot of issues, it's likely not going to address *everything*. Something else could be going on that isn't related to diet. Stress, sleep, hormones, thyroid, and so many other issues can affect weight loss. Be sure to check out chapter 4, which dives into the other metabolic health factors that you need to consider.

Now that you have a better understanding of the different versions of carnivore, pick which version is right for you and your Whys. Write down your choice on your prepping worksheet. Remember, you can always start at one level of strictness and increase or decrease strictness as you go. You are not stuck with your choice. How you feel is going to dictate how you approach the carnivore way of eating as you continue.

SHOULD YOU GO COLD TURKEY OR EASE INTO CARNIVORE?

Whether you are going to go cold turkey or ease into carnivore is a big decision. The following are some considerations that will help you make that choice. If you decide to ease into carnivore, I have laid out a gradual carbohydrate reduction guide for you on page 84. Otherwise, you'll start with the section "Month 1" that begins on page 88.

HOW MANY CARBS ARE YOU CURRENTLY CONSUMING PER DAY?

If you are currently consuming 200 to 500-plus grams of carbohydrates every day, easing into carnivore will minimize the amount of keto flu you experience. If you are already eating low carb or keto, going cold turkey likely won't cause many issues.

ARE YOU EATING A SAD OR A WHOLE-FOOD DIET?

Are you currently following a standard American diet (SAD), with 45 to 65 percent of your daily calories coming from carbohydrates? Are you consuming large amounts of ultra-processed foods like bread, cereal, pasta, cookies, chips, juices, and sugary sodas and coffee drinks, or are you already eating mostly whole, real foods such as meat, dairy, vegetables, fruits, legumes, and whole grains? A person who is eating a SAD would likely experience severe keto flu going cold turkey into carnivore and would benefit from slowly replacing ultra-processed foods with whole foods first, and then gradually reducing their carbohydrate intake while upping fats and protein. If you are already consuming whole, real foods most of the time, it may be easier for you to go cold turkey into carnivore, depending on which whole foods you have been eating.

ARE YOU EATING A LOT OF HIGH-OXALATE FOODS?

While you may be eating a whole-food diet, which foods you are eating can determine whether you should go cold turkey or ease into carnivore. Earlier I touched on phytotoxins, or plant toxins, one of which is oxalate. If you have been consuming some of the high-oxalate foods listed below, going cold turkey into carnivore is not advised. Slowly easing into carnivore will minimize oxalate dumping.

- Spinach
- Almonds
- Rhubarb
- Sweet potatoes
- Beets
- Chia seeds
- Chocolate
- Plantains
- Quinoa
- Buckwheat
- Whole grain bread
- Blackberries
- Raspberries
- Kiwis
- Apricots
- Dried figs

Look at this list of high-oxalate foods and put a little mark next to the ones you eat regularly. If you check off more than three to five, I recommend following the gradual carb reduction guide as opposed to going cold turkey into carnivore. If you decide you still want to go cold turkey into carnivore, be sure to drink a cup of black tea every day. Black tea is high in oxalates, and it will slow the oxalate dumping that will occur if you stop eating oxalates suddenly.

I have personal experience with this issue. I didn't know anything about oxalates before starting carnivore. I went cold turkey, and my keto flu lasted six weeks. Little did I know that it was likely severe oxalate dumping on top of the two to three weeks of keto flu. Trust me, it was not fun, and I want you to avoid a similar situation.

ARE YOU AN ABSTAINER OR A MODERATOR?

An abstainer is a person who can't have just one: just one chip, just one cookie, just one drink. If it is in the house, you will eat or drink it. A moderator, on the other hand, can easily say no. Having high-carb snacks in the house doesn't bother them. They can have one alcoholic beverage and then stop. If you are more of an abstainer, going cold turkey into carnivore can be beneficial because it may be harder for you to slowly ramp down your carb consumption. Cutting the cord is sometimes a better solution for an abstainer. If you are a moderator, you could choose either approach. Gradual carb reduction is not as much of a struggle for a moderator. You may become more of a moderator as you break your sugar and carb addiction, or you may remain an abstainer forever. Only time will tell.

DO YOU FATTEN EASILY?

Have you always had a hard time with your weight? Do you seem to gain weight readily while others around you eat the same things and stay thin? For those who have always struggled with their weight, going cold turkey into carnivore is sometimes less frustrating.

WHAT TIME CONSTRAINTS DO YOU HAVE?

Do you have a big event coming up, like a wedding or a vacation? Are you working on a difficult project at your job? Going cold turkey into carnivore is like ripping off a bandage. You may have some keto flu for a few weeks, but then it is over, and you can move on. But if you have important things ahead of you on your calendar, it may be better to ease into carnivore so you can minimize keto flu symptoms, which can be disruptive.

WHAT IS YOUR TOLERANCE FOR PAIN?

Do you have a high or a low tolerance for discomfort? When you are under the weather, are you able to soldier on and get done what you need to get done, or do you need to lie in bed all day? If you can handle a bit of pain, going cold turkey into carnivore won't be as much of a struggle for you. If not, easing into it is a better route.

WHAT ARE YOUR WHYS?

Are your Whys related to a serious metabolic health condition that is affecting your quality of life? If so, going cold turkey into carnivore may be a better option for you than living with the daily symptoms you are already experiencing. Yes, there may be some keto flu or oxalate dumping, but that will still be better than how you are living now. If your Whys are more about weight loss, longevity, and increased energy levels, you are not in such a dire situation as, say, someone who has to run to the bathroom thirty times a day. Easing into carnivore to avoid the worst of the keto flu may be a better option for you.

After reading through all of these considerations, do you think cold turkey or easing into carnivore would be the better choice for you? These are just guidelines; you can choose either approach. But hopefully now you are leaning toward one option over the other. Mark down your choice on your prepping worksheet, and remember, you can always change your mind.

SPECIAL CONSIDERATIONS

Before we get into your prep for day 1 of carnivore, there are some special considerations to keep in mind. Reading this section will help you transition to carnivore more easily and minimize some of the difficulties that could arise.

MEDICATIONS

If you are on any type of medication, *do not stop taking it*. Work with your doctor to adjust your dosages if needed. I do advise you to let your doctor know that you are going to be doing a low-carb diet and you will want them to pay special attention to your dosage levels, especially for blood pressure medications, insulin and other diabetes medications, and psychiatric meds. After some time on carnivore, many people find that their blood pressure levels go back to normal, and they no longer need high doses of blood pressure medication. Some can come off blood pressure medications completely. Same with insulin: You may find that you need lower daily doses to regulate your blood sugar. This is common. The carnivore diet is excellent for regulating blood sugar, and you may see your A1c and fasting glucose levels return to normal relatively quickly. Pay close attention to the amount of insulin you are taking and work with your doctor to adjust the dosages as needed.

The same advice goes for psychiatric medications. Please *do not* take yourself off your meds. Many of these medications need to be titrated down slowly, as any abrupt changes in dosage may cause serious setbacks. There is no shame in taking psychiatric medications. What is most important is your health and quality of life. You may eventually be able to reduce or eliminate your psych meds with the carnivore diet, but you may not. And that is okay!

BARIATRIC SURGERY

If you have had any kind of bariatric surgery, you can still successfully go carnivore, but you will want to use the following tips:

- Ease into carnivore instead of going cold turkey.
- Consume three to six smaller meals in an eight- to ten-hour feeding window.
- Stay away from liquid or rendered fats.
- Chew your food slowly and thoroughly.
- Take a sip or two of water during each meal to help with digestion.
- You may need HCL supplements, ox bile, or other digestive aids.
- Your protein minimums will be the same as everyone else's, but you may have a tough time consuming it. Using protein powders in shakes works for some but runs right through others. You could incorporate protein powder into eggs, pancakes, meatloaf, and other foods to increase the amount of protein you are consuming without increasing the volume of food. Powdered dehydrated meats can work as well.
- Vitamin and nutrient deficiencies can be a real issue for you. Continue taking your supplements and/or getting vitamin infusions as needed. Get regular blood work to test vitamin and mineral levels.

I have several videos on this topic on my YouTube channel, so feel free to check those out if you would like more information on your unique circumstances.

NO GALLBLADDER

You can still do carnivore if your gallbladder has been removed, but you may benefit from easing into it. Gradually increasing your fat consumption will give your body time to adjust. Avoid liquid or rendered fats. Some people see success with digestive enzymes and/or HCL supplements.

LIPEDEMA

Lipedema is a chronic condition that occurs almost exclusively in women. It is characterized by abnormal fat deposits that accumulate in the extremities. These deposits are symmetrical and can make the legs look like columns. They can be quite painful, with pain building throughout the day. Until recently, many doctors did not recognize lipedema as a real condition. But it is very real and can greatly affect a person's quality of life.

Carnivore can help with lipedema symptoms, but for some people, a higher-protein version is most effective. For more information on this condition, check out Linda Salant's Instagram account or YouTube channel, *The Carnitarian*. She has been very open about how she is healing her lipedema with the carnivore diet.

GLP-1 AND CARNIVORE

GLP-1 receptor agonists have become extremely popular, and carnivore is one of the best diets to follow while taking them. The key is to preserve lean mass—since the goal of weight loss is to lose fat, not muscle. Most side effects come from starting doses that are too high and from failing to adjust diet and exercise. To stay healthy and maximize results:

- Eat 1 gram of protein per pound of body weight daily.
- Strength train two or more times per week (30-plus-minute sessions).
- Start at the lowest dose and increase slowly (compounded GLPs make this possible with the right practitioner).
- Get a DEXA scan before starting and retest every 1 to 3 months to track muscle versus fat changes.
- Aim to lose 1 to 3 pounds of weight per week to protect lean mass.

As you can see, carnivore is not one size fits all. It's going to be a little different for each person. As you continue your carnivore journey, you will figure out how to tailor it to you.

Now that you've made it through the weeds, let's get into some action steps. You are going to do the work needed to prepare for your first month on carnivore. Let's go!

PREPPING MENTALLY FOR CARNIVORE

This section gives you everything you need to hit the ground running on day 1 of the carnivore diet. Don't skimp on any of these steps; try to complete as many as you can.

GETTING INTO THE RIGHT MINDSET

I will argue that mindset is the most important part of this entire process. If you can't get your mind right, everything you do will eventually be defeated by your own negative thoughts. Simply making the decision to do carnivore and committing to at least thirty days is a huge step, and I commend you for it!

Manage your expectations. Carnivore is not an overnight fix. It is not a get-out-of-jail-free card. How long did it take you to get to where you are today? You are not going to get back to perfect health and a perfect weight in a month. One of the top mistakes newbies make on carnivore is expecting dramatic results in too little time. It is normal to lose a lot of weight in the beginning, but it is also normal to lose only a little, or even to gain. You need to practice loads of patience.

Switch from a weight-loss focus to a metabolic health focus. If you have weight to lose, it will come off as your metabolic health improves. But if weight loss is your sole concern, you will be disappointed when you run into an inevitable stall. Yes, weight-loss stalls can occur on carnivore. If you accept that, it will not be so much of a surprise when you run into one. If you focus on metabolic health gains instead, you won't be as disappointed if and when your weight loss slows.

Don't compare yourself to others. When we compare ourselves to influencers online or people on TV, we do ourselves a disservice. Every individual has a unique lived experience. Your age, gender, race, ethnicity, socioeconomic status, where you grew up and currently live, education levels, trauma, genetics, health status, sexual orientation, and so much more influence who you are today, and you should embrace that history. You can only truly compare yourself to yourself. What improvements have you seen in *your* health over the past month? How much weight did *you* lose? How are *your* clothes fitting? You will never be that other person you are comparing yourself to, and you don't want to be! How boring it would be if we were all alike. You are a beautiful and unique person, and when you start believing that, your mind will begin to change.

Remember that carnivore is not a magic bullet. While improving your nutrition is a necessary component to healing, it's not going to fix every ailment, ache, and pain. There may be another root cause issue that is responsible for your condition, and going carnivore will help to reveal if that is the case. If you are still not feeling great after six months of strict carnivore, there is something else going on that you need to address. I discuss this more in chapter 4.

Stay positive and believe that you will see improvements. There have been many studies on the placebo effect and how, if you are taking or doing something that you believe is going to help, it *will* help. The mind is a powerful thing. Don't discount the value of positive thinking and believing you will achieve your goals. One way elite athletes do this is **visioning**. They imagine themselves winning that race, breaking that world record, or completing a stunt perfectly. You can do the same in your life by closing your eyes and painting a picture of success in your head. You can see yourself walking without pain. You can see yourself playing with your grandkids. You can see yourself 50 pounds thinner and feeling healthy. I practice visioning every day! My visioning is usually centered around being healthy, toned, and energetic and having abundance flow into my life, and it's been a game changer for my mindset. Take a moment to close your eyes and give it a try. Write out your vision on the prepping worksheet.

Repeat positive affirmations daily to bolster your positive thinking. Here are some examples to get you started:

- I am brave and strong.
- I succeed at everything I put my mind to.
- I am an amazing person, and people love me.
- I am healthy, wealthy, and intelligent.

Write down a few positive affirmations on your prepping worksheet and on a sticky note to post in a place where you can read them every day. You will be surprised at the effect that positive affirmations will have on your mindset over time.

This is not a diet; it is a complete lifestyle shift. So many people get stuck on the yo-yo diet train because they keep thinking they can change their diets for a short time and then return to their previous way of eating after losing weight. Don't fall into that trap. Instead, see this as a completely new lifestyle that you will be maintaining for the long term.

You don't necessarily have to stay carnivore forever, but you can never go back to ultra-processed foods. Ultra-processed foods will keep you alive, but they will not keep you healthy. You need to see those foods for what they are: slow-acting poisons that rob you of health. You will start to view them this way if you eat an ultra-processed cheat meal after doing carnivore for some time. Those "foods" will make you feel terrible physically and maybe mentally, and you will wonder how you ever got away with eating them every day. Once your body is used to real food, it will begin to reject imitations.

SETTING REALISTIC GOALS AND MANAGING EXPECTATIONS

Now that we have discussed mindset, let's move on to goal setting. I want you to use your Whys to inform your goals. What is it going to take to get you to those Whys? When I am setting goals, I focus on short-, medium-, and long-range goals. Shorter goals are less difficult, while long-range goals involve many steps and take more time to accomplish.

The first goal should be, "I am going to do strict carnivore for thirty days." Starting with a thirty-day commitment and then recommitting to another thirty after you reach that goal makes ninety days seem less intimidating, and one month is a great short-range goal. Come up with another short goal that you can reach in thirty days in addition to staying carnivore. This could be something like, "I will try a new type of meat," or, "I will go to sleep one hour earlier." It doesn't have to be related to carnivore per se.

An ideal medium-range goal will take three to six months to accomplish. Come up with one or two that you can reach in this period. Perhaps a goal could be gradually increasing your daily movement in some way. If you are starting from a sedentary lifestyle, it could be as simple as walking around the block once a week or parking your car farther away from the store entrance so you must walk more.

After that, think of one or two long-range goals that will take at least a year to achieve: maybe improving a serious health condition, prepping for a marathon, or fitting into an outfit you haven't worn in years.

Once you have determined your goals, jot them down on your prepping worksheet. You may want to post them alongside your Whys and your positive affirmations. You will be surprised at how effective revisiting these goals daily can be in achieving them.

When it comes to weight loss, every individual is going to have a different lived experience. This also applies to the amount of weight each person will lose their first month on carnivore. Some people lose a ton of weight. Some lose only a little. And some gain weight. Going carnivore is not a guarantee that you will lose a massive number of pounds in a short time, although many people have that experience.

If you have been undereating for many years, you may gain weight in the beginning. This makes sense, because if you've been undereating, your metabolism has slowed down to compensate for the lack of nutrition. Early weight gain after years of restriction does not mean that carnivore "isn't working." It means that you are finally giving your body the nutrients it needs, and it is going to hold on to every ounce of fat you give it until it feels safe enough to release it. It's an evolutionary response, and there isn't much you can do about it. Your body is trying to protect you from famine and death. So, for the time being, gaining a little bit of weight is the best thing you can do. Once you have replenished the nutrients and shown your body that it is not experiencing a famine, your metabolism will adjust, and you will begin to burn more energy. But it's a process, and it takes time. That is just the reality of the situation.

Also, weight loss is never linear, meaning it is never a straight path downward. It has always been a series of ups and downs, for every single person since the beginning of time.

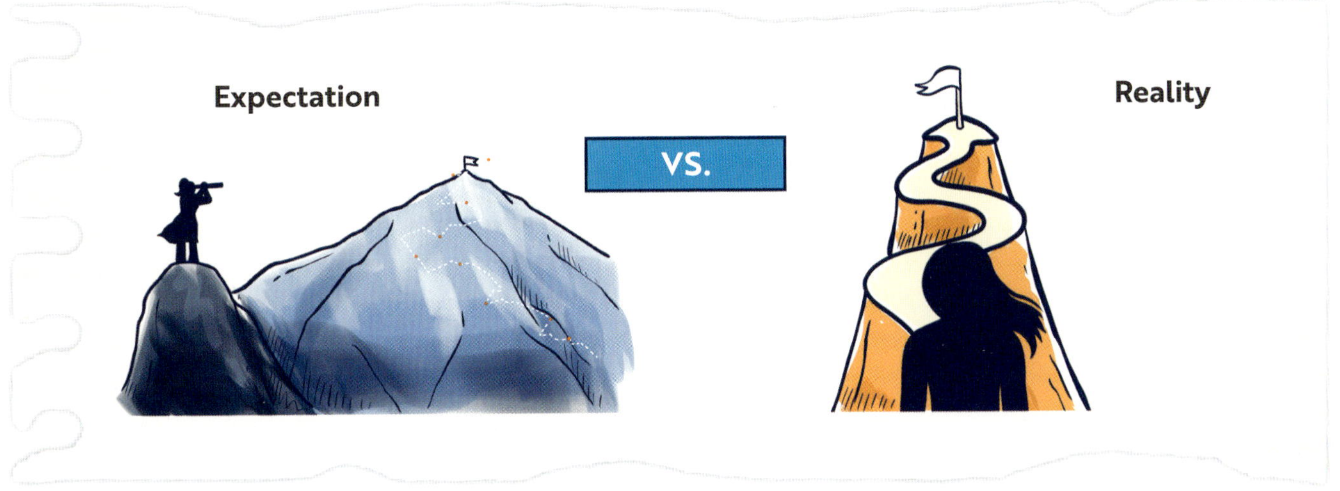

Chronic overexercising can overstress the body, which can lead to a slowdown in weight loss. Do not go carnivore and then add six days a week of high-intensity cardio, or you will tank your energy levels and your progress. A better way to boost your metabolism is low-impact walking paired with strength training. Building muscle is one of the most effective ways to increase weight loss over time. Muscles need energy to function, so you will burn more calories overall when you have more muscle on your body. Muscles are also a great place for excess glucose to go. You don't have to be a bodybuilder to see these benefits. People of all ages and backgrounds benefit from strengthening their muscles.

I think it is best to have *zero* weight-loss expectations for the first month of carnivore and just see what happens. You will likely be pleasantly surprised. But even if you gain weight, that doesn't mean you failed. It means there is something else going on. And don't worry, we will talk about troubleshooting carnivore later on in this book.

TAKING BASELINE MEASUREMENTS

I just told you not to think too much about the number on the scale, but in order to measure your progress, you do need to have a baseline. You will want these measurements down the road to see how far you've come.

First, step on a scale and get a baseline weight. Make sure you do so in the morning after using the bathroom but before drinking or eating anything. Mark the weight down on your prepping worksheet.

Next, get a fabric measuring tape and take at least three measurements: chest, waist, and hips. I also like to do a belly measurement, which falls between your natural waist and your hips, right around your belly button. I held a lot of my post-pregnancy weight gain there. You can also measure your upper arm, thigh, and calf circumference if you like. Write all of these measurements on your worksheet.

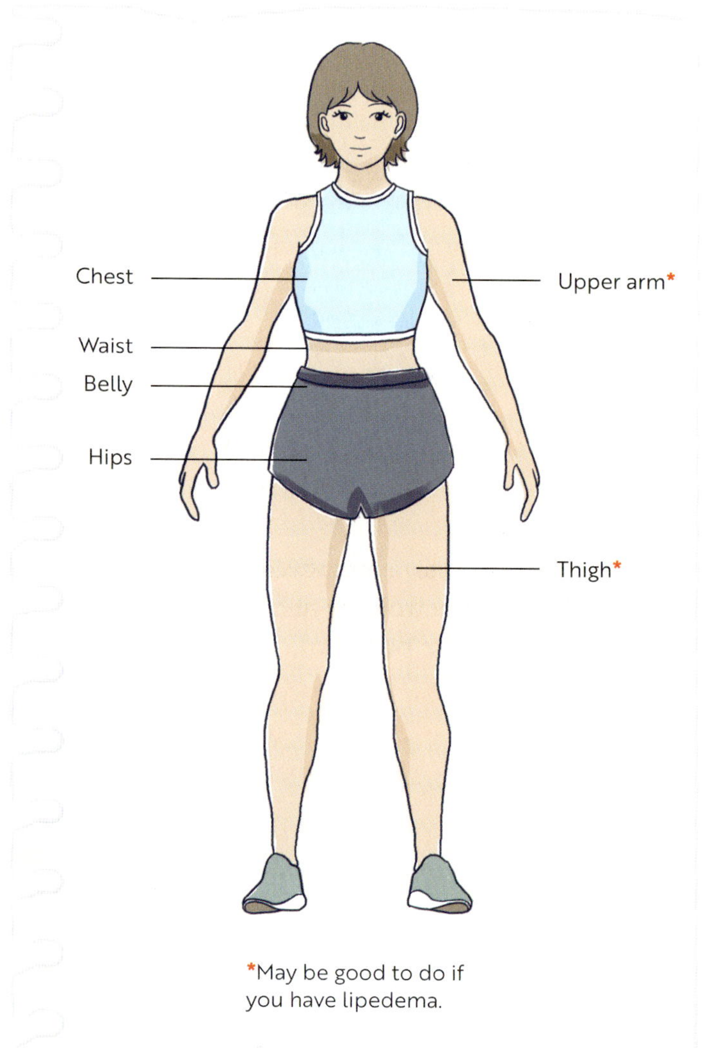

*May be good to do if you have lipedema.

Next, take some photos in whatever clothing you feel comfortable wearing. Bra and underwear, boxers, workout clothes, or regular clothing is fine. Take at least one front-facing and one side-facing photo. You can print them and attach them to your prepping worksheet or just store them on your phone to compare with your after photos later. Be sure to take these photos, even if you're not happy with how you currently look. Sometimes you will see changes in your photos before you see any movement on the scale or in your measurements. You will want these photos down the road, trust me.

If you have time and a little bit of money, it is worth it to do two more baseline measurements. The first is blood work. Everyone should be getting blood work done at least once a year. If you get these tests *before* starting carnivore, you will be able to see metabolic health improvements that don't show up on the scale. Improvements in these numbers can be very encouraging, especially if the scale is not moving as fast as you would like. You can also make tweaks to the diet or know when to reintroduce foods based on these numbers. Here are the blood tests I recommend:

- **Standard lipid panel:** Total cholesterol, triglycerides, HDL cholesterol, and LDL cholesterol
- **Comprehensive metabolic panel:** Fasting glucose, electrolytes, and some kidney and liver function numbers
- **Fasting insulin:** Elevated fasting insulin levels are better indicators of pre-diabetes risk than A1c and fasting glucose. Typically, if your fasting insulin levels are elevated, you have some insulin resistance.
- **A1c:** Average glucose levels over the last three months
- **hs-CRP:** An easy-to-measure systemic inflammation marker
- **Vitamin D:** Normal levels of D are an indicator of metabolic health and a well-functioning immune system. Most people are deficient in vitamin D.
- **GGT:** A liver function marker

You can either ask your doctor to order these tests or order them online in most US states. In most other countries, you will have to go through your doctor to get them done. (For more information on how to order blood tests online and how to interpret them, head to chapter 8.) Staple or paperclip your results to your prepping worksheet so everything is in one place for future reference.

Another test I find helpful as a baseline to measure progress is a body composition DEXA (dual-energy X-ray absorptiometry) scan. It measures bone density, visceral fat levels, and body composition and costs anywhere from $39 to $200. There is more info on DEXA scans on pages 175–176. Once you get the printout of your results, put it with your prepping worksheet as well.

While I do want you to take a baseline weight on a scale, I don't want you to use the scale as your main measurement tool. Instead of focusing on losing a specific amount of weight the first month, I want you to focus on non-scale-related goals. Find an article of clothing that does not fit you right now, try it on, and take some pictures. At the end of the first month on carnivore, try on that garment again. How the fit has changed is a much better indicator of your progress than the number on the scale.

Finally, on your prepping worksheet, make notes on how you feel physically most of the time. Any aches, pains, ailments, chronic conditions, brain fog, fatigue...whatever it is that ails you, write down those symptoms. After a month on carnivore, come back to that list and write down how you feel again. Improvements in your health are among the best indicators of progress. It is going to be very interesting to see how you feel at the end of the first month, the first ninety days, and beyond!

GETTING SUPPORT

Next up is getting your partner, family member, roommate, or other important person in your life on board with you. The best-case scenario is that they do carnivore with you for the ninety-day period. It is so much easier when everyone in the house is eating the same food. At the very least, having their support and understanding will go a long way toward helping you stay consistent.

If your partner is eating a SAD and refuses to change their ways, don't worry! It may be a bit more challenging for you with all that food around, but when they see your results, they might change their mind and join you. Actions and results speak louder than words, and maybe you can lead by example!

There are many low-carb and carnivore communities out there, so if you cannot find support at home, seek out one or many of these communities! You will find your people there. There are also many in-person "Meatups" that you can attend and many low-carb conferences that are open to the general public. Get plugged in!

PREPARING FOR THE KETO FLU

Yes, it's real! Keto flu is sugar or carbohydrate withdrawal, and it is very similar to drug withdrawals. If you are going cold turkey into carnivore, you will likely experience some keto flu symptoms. If you are easing into it, you will hopefully avoid the worst of it. Keto flu typically lasts two to three weeks at most. Symptoms include

- Fatigue
- Brain fog
- Nausea
- Irritability
- Muscle cramping
- Sugar cravings
- Diarrhea or constipation
- Headaches
- Racing heart/heart palpitations
- Sleep disturbances, such as restless legs, cramping, difficulty falling or staying asleep, and frequent urination

Why does keto flu happen? Well, your body is transitioning to a new fuel source: fat. When you're eating a typical American diet, your primary fuel is glucose. It is a fuel that the body uses very efficiently. When you switch to eating close to zero carbs, you are no longer providing your body with quick shots of glucose, so you're going to go through some withdrawal. It's nothing to fear.

These symptoms are common, but there are ways to avoid them or lessen their severity. I recommend electrolytes for new carnivores. These are essential in the early stages because you will be losing some water weight, and with that water goes electrolytes. There are many brands you can try; just make sure to get one without added sugars, dyes, flavors, or fillers. You want a product that contains at least sodium, magnesium, and potassium. You can also make your own; just search online for a recipe. Unrefined salt like Celtic sea salt is another electrolyte option because it retains all its minerals. Regardless of the electrolyte you choose, make it a part of your morning routine to mitigate the worst of your keto flu symptoms. Even if you are not experiencing symptoms, be sure to take some electrolytes in the morning for at least the first month on carnivore.

Another way to keep keto flu symptoms in check is to drink bone broth or meat stock. Eating enough food can help with fatigue and weakness. And rest is important during this first month because your body is doing the hard work of transitioning from primarily glucose as fuel to fat. Give your body a break and take it easy when you can.

And of course, gradually reducing your carbohydrate intake as opposed to going cold turkey into carnivore is always an option. This approach can help lessen the worst of the keto flu symptoms because you are weaning your body off carbs slowly while increasing your fat intake.

Obsessed with Purity: Dealing with Orthorexia

Orthorexia is an obsessive preoccupation with eating only "healthy" foods. What those healthy foods are is defined by each individual. I think that some people, in their quest to improve their health, can start veering toward orthorexia if the quest starts to consume their life and thoughts. If you are experiencing severe anxiety or depression around your food choices, it could be orthorexia. On the other hand, wanting to consume only foods that are healthy and nutritious is not a bad thing. I think it becomes a negative when it is all you think about, to the detriment of your daily life.

Here's my advice: There is only so much you can do. You can't avoid every toxin, especially in this modern world. But you can filter your tap water. You can cook with stainless-steel or ceramic pans rather than nonstick. You can purchase the highest quality whole, real foods you can afford and avoid fillers and additives. You can set up a high-quality air filter. Just do what you can, and move on.

PREPPING YOUR KITCHEN FOR CARNIVORE

Now let's work our way into the kitchen. The next big job when prepping for carnivore is to clear your pantry, refrigerator, and freezer of all non-carnivore foods, including ultra-processed foods and drinks. If they are in the house, they can be a temptation. I recommend boxing everything up and storing it in the garage or at a friend's or family member's home so that it is not easily accessible to you. If you really want to take the plunge, you can throw away or donate all of the food.

If you are unable to clear the shelves completely because you are the only person in your household who is going to be doing carnivore, try to get rid of the food items that are most tempting to you. You may have a weakness for cookies and popcorn but have no desire for cereal and chips, for example. If you are living with people who will not be following carnivore, this is about the best you can do.

RESTOCKING YOUR KITCHEN WITH CARNIVORE FOODS

You're going to want to go to the grocery store before day 1, especially after getting rid of all of the non-carnivore foods in your kitchen. You don't know how many people I've talked to who decided to go carnivore and then woke up in the morning and realized they had nothing to eat.

The biggest question in the beginning is, "What can I eat and drink?" Well, a lot more than you might think. In general, if it is an animal, you can eat it. That means any kind of meat is fair game. Food products that are produced by animals, such as eggs and milk, are generally okay as well, depending on which version of carnivore you have chosen to follow (refer to pages 58–60). To give you a better idea of the possibilities, I have a complete grocery list that you can print out at JennyMitich.com. I have also provided a sample two-week meal plan that you can follow on page 82.

Spring for the highest-quality meats and animal products you can afford. The lists on the next two pages give you a few things to look for.

Bare Minimum Items

- [ ] Eggs (pastured organic if possible)
- [ ] 80/20 ground beef (grass fed if you can)
- [ ] Chicken
- [ ] Bacon
- [ ] Pork
- [ ] Grass-fed butter

Beef

- [ ] Steak of any kind: ribeye, New York strip, sirloin, skirt, flank, etc.
- [ ] Ground beef
- [ ] Beef ribs
- [ ] Organ meats: liver, heart, kidneys, etc.
- [ ] Tongue
- [ ] Stew meat
- [ ] Sausage (avoid dextrose/corn syrup/ carbs above 1g per serving)

Pork

- [ ] Bacon
- [ ] Chops
- [ ] Sausage (avoid dextrose/ corn syrup/carbs above 1g per serving)
- [ ] Tenderloin
- [ ] Loin roast
- [ ] Shoulder
- [ ] Ribs
- [ ] Pork rinds
- [ ] Belly
- [ ] Ham
- [ ] Ham hocks

Other Red Meats

- [ ] Veal
- [ ] Bison
- [ ] Lamb: chops, steaks, roasts
- [ ] Mutton
- [ ] Venison
- [ ] Goat
- [ ] Elk/Moose/Bear

Chicken

- [ ] Wings
- [ ] Thighs (skin on and bone in)
- [ ] Drumsticks
- [ ] Whole chicken
- [ ] Breast
- [ ] Organ meats: liver, heart, kidneys, chitlins
- [ ] Sausage (avoid dextrose/corn syrup/ carbs above 1g per serving)

Seafood

- [ ] Fish (wild-caught if possible; farmed mollusks are fine)
- [ ] Tuna
- [ ] Salmon
- [ ] Walleye
- [ ] Red snapper
- [ ] Anchovies
- [ ] Bass
- [ ] Catfish
- [ ] Cod
- [ ] Grouper
- [ ] Trout
- [ ] Shrimp
- [ ] Scallops
- [ ] Mussels
- [ ] Oysters
- [ ] Lobster
- [ ] Crab
- [ ] Sardines (tinned or fresh)

Other Birds/ Waterfowl

- [ ] Turkey
- [ ] Duck
- [ ] Goose
- [ ] Pheasant
- [ ] Quail

Eggs of any kind are acceptable on carnivore.

Animal Fats

- [ ] Bacon grease
- [ ] Beef tallow (fat from cows)
- [ ] Mutton tallow (fat from sheep)
- [ ] Butter
- [ ] Suet (fat around kidneys and loins of beef, lamb, and mutton)
- [ ] Lard (fat from pigs)
- [ ] Ghee
- [ ] Duck tallow
- [ ] Schmaltz (rendered fat from chickens or geese)
- [ ] Bear fat
- [ ] Goose tallow

Dairy

- [ ] Heavy cream
- [ ] Half-and-half
- [ ] Cheese (I always grate my own from a block to avoid anti-caking agents)
- [ ] Butter (I always use butter, even if I am not eating other dairy)
- [ ] Full-fat Greek yogurt
- [ ] Full-fat cottage cheese
- [ ] Full-fat sour cream
- [ ] Full-fat cream cheese

Processed Meats

- [ ] Bacon
- [ ] Sausage
- [ ] Kielbasa
- [ ] Knockwurst
- [ ] Beef hotdogs
- [ ] Lunch meat
- [ ] Brats
- [ ] Pepperoni
- [ ] Jerky
- [ ] Ham
- [ ] Canned meats
- [ ] Smoked or dried meats
- [ ] Corned beef

Tip: Always read the label, avoid dextrose/corn syrup/carbs over 1g per serving, and get the highest quality you can.

Grocery Shopping Guidelines:

- **Bacon:** Try to get a brand with the fewest additives possible. But I don't freak out if there is a bit of dextrose or sugar in the bacon I am eating as long as the nutrition label reads "0g carbs." I don't worry about getting uncured bacon; I eat regular bacon most of the time. Do what works best for you.
- **Ground beef:** The fattier, the better; 80/20 is a good place to start.
- **Steaks:** I shop the sales and freeze what I am not going to use immediately.
- **Pork:** Pork shoulder and pork chops are my go-to pork products (besides bacon, of course). But if I see tenderloin or other options on sale, I will purchase it.
- **Hotdogs:** I buy all-beef hotdogs and avoid any product with corn syrup in it.
- **Sausages:** Be sure to read the ingredient list and avoid anything that has corn syrup in it. If there is dextrose, make sure the carbs per serving are under 2 grams.
- **Seafood:** Wild-caught over farmed. (This doesn't apply to mussels or oysters.)
- **Chicken:** I typically purchase drumsticks and bone-in, skin-on chicken thighs. I also really love wings. I use chicken breast only when a recipe calls for it or if I'm doing a higher-protein version of carnivore because it is very low in fat.
- **Eggs:** Preferably pastured organic, but cage-free eggs are also great. If these options are too expensive, regular eggs will work just fine.
- **Butter:** Preferably grass fed. I always get salted butter, but get what you prefer.
- **Other fats:** You can use tallow, bacon grease, lard, or suet. The important thing is that the fat is animal based.

GRASS-FED VERSUS GRAIN-FED BEEF

There are conflicting opinions on this top ic. Nutritionally, there are marginal benefits to eating grass-fed beef over conventionally raised, grain-fed beef. Grass-fed beef has a slightly better omega-6 to omega-3 ratio and a slightly better nutritional profile. One major difference between the two is that grass fed typically has less fat and a slightly gamier taste, and cooking a grass-fed steak is a little different. Environmentally, grass-fed cows on a regenerative farm can be a carbon sink, meaning they lock up carbon from the atmosphere over time. But here's the thing: All cows are mostly grass fed for most of their lives. Conventionally raised cattle only eat grain for the last few weeks to few months of their lives to fatten up before slaughter. There are lots of ethically raised cows that eat grass for most of their lives and then are finished with grain to improve their fat profile.

Here's my opinion: Get what you prefer and can afford. I personally eat conventionally raised beef most of the time. I buy a whole ribeye from Costco every four to six weeks and then, at my local grocery store, I pick up any ribeyes that are 50 percent off that I find. I do purchase American Wagyu ground beef from a ranch in Minnesota because the flavor is out of this world. And I get a monthly delivery of grass-fed, grass-finished beef from ButcherBox. (If you would like to try these meats, head to JennyMitich.com for links and coupon codes.) There are a few regenerative farms that I support as well. But the bottom line is that all beef, whether it is grass or grain fed, is a nutrient-dense food, and you need to include as much of it in your carnivore diet as you can afford.

PROCESSED MEATS

This is another contentious topic. Can you eat processed meats on the carnivore diet? In my opinion, yes, but with some caveats. First, you need to read the ingredient list, just as you would with spices and seasonings. You want to avoid dextrose, corn syrup, and other added sugars, along with vegetable seed oils such as canola, soybean, and sunflower. You want the list to be as short as possible. And when looking at the nutrition label, try to keep it to 2 grams of carbs or less per serving.

Would you want to make processed meats the focus of your diet? No. But if you want to include some, I think that is fine. If processed meats are all you can afford, then get processed meats! They are still infinitely better than ultra-processed carbs, seed oils, and sugar.

My twins and I eat Bob Evans breakfast sausage and Kirkland thick-cut bacon every morning. I eat some deli meats on a charcuterie board a couple of times a month. I also use some deli meats in recipes. Typically, making your own sausages or deli meats is your best bet if you have the time, because then you can control the ingredients. Purchasing from a local farm or butcher is another great option because they typically don't add a ton of ingredients.

Nutrition Facts

Varied servings per container

Serving size	**2oz (57g)**
Amount per serving	
Calories	**50**
	% Daily Value*
Total Fat 1g	2%
Saturated Fat 0g	0%
Trans Fat 0g	
Polyunsaturated Fat 0g	
Monounsaturated Fat 0g	
Cholesterol 25mg	9%
Sodium 560mg	24%
Total Carbohydrate 0g	0%
Dietary Fiber 0g	0%
Total Sugars 0g	
Includes 0g Added Sugars	0%
Protein 9g	
Vit. D 0.1mcg 0% · Calcium 10mg 0%	
Iron 0.3mg 2% · Potas. 150mg 4%	

*The % Daily Value (DV) tells you how much a nutrient in a serving of food contributes to a daily diet. 2,000 calories a day is used for general nutrition advice.

Tips

- Try to keep carb count below 2g per serving.
- Avoid added sugars and vegetable seed oils.
- Avoid dyes and colorings.
- Some preservatives are okay; I'm not as militant with those, but I do avoid BHT and BHA.
- It boils down to price and preference. Use the tips below as guidelines.

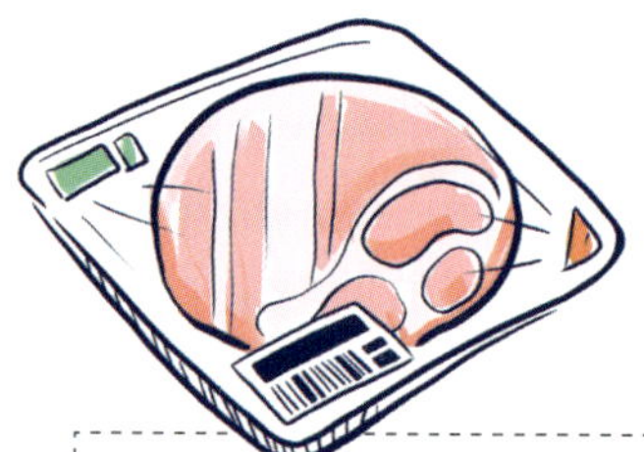

Aim for the shortest ingredient list possible

Avoid preservatives like BHT and BHA

INGREDIENTS: PORK HAM CURED WITH WATER, SALT, SUGAR, CORN SYRUP, BHT, AUTOLYZED YEAST EXTRACT, SODIUM ERYTHORBATE, SODIUM NITRITE, SOY PROTEIN CONCENTRATE.

GLAZED WITH: SALT, DEXTROSE, MOLASSES POWDER (MOLASSES MALTODEXTRIN), CARAMEL COLOR, COTTON SEED OIL.

CONTAINS: SOY
CARAMEL COLOR ADDED

Avoid vegetable seed oils such as canola, soybean, and sunflower

Avoid food colorings and dyes

Avoid dextrose, corn syrup, and other sugars

Avoid soy

SPICES AND SEASONINGS

Some carnivore purists argue that if you consume any plant material, you are no longer doing carnivore. But I disagree. Plenty of carnivores add some spices to their meats. In my opinion, it's only when you are chewing the leaves or fruit of the plant that you are no longer eating carnivore. A little bit of garlic powder isn't the end of the world for most people.

There are exceptions, though. If your Why is a severe autoimmune condition, allergies you can't seem to pin down, or a condition that is severely impacting the quality of your life, I suggest avoiding all spices and seasonings except salt for the first ninety days of carnivore. You may be highly sensitive to some or all plant materials, and you will have to reintroduce them one at a time down the road. I go over the reintroduction process on page 100.

When you are looking for spices and seasonings, there are a few things to watch out for. In general, I spring for organic. I look at the ingredient list and avoid anything with anti-caking agents (they are typically labeled as such), dextrose or other sugars, or any kind of filler. But these spices can be a bit pricey, so get what works best for your budget. You are only going to be using a little bit here and there, so it's okay if you can't get the highest-quality spices.

ARTIFICIAL OR NATURAL SUGAR SUBSTITUTES

This is yet another topic that has a lot of opinions floating around about it in the carnivore world. Here's the thing: Plenty of long-term carnivores use artificial or natural sugar substitutes and experience success. And then there are others who can't touch the stuff because it triggers a previous sugar addiction or gives them gastrointestinal distress. You are going to figure out what works best for you, but here are some tips to get you started.

I advise cutting all sugar substitutes, natural or artificial, from your diet for at least the first ninety days. After that, you can reintroduce them one at a time to see if they cause any sugar cravings or gastrointestinal distress. Personally, I do not use many sugar substitutes, artificial or natural. Occasionally I have an LMNT electrolytes packet that is sweetened with stevia or have one of their sparkling water drinks. If I am making an egg pudding or a carnivore cheesecake for the holidays, I sweeten it with allulose. But otherwise, I avoid sugar substitutes.

The following are common artificial and natural sweeteners. I would stick to the natural ones if you decide to use sweeteners.

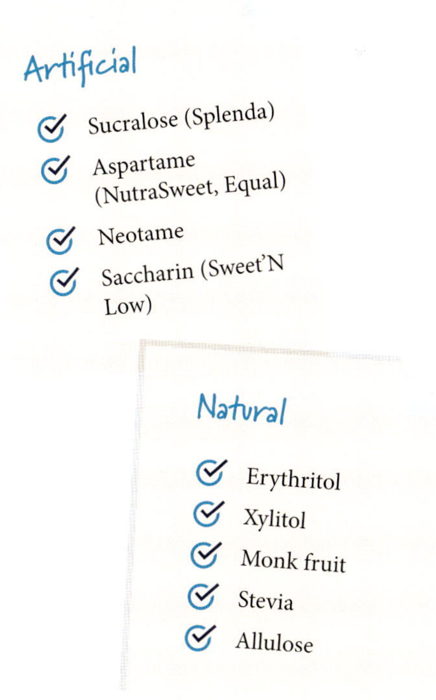

KNOWING WHAT YOU CAN DRINK

In general, plain water is going to be your main beverage. Sparkling water is good, too. Sugar-free electrolyte drinks are allowed. But what about tea, coffee, diet soda, and energy drinks? Can you have that stuff on carnivore? There are many arguments over this topic in the carnivore space.

In general, I think coffee is fine. Many carnivore experts avoid coffee because of the pesticide loads on the beans and phytochemicals within the beans, but I continue drinking it because I enjoy the taste and the morning ritual. You must make that decision for yourself. I would steer clear of black and green teas because of the high oxalates, but a cup here and there won't kill you. Herbal teas are generally fine. Some carnivores can drink diet soda or other sugar-free beverages without triggering sugar cravings. I would definitely stay away from energy drinks, though, because there are way too many ingredients in them. I think you will discover that you no longer need heavily caffeinated drinks because your energy levels are going to go up on carnivore.

As far as how much water to consume, take your current weight and divide it by 2. Drinking at least that number of fluid ounces is a good starting point. If you weigh over 200 pounds, you can divide your weight by 2.5 or 3 instead. If you're a coffee drinker, know that caffeinated coffee is a diuretic, which means it dehydrates you. So, for every 8-ounce cup of regular coffee you drink, you will need to add 12 ounces of extra water to your daily hydration goal. Decaffeinated coffee does not have the same diuretic effect.

A good way you can tell if you are sufficiently hydrated is to check the color of your urine. You don't want it to be colorless. Instead, you are looking for a light straw to light yellow color. Sometimes supplements can discolor your urine, so keep that in mind.

YES	MAYBE	NO
Water	Tea	Energy drinks
Sparkling water	Diet soda	Juices
Electrolytes (sugar free)		Coconut water
Coffee		Drinks with sugar

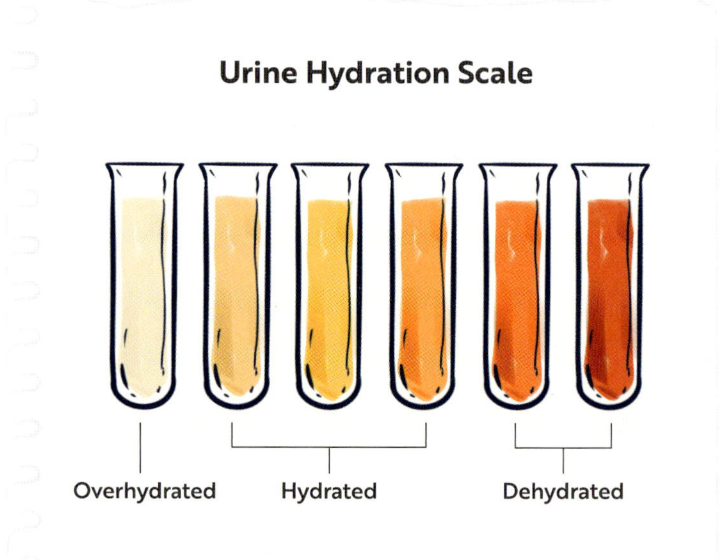

IS ALCOHOL ALLOWED?

Alcohol is not carnivore, and I do not recommend drinking during your first ninety days on the diet—for several reasons. First, when you consume alcohol, your body must stop what it is doing and process the alcohol first, before glucose, ketones, or the food you just ate. Second, alcohol can trigger sugar and carb cravings. Third, if you include alcohol, you will not reap the full benefits of the diet. So, for the first ninety days at least, it's best to not drink any alcohol.

If abstaining is not a possibility for you, keep it to one drink and pick something that is as low in carbs as possible, like a vodka soda or a whiskey on the rocks. If you are in a social situation and you want to feel included but not drink, ask the bartender to make you a sparkling water in a lowball glass with a lime. No one will notice you are not drinking.

If you continue carnivore for the long term, having a drink once in a while is a possibility. I was a bit of a partier in my teens and twenties, but now, in my forties, I have a drink or two every six to eight weeks. I typically keep it low carb, but I will admit to enjoying a couple of beers in the summertime or a margarita at a Mexican restaurant. You will figure out what works best for you. But in the beginning, it's best to avoid alcohol.

CARNIVORE ON A BUDGET

Let's address the elephant in the room and talk about the costs of a carnivore lifestyle. After the pandemic and the subsequent inflation, meat prices have gone up significantly. In today's economy, finding affordable foods can be a struggle. But that doesn't mean carnivore has to break the bank. In fact, there are many money-*saving* benefits that you may not have considered.

First, think about all of the foods you will *not* be purchasing anymore. Snacks, sodas, ice cream, cookies, vegetables, fruits...eliminate whatever non-animal products you regularly used to include on your grocery list. I am saving money on carnivore because of that fact alone. Also, food waste goes way down. You won't have fruits and vegetables going bad in your fridge anymore. I used to spend $5 to $6 for a little package of greenhouse-grown organic lettuce, and half the time, it went bad before I got to it. Now, I eat most of the food I purchase right away, and if there are leftovers, I eat them within a day or two.

Another factor that you may not have considered is that you will not be eating as often. Many carnivores eat two meals per day with no snacks in between, so the total volume of food is much less. Carnivores also tend to eat at home more of the time, which saves a ton of money compared to eating out.

The amount of money saved because of health improvements will be different for each person. You may not be getting sick as often, you may be able to reduce or eliminate medications you are taking, and it may be less expensive for you to get health or life insurance if you can get your weight and health back to normal ranges.

There are ways to save money at the store as well. You can talk to the meat manager and ask when they do their daily markdowns. Every day, the store must get rid of the meat that has to be sold by that day. My local grocery store does markdowns first thing in the morning of between 30 and 50 percent. I hit the store several times a week and purchase reduced-price meat. Sometimes I find a lot, sometimes a little. But I scoop it up and freeze it right when I get home if I am not going to cook it right away.

My grocery store also has weekly sales on certain cuts of meat. I have gotten great deals on pork tenderloin for $1 per pound. I have found pork shoulder for $0.49 per pound. Recently, the store was selling bone-in choice ribeye for $8.99 per pound, and I found some that were marked down 50 percent. I'm telling you, there are deals to be had, so search all of the stores in your area and figure out which ones have the best sales.

Another way to save money is by buying bulk meat and butchering it yourself. I love doing this with the whole ribeyes and whole sirloins from Costco. The whole ribeye typically weighs between 12 and 22 pounds and is almost always at least $2 to $4 cheaper per pound than precut ribeyes. Also, the whole ribeye is not blade tenderized, so it may be safer to consume in the long run. Blade tenderization is a process where a device pierces the meat with needles or blades to make it more tender. The problem is that it can introduce bacteria into the meat. I personally have never had issues with blade-tenderized meat, but I have gotten plenty of comments on YouTube about this problem. Just another reason why cutting your own meat is a better option.

A lot of people invest in a deep freezer and order a quarter, half, or whole cow from a local farm or ranch. This is an excellent way to save money. Perhaps you can team up with a few other families and go in on a whole cow to maximize savings.

After a couple of months on carnivore, you are going to be a deal-scouting expert! It just takes practice. If you are living on an extremely limited budget, I created two videos for you over on my YouTube channel: One is how to do carnivore on a $100 monthly food budget for one person, and the other is a $300 budget for a family of four. I posted an updated low-budget carnivore video in June 2025, and I was *still* able to do carnivore on an ultra-low budget, despite high prices. While it sounds impossible, I was able to do it. You can, too!

CARNIVORE ON A BUDGET

- Shop sales.
- Deep freezer—buy in bulk.
- Buy 1/4, 1/2, or whole cow from a local ranch or farm.
- Talk to the meat manager at your local grocery store and see when they do their markdowns.
- Bulk meat is typically a few dollars cheaper per pound than precut. Cut it yourself!

Remember: You've eliminated a lot from your grocery list, so you may be saving money right off the bat!

CARNIVORE KITCHEN SUPPLIES & TOOLS

There are endless kitchen gadgets and tools on the market, but you don't need most of them. You can get away with a single frying pan, a stove or microwave, and a spatula. But having more tools to play with is always fun and will allow you to prepare some amazing dishes. Here are the tools that I use every week, along with some that I would categorize as luxuries.

Must-haves:

- Cast-iron skillet (10- to 15-inch)
- Frying pan (stainless steel or ceramic coated)
- Saucepan (stainless steel or ceramic coated)
- Sauté pan (stainless steel or ceramic coated)
- Air fryer (ceramic coated or glass)
- Microwave
- Meat thermometer (manual or Bluetooth)
- Parchment paper
- Half and quarter sheet pans
- Wire racks for baking sheets
- Slow cooker
- Vacuum sealer
- Kitchen scale
- 6-inch boning knife (for butchering other bulk meats)
- 10-inch breaking knife (for breaking down whole ribeyes)
- Immersion blender (for making mayo and blending up eggs)
- Regular blender
- Tongs
- Spatula

Luxuries:

- Stand mixer
- Instant Pot
- Ice cream maker
- Crepe pan
- Crepe flippers
- Oyster shucker

When it comes to the pans you use, I suggest a high-quality set of either ceramic-coated or stainless-steel cookware. Nonstick coatings are highly toxic and can leach chemicals into your food. PFOA, PTFE, BPA, and other potentially toxic materials are present in a lot of the cheaper, low-quality cookware on the market.

MEAL PREP

After you get back from the grocery store, it's a good idea to do some meal prep. This is especially important because if you get hit with the keto flu, you are not going to feel like cooking. Getting into the habit of meal prepping early on is also important because your hunger cues are going to be a bit out of whack, and it's better to have something ready to eat than to have to take the time to cook.

Grilled meats, hard-boiled eggs (page 236), pot roast (page 219), Breakfast Casserole (page 228), and some steaks are my go-tos for meal prepping. If you want to do a bit more work, my Taco Balls (page 294) and Beef Stroganoff (page 276) are *excellent* when reheated. If you decide to follow my meal plan, prep a few of the meals before day 1, and you will be ready to hit the ground running!

OPTIONAL CARNIVORE MEAL PLAN

For the most part, your carnivore diet is going to be made up of meats, eggs, and butter. But if you need a bit more structure or are super confused about how to eat in the beginning, I have a two-week meal plan for you. This plan includes recipes from this book (marked with an asterisk) to provide a bit of variety so you don't get bored (which is common in the first few months on carnivore) and is simple to follow. If you would like to build your own meal plan, I have a free template that you can print out at JennyMitich.com.

This plan specifies two meals per day, but you can break it up into three meals, or even more if you have a unique situation, like having undergone bariatric surgery. Or you can do one meal a day (OMAD) if you prefer. If there is something here that you don't eat, switch it out for an animal product that you do consume. Make it your own!

WEEK 1	DAY 1	DAY 2	DAY 3	DAY 4	DAY 5	DAY 6	DAY 7
	Ground Beef and Eggs*	Breakfast Casserole*	Eggs and bacon	*Leftover* Breakfast Casserole*	Air Fryer Egg Bites*	Eggs, sausage, and smoked salmon	Air Fryer Egg Bites*
	16- to 24-oz. steak of your choice	Hearty Meat Soup*	Beef Stroganoff with Carnivore Noodles*	Wings*	16- to 24-oz. steak of your choice	Burger patties with bacon	Taco Balls*

WEEK 2	DAY 1	DAY 2	DAY 3	DAY 4	DAY 5	DAY 6	DAY 7
	Eggs, bacon, and sausage	Flanken short ribs and eggs	Air Fryer Egg Bites*	Steak and eggs	Ground Beef and Eggs*	Air Fryer Egg Bites*	*Leftover* steak and eggs
	Walleye* with butter and 8 oz. sirloin	Carnivore Quesadilla*	16- to 24-oz. steak of your choice	Carnivore Mac & Cheese Casserole*	Taco Balls*	*Leftover* Ground Beef and Eggs	Slow Cooker Pot Roast*

YOU ARE READY TO START CARNIVORE!

Go over your prepping worksheet and make sure you haven't forgotten anything. If you did, I strongly suggest you complete each step so that you will have the best chance of success. Once your worksheet is complete, pick a day to get started and head to the next chapter: Carnivore Timeline.

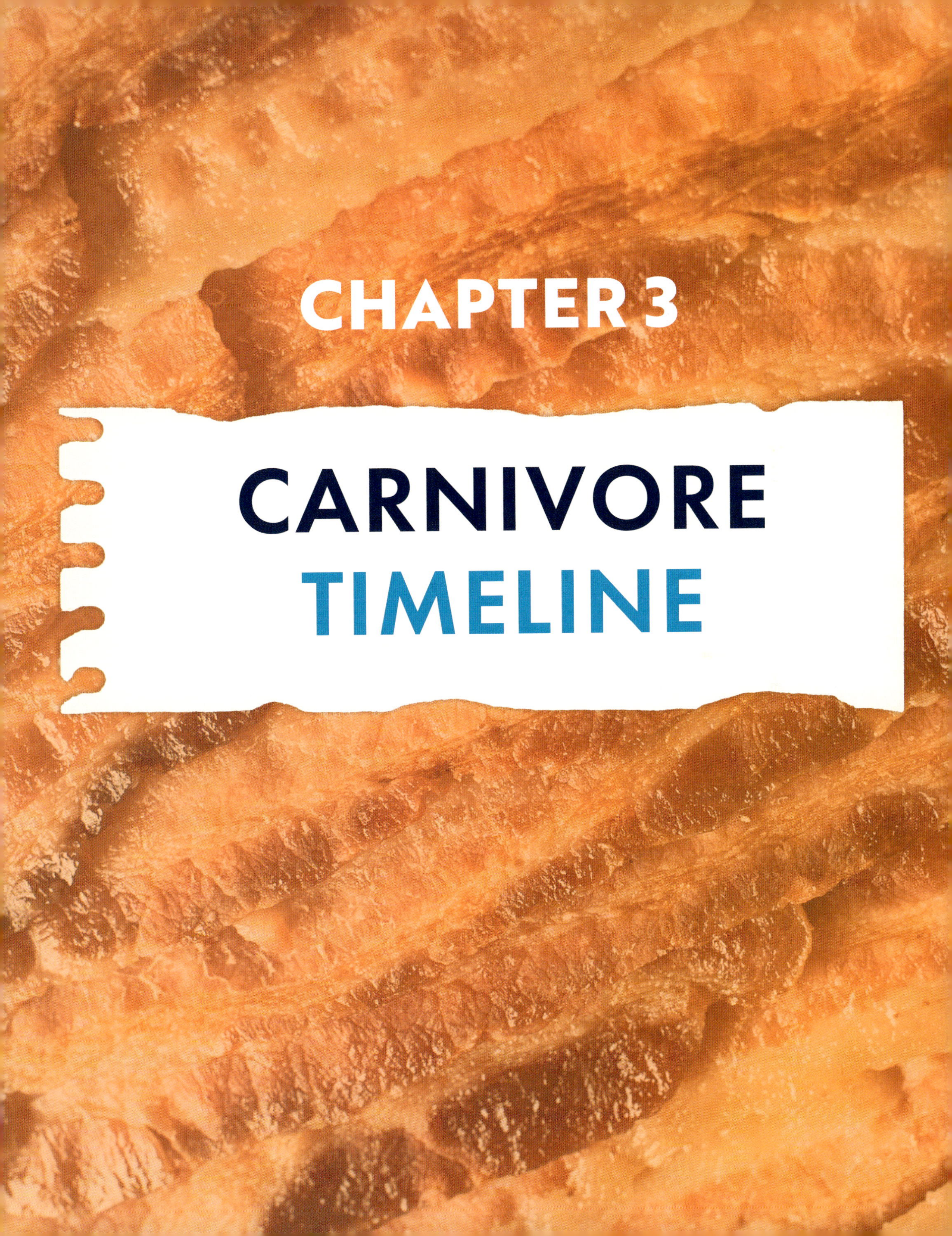

CHAPTER 3

CARNIVORE TIMELINE

You have done all of the preparation, and now it's time to get started! If you are easing into carnivore, use my gradual carbohydrate reduction guide to begin. Otherwise, head to "Month 1" on page 88.

FOUR-WEEK GRADUAL CARBOHYDRATE REDUCTION

WEEK 1

- ☑ Cut ultra-processed foods
- ☑ Eat only whole, real food
- ☑ Replace 1–2 high-oxalate foods w/ low-oxalate ones (see lists)
- ☑ Increase amount of fatty meats
- ☑ Track your food intake

WEEK 2

- ☑ Reduce daily carbs by 25–50g
- ☑ Increase amount of protein and fat
- ☑ Replace 1–2 more high-oxalate foods with low-oxalate ones

WEEK 3

- ☑ Reduce daily carbs by another 25–50g
- ☑ Replace 1–2 more high-oxalate foods with low-oxalate ones

WEEK 4

- ☑ Reduce daily carbs by another 25–50g
- ☑ Continue switching out high-oxalate foods for low-oxalate ones

WEEK 1

The focus this week is to stop eating ultra-processed foods, grains, seed oils, and added sugars. I also want you to clear out any artificially sweetened items or keto desserts. You are going to be focusing on eating only whole, real foods in the form of fattier cuts of meat, vegetables, fruits, and dairy if you tolerate it. The goal is to get your body used to using real food as fuel.

I want you to track your food this week so you can get an idea of how many grams of protein, fat, and carbs you are eating. That information is going to be helpful when you begin reducing carbs. You can use any free food-tracking app such as MyFitnessPal, Chronometer, or Carb Manager. This first week, try to get your carb count down to between 100 and 150 grams per day. Aim for a *minimum* of 100 grams of protein and 100 grams of fat per day, but you can always eat more than that. Remember that protein is the building block and fat is the fuel. You want to start getting used to consuming more animal proteins and fats.

As far as what to eat, take a look at the Complete Carnivore grocery list on pages 73–74 and pick the meats and animal products that you enjoy. You can cook a recipe from this book as your main dish and then add some fruits and/or vegetables on the side. Experiment with preparing different meats, because it takes some practice. It took me a few tries to cook a ribeye to my desired temperature in a cast-iron or stainless-steel pan.

As far as which fruits and vegetables to choose, check out the lists below for some great options. If you have been consuming a lot of high-oxalate foods (see page 61), I recommend replacing one or two of them this week with lower-oxalate options.[1] I wouldn't cut all high-oxalate foods at once because that can cause very unpleasant oxalate-dumping symptoms, and you don't want that. You can cut more high-oxalate foods in the coming weeks. All of the options listed here are low in oxalates. Another way to avoid oxalate dumping is to consume one cup of black tea daily during this carb reduction phase.

Low-Oxalate, Low-Lectin, Lower-Carb Fruits

- Apples
- Blueberries
- Cantaloupe
- Coconut
- Cherries
- Cranberries
- Honeydew
- Lemons
- Oranges
- Peaches
- Pears
- Papayas
- Plums
- Ripe avocados
- Strawberries
- Watermelon

[1] Ryan Andrews, "All about lectins," PrecisionNutrition, https://www.precisionnutrition.com/all-about-lectins, accessed July 8, 2025. Cynthia Demarco, "Should you eat a lectin-free diet?" MD Anderson Cancer Center, February 12, 2024, https://www.mdanderson.org/cancerwise/should-you-eat-a-lectin-free-diet.h00-159695178.html.

Low-Oxalate, Low-Lectin, Lower-Carb Vegetables/Legumes

- Alfalfa sprouts
- Arugula
- Asparagus
- Bell peppers (peeled and seeded)
- Black-eyed peas
- Bok choy
- Broccoli sprouts
- Broccoli
- Brussels sprouts
- Chives
- Cabbage
- Carrots
- Cauliflower
- Cucumbers (peeled and seeded)
- Endive
- Escarole
- Garlic
- Kale
- Kimchi
- Lettuce (romaine, Bibb, butter, iceberg)
- Mushrooms
- Mustard greens
- Onions
- Radishes
- Rutabaga
- Turnips
- Winter squash (peeled and seeded)
- Watercress
- Water chestnut
- Zucchini (peeled and seeded)

Low-Oxalate, Low-Lectin, Lower-Carb Seeds/Nuts

- Chestnuts
- Flax seeds
- Pumpkin seeds (roasted)
- Sunflower seeds (roasted)

WEEK 2

By the start of this week, you should no longer be eating ultra-processed foods, grains, seed oils, or added sugars. Your meals should be made up of meat, vegetables, fruits, and perhaps dairy. Taking the information from your food-tracking app, reduce your carb intake by 25 to 50 grams to end up somewhere between 75 and 125 grams of carbs per day. To do so, switch to lower-carb fruits and vegetables and reduce your plant intake in general. You don't want to drop carbs too quickly. Ease into it nice and slowly. You have another few weeks to get down into the single digits.

At the same time you are reducing carbs, increase your protein and fat intake by eating more fatty cuts of meat (maybe going from an 8-ounce steak to a 12-ounce one), cooking everything in animal fats, or adding some butter. Start to increase the amounts of proteins and fats you consume by a little each day. Protein is highly satiating, so this can be difficult in the beginning.

If you had been eating a lot of high-oxalate foods prior to week 1, pick another one or two of them to replace with lower-oxalate options this week.

Even though you're taking the carb reduction slowly, you may begin to feel some keto flu symptoms. Be sure to have electrolytes on hand and take some first thing in the morning to help counteract any keto flu symptoms that may pop up—or even prevent them. Refer to pages 70–71 for more information on keto flu.

If you feel extremely wiped out at this lower level of carb consumption, up your carbs by 25 grams and see how you feel. You may need to take the carb reduction a bit slower, and that's okay! This is not a race.

WEEK 3

Reduce your carb intake by another 25 to 50 grams to end up somewhere between 50 and 100 grams per day. Continue increasing your protein and fat consumption to make up for the reduction in carbs. If you were eating a lot of high-oxalate foods, pick another one or two to switch out for lower-oxalate options.

Listen to your body. How are you feeling? Pay attention to any keto flu symptoms you are experiencing. If you feel generally good, keep doing what you're doing. If you are not feeling good, up your carbs by 25 grams and see how you feel.

WEEK 4

This week, let's get those daily carbs down to 25 to 50 grams. You are going to be choosing the lowest-carb plant options available, and the bulk of your calories will be coming from protein and fat. Continue taking your electrolytes and listening to your body. If you get down to this level of carb intake and are feeling terrible, bump it up by 25 grams and see how you feel. While this is a four-week guide, you can take longer to transition if needed. This is important if you have been consuming a lot of high-oxalate foods when you start, because you want to gradually reduce your intake to slow the oxalate-dumping process. The key is to continue reducing the amount of plant material you eat while upping the animal products.

When you've reached the end of week 4, you are ready to transition to full carnivore. Great work! Now, you will eliminate the remaining fruits and vegetables and consume only animal foods. Cutting all carbs may still cause some keto flu symptoms, but again, drink your electrolytes and make sure you are eating enough food, and you will get through it quickly.

MONTH 1

It is finally time to start carnivore! It may have taken a lot of preparation to get to this point, and I am proud of you. So many people don't make it this far, and it is a testament to your hard work and tenacity that you are here today. Remember that this is mostly a mental game, and believing in yourself is half the battle. Let's get started!

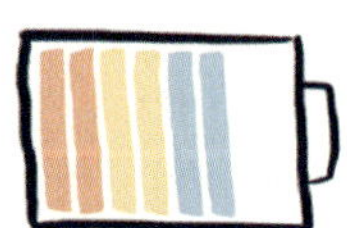

Eat until comfortably stuffed.

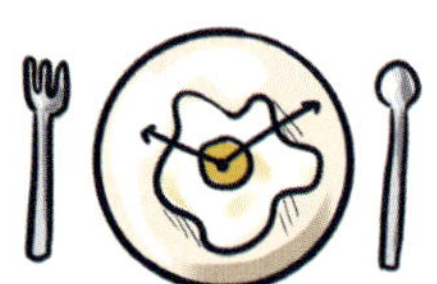

Only eat again when truly hungry.

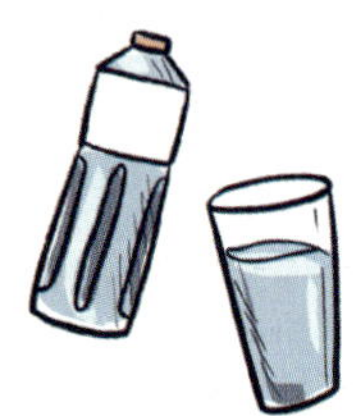

Drink enough water.

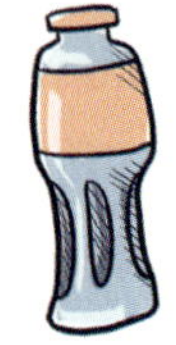

Drink electrolytes first thing in the morning to help with keto flu.

On day 1, I want you to eat a carnivore meal until you are comfortably stuffed. Don't limit yourself to a certain number of calories or a certain amount of food. Just eat until you are comfortably stuffed—meaning that you have eaten enough to feel satisfied, but if you were to take another bite, you would not feel good. It may take a little practice to find that sweet spot, but there is a reason why you need to eat this way. If we think back to our hunter-gatherer ancestors, they didn't have refrigerators, and they weren't storing food in cabinets. They lived off the land. Several times a week, they killed an animal and then consumed it quickly while it was fresh: feast or famine. So you are mimicking that. Eat until you're comfortably stuffed, and then don't eat again until you're truly hungry. Dr. Anthony Chaffee, a long-term carnivore and influencer in this space, says to stop eating when the food stops tasting good. That is a good way to describe that "comfortably stuffed" feeling.

Your goal in this first month is to follow your hunger. This is going to take some time to get used to. In today's world, you are programmed to eat three meals a day plus snacks, so you're constantly eating. You don't *know* when you're truly hungry. On carnivore, you're going to break that cycle.

What should you eat? You can follow the meal plan I laid out for you (see page 82). You could meal prep a bunch of recipes from this book and have them ready to go. You could eat steak and eggs for every meal. The world is your oyster! It's a good idea to plan a few things to eat in the first few days so you don't have to think about it too much. Once you do carnivore for a couple of weeks, you will start to figure out what your preferences are. I eat beef, butter, bacon, and eggs 90 percent of the time, and that works for me. You will figure out what works for you.

One thing I love about carnivore is that I don't have the sugar crashes I used to get when I ate a lot of carbs. Now, my hunger is different. After eating, I am completely satisfied, I don't have sugar spikes or crashes, and I don't have to take a nap. When I'm truly hungry again, it's not a lightheaded kind of feeling; it's just, oh, it's time to eat. And then I listen to my body and eat until I'm comfortably stuffed.

In the beginning of carnivore, your hunger cues are going to be out of whack. So, if you are hungry again in four hours, eat until you are comfortably stuffed again. As you continue, the intervals between meals are going to get longer and longer. For this first month, though, feed your body every time you feel truly hungry. This technique is known as "intuitive eating" and works for a lot of people starting carnivore.

Some people try this intuitive eating approach but find that after a week or two, their appetite tanks, and if they were to follow their hunger, they would only be eating every few days. If you experience this lack of appetite, I would schedule two or three mealtimes per day and eat at those times until you are comfortably stuffed. You need to eat enough food so that you don't slow down your metabolism. Set alarms if you find yourself missing meals.

Make sure you are drinking enough water by following the calculation you did earlier (divide your current weight by 2 or, if you weigh over 200 pounds, by 2.5 or 3). I advise drinking electrolytes every morning, right when you wake up, to mitigate the worst of the keto flu symptoms that could arise. You can take more electrolytes throughout the day if you like. Anytime I felt weak or fatigued in the beginning of carnivore, I would have another packet of the raw unflavored LMNT drink mix, up to three packets per day.

And that's it! Eat until you're comfortably stuffed, and eat again only when you are truly hungry. If you experience a loss of appetite, schedule your meals. Drink enough water, and take electrolytes.

Over the next month, your body will become fat adapted, meaning more efficient at using fat as fuel. If you end up experiencing keto flu symptoms, they typically last only two to three weeks.

HOW MUCH TO EAT PER DAY

Intuitive eating is great, and I always advise people to start that way, but I get hundreds of questions per week about how much to eat per day, what macros to aim for, minimum protein and calorie goals, etc. Also, some people never reach a point where they feel full, even on carnivore, so eating to satiety doesn't work for them. So, while I advocate for intuitive eating, I want to touch on some guidelines to ensure you are getting adequate nutrition on carnivore. The general guidelines are as follows:

- Women should eat a minimum of 1½ pounds of meat per day; men should eat at least 2 pounds.
- Be sure to meet your minimum protein goal on most days. (You will calculate this in the next section.)
- Make up the rest of your calorie intake with fat or a combination of fat and more protein.

But what should your protein goal be? How much fat should you consume? What about calories—are they important? Let's start by discussing how much fat, protein, and calories you should eat per day. I think there is value in meeting some bare-minimum goals to ensure you are eating enough food and fueling your body appropriately.

FAT-TO-PROTEIN RATIO

On carnivore, most of your calories are going to come from fat and protein. If you are consuming dairy, you may get a few carbs. An egg has 0.7 gram of carbs, and some processed meats have a few grams. But in general, most of the food coming into your body is going to be either fat or protein, and both macronutrients are important for different reasons.

Your body is a vehicle. Protein makes up the building blocks or structure of the vehicle. Fat is the fuel that runs the vehicle. Protein is broken down into amino acids: histidine, isoleucine, leucine, lysine, methionine, phenylalanine, threonine, tryptophan, valine, alanine, arginine, asparagine, aspartic acid, cysteine, glutamic acid, glutamine, glycine, proline, serine, and tyrosine. Fat is broken down into free fatty acids, which can then be converted to triglycerides and ketones.

Consider the charts below. Both protein and fat have a part to play in getting your vehicle—your body—where it needs to go. Not getting enough fat and/or protein will make the vehicle inefficient at best and inoperable at worst.

The carnivore diet is typically a high-fat, moderate-protein way of eating. But you can do higher-fat carnivore or higher-protein carnivore depending on your needs.

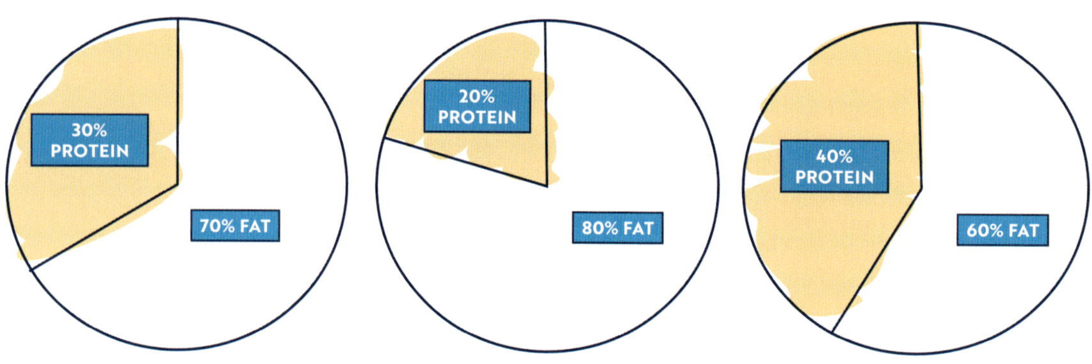

A lot of people starting carnivore just eat fatty meats and do not worry too much about the macronutrients they are consuming. But I think it is important to understand the composition of your diet in a general sense. Plenty of beginners make the mistake of consuming too many lean meats and not enough fat, or way too much fat and not enough protein.

If you need goals to aspire to, I advise new carnivores to aim for a macro split of 70 percent fat to 30 percent protein. That sounds like a lot of fat, but it's about the same amount of fat and protein in grams. Why is that?

1 gram of protein has **4 calories.**

1 gram of fat has **9 calories.**

So, if you eat 150 grams of protein, it equals 600 calories, which would make up about 30 percent of a 2,000-calorie daily diet. Meanwhile, 150 grams of fat equals 1,350 calories, or nearly 70 percent of a 2,000-calorie diet. (You'll be skipping the carbs, of course.) The difference in the number of calories per gram is the reason 150 grams of fat makes up 70 percent of your calorie intake while 150 grams of protein is only 30 percent.

I know this can be a bit confusing, and that is why I advocate for using food-tracking apps if you want to keep track of your fat-to-protein ratio. This can be helpful in the beginning because it is low effort and allows you to estimate your actual food intake instead of guessing. Plus, if you run into issues, you can look back at this data and identify patterns. The data will be helpful when it comes to tweaking carnivore to your situation.

The most popular tracking apps within my carnivore community are MyFitnessPal, Carb Manager, and Chronometer. The free versions of these apps are sufficient—no need to pay for the premium versions unless you really want to. I use MyFitnessPal and find it to be the simplest of the three. Download the app you want to use and then input your daily meals. Each of these apps has a robust food database, so it's easy to find what you are eating.

Tips for using a food tracker:

- Use the raw weight for meat.
- Save the staple foods you eat every week in your "recent meals" so you don't have to search for them each time.
- Don't bother inputting macro or calorie goals; just log your food daily.

I recommend tracking your food for at least the first few weeks of carnivore, until you have a better understanding of the composition of your diet. This awareness will be important as you continue living a carnivore lifestyle. You don't have to track your food forever, but doing it in the beginning will lay the groundwork for success down the road.

Who would benefit from higher-fat carnivore?

While most people start with a 70/30 fat-to-protein ratio, there are those who would benefit from a higher percentage of fat, such as 75/25 or 80/20. This includes some perimenopausal and postmenopausal women, along with adolescents. Some people simply feel better when they eat more fat. If you fall into one of those categories, feel free to start with one of those higher fat ratios. Remember, you can adjust this ratio whenever you want based on how you are feeling, how much weight you are losing, etc.

Who would benefit from higher-protein carnivore?

On the other end of the spectrum, some people benefit from lower fat and higher protein, such as 65/35, 60/40, or even 50/50. Athletes who have high protein needs may fall into this category. Some women experiencing lipedema (an abnormal buildup of excess fat in the lower body) have seen benefits from a higher-protein version of carnivore. Also, if you have a lot of weight to lose, higher-protein carnivore could be beneficial for a time to allow your body to tap into its own fat stores. If you fall into one of these categories, feel free to start with a higher protein ratio. The more active you become, the more protein you may need, so again, feel free to adjust the amount of protein you consume as you continue on carnivore.

HOW MANY CALORIES SHOULD YOU CONSUME?

There are varying schools of thought about calories on carnivore. Some experts say calories don't matter, while others beg to differ. The science behind "calories" is a bit antiquated; it's a lot more complicated than calories in, calories out. First, it is impossible to know exactly how many calories you consume in a day because it is always an estimate. Calorie counts on nutrition labels are allowed a variability of plus or minus 20 percent, so there is no way to determine just how many calories are in anything you eat because there is so much variability from item to item. Also, the nutrient density of a whole food depends on many factors. For example, if a tomato plant is grown in soil that is deficient in nitrogen and phosphorus, then its tomatoes will be deficient in those nutrients. A steak from one cow is going to have a slightly different fat-to-protein profile than the same cut of steak from another cow. Food-tracking apps do their best to take the calorie range for each food and boil it down to an average. But just know that the number of calories in each food you are tracking is an estimate.

Another thing to consider is how your body metabolizes the food you consume. Your metabolism is influenced by many factors, such as your age, health status, exercise habits, history with dieting, and so much more. If you have lived on 700 calories a day for years, your metabolism is much slower than someone's who has properly nourished their body. You may process a 10-ounce ribeye differently than another person. If you have low stomach acid, you may not absorb all of the nutrients from the food you are eating. Nutrient absorption rates vary greatly from individual to individual.

Another wrinkle in this discussion is that not all calories are created equal. Calories from an ultra-processed snack cake are going to be metabolized completely differently than calories from a steak.

I do not say all this to discourage you, but to inspire you. Tracking calories is not an exact science. I hope these insights will help shift your views on calories a bit. But with all that said, I do think there is a bare minimum number of calories you should be consuming every day.

Over the past few decades, we have heard 1,200 or 1,400 calories floated as a daily goal. I am here to tell you that that is a ridiculously low number for a healthy adult. That is the minimum number of calories a child should be consuming. I recommend at least 1,600 to 1,800 calories per day for women and 2,000 to 2,200 calories per day for men on carnivore to meet all your nutritional needs.

Calorie maximums are dependent on several factors. Some people eat 3,000 to 4,000-plus calories per day on carnivore and reach their goals.

For now, I don't want you to get bogged down with specific calorie goals. Just make sure you are eating the *minimum* amounts listed previously, and after the first month or two on carnivore, you can tweak your calorie intake if needed. For now, you want to let your body adjust to carnivore and make sure you are eating enough to keep it nourished and running efficiently.

The charts on the next page present conventional calorie estimates for children and adults based on age, gender, and activity level.

DAILY RECOMMENDED CALORIE INTAKE IN CHILDREN (kcal)

Age (years)	Male		Female	
	Sedentary	Active	Sedentary	Active
2	1000	1000	1000	1000
3	1000	1400	1000	1200
4–5	1200	1400	1200	1400
6	1400	1600	1200	1400
7	1400	1600	1200	1600
8	1400	1600	1400	1600
9	1600	1800	1400	1600
10	1600	1800	1400	1800
11	1800	2000	1600	1800
12	1800	2200	1600	2000
13	2000	2200	1600	2000
14	2000	2400	1800	2000
15	2200	2600	1800	2000

Made by Unaiza Faizan

DAILY RECOMMENDED CALORIE INTAKE IN ADULTS (kcal)

Age (years)	Male		Female	
	Sedentary	Active	Sedentary	Active
16–18	2400	2800	1800	2000
19–20	2600	2800	2000	2200
21–25	2400	2800	2000	2200
26–40	2400	2600	1800	2000
41–45	2200	2600	1800	2000
46–50	2200	2400	1800	2000
51–60	2200	2400	1600	1800
61–65	2000	2400	1600	1800
66 and older	2000	2200	1600	1800

Made by Unaiza Faizan

SETTING A MINIMUM PROTEIN GOAL

Now that you have a minimum calorie goal, it's time to figure out your minimum protein intake for the day. You would be surprised at how many people drastically undereat meat-based protein, and once you go carnivore, you may think you are overeating it! But protein is difficult to overeat, and our bodies are built to use it. Protein is an essential macronutrient, and without it, you would eventually die.

If your body is a vehicle, then protein is the chassis. If you are not getting enough protein, your body will start to utilize the protein from your hair, nails, and muscles to meet its daily demands. You don't want that, so let's do a quick and easy calculation to figure out your minimum daily protein needs.

There are many ways to calculate this number, but the way I like to do it is 1 gram of protein per pound of ideal body weight. For example, I would like to weigh 130 pounds, so I need a minimum of 130 grams of protein per day. Keep in mind that your minimum protein goal is just that: a minimum. I almost always eat more than 130 grams. Some days I even go over 200 grams—it just depends on the day.

This calculation works for a lot of people, but there are exceptions. Say your ideal weight is 200 pounds, and 200 grams of protein daily seems a bit overwhelming. That's okay! Instead of multiplying by 1 gram, multiply by 0.6 or 0.8 gram. This is not an exact science; you are just trying to determine a goal.

PROTEIN CALCULATIONS

Body Weight	Daily Protein			
	0.6 g/lb	0.8 g/lb	1 g/lb	1.5 g/lb
100 lbs	60g	80g	100g	150g
120 lbs	72g	96g	120g	180g
140 lbs	84g	112g	140g	210g
160 lbs	96g	128g	160g	240g
180 lbs	108g	144g	180g	270g
200 lbs	120g	160g	200g	300g
220 lbs	132g	176g	220g	330g
240 lbs	144g	192g	240g	360g

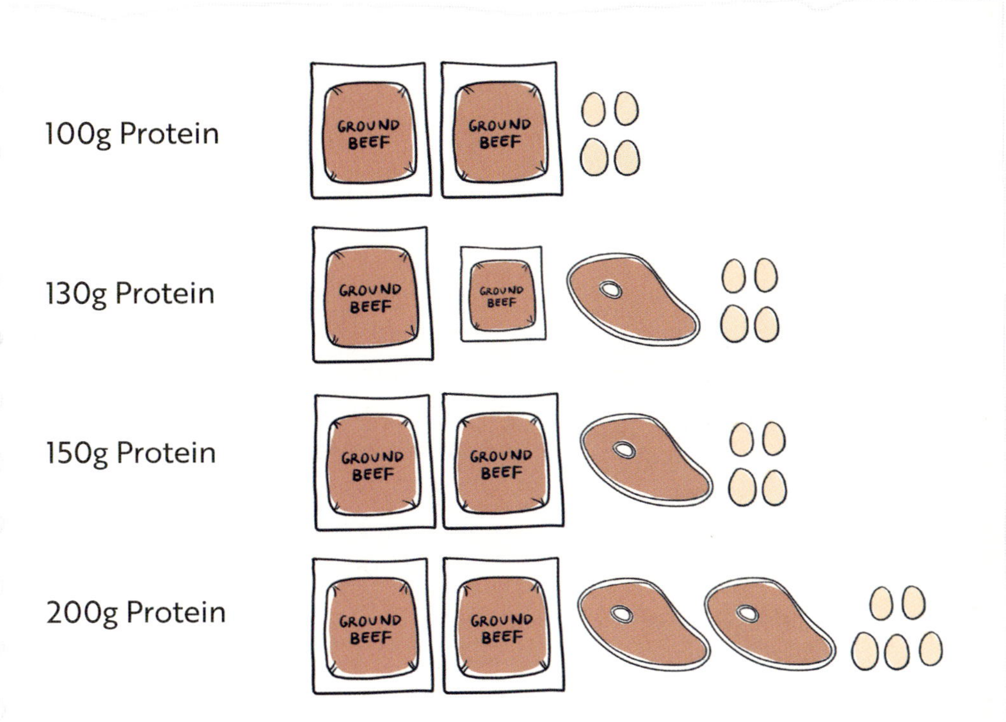

HOW MUCH FAT SHOULD YOU CONSUME?

Once you have your calorie and protein goals, you'll make up the rest of your calories with fat or more protein. For example, if you have a daily calorie goal of 1,800 and a protein goal of 150 grams (600 calories), you need to eat at least 1,200 calories of fat or fat plus protein.

Making up the rest of your calories with fat doesn't mean you have to eat sticks of butter or liquid beef fat. Most of the fat you are going to consume will be part of the meat. That is why fattier cuts are recommended: They make it a lot easier to eat high fat. If you want to eat a stick of butter, that's okay! "Steak and Butter Gal" Bella Ma craved frozen butter in the beginning because she'd been a vegan for years, and her body needed the additional fat. She still eats butter from the stick, but you don't have to do that if you don't want to. And if you have extra weight, let your body use its own fat for fuel now—the extra butter can come later when you're closer to your goal. You will figure out what works best for you.

My favorite way to hit my fat and protein goals for the day is to eat a ribeye steak, which has the perfect fat-to-protein profile of 70/30 and is full of vitamins and minerals. Most carnivores try to include ribeyes in their diets as often as possible.

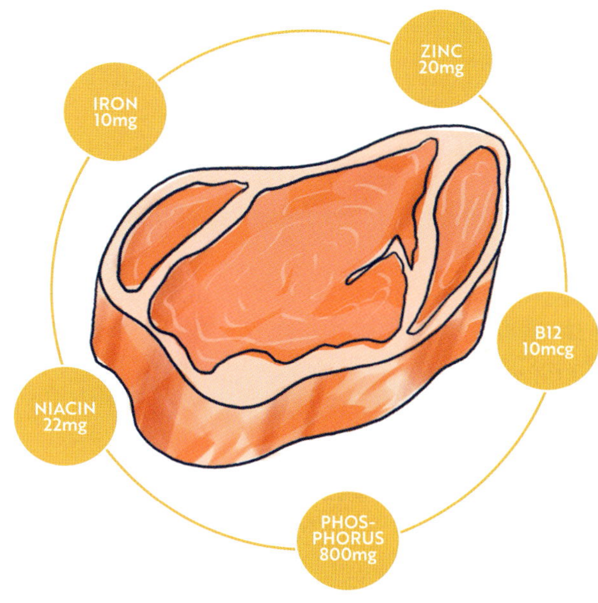

MEAL FREQUENCY/TIMING/FASTING

How many meals a day will you eat on carnivore? Well, that depends on the individual. For the first month, I want you to have two or three meals per day. It is very hard to get all of the nutrients you need from just one meal. Your digestive system can only break down and absorb so many nutrients at a time, so eating two or three meals per day is a better bet. After a month or two on carnivore, you might adjust your meal frequency a bit. Most carnivores eat two meals per day, but some thrive on one or three. Carnivores who have had bariatric surgery may need to eat up to six times per day.

What time you should eat each meal depends on your hunger cues and your schedule. Some people eat lunch and dinner. Others eat breakfast and lunch or breakfast and dinner. But I do think you should keep all your food consumption to a specific feeding window. I recommend starting with a twelve-hour window and slowly reducing it to eight to ten hours. So, if you have a twelve-hour feeding window, maybe you start eating at 8 a.m. and have your last meal by 8 p.m. An eight-hour window could start at 10 a.m. and end at 6 p.m. Play around with it and figure out what works best for you.

Keep in mind that eating earlier in the day is often recommended because your body handles glucose and insulin more efficiently in the morning. This is due to natural fluctuations in hormones and your circadian rhythm, which support better metabolic function earlier in the day.

You may have heard about intermittent fasting or regular fasting. Fasting just means going a period of time without eating, and there are lots of different techniques. I don't think you should fast in the first month or two on carnivore. You need to give your body time to get used to this way of eating. You will know you are ready to play around with fasting when you naturally are going at least sixteen hours between meals and not even noticing. Until then, focus on relearning your true hunger cues and getting used to carnivore. Fasting is discussed in more depth in chapter 5.

I eat two meals per day most days. I eat at around 8 to 9 a.m. with my twins, and then I like to have my final meal of the day at around 3 or 4 p.m. That allows me a solid sixteen-hour fast between meals. Some days I eat lunch, too, if I feel hungry. If I am attending a social event, I either eat beforehand or push my dinner later. But I almost never eat past 8 p.m. I don't like to eat that close to bedtime because my body would still be focused on digestion as opposed to preparing for sleep, and eating that late always affects my sleep.

WHAT ABOUT SNACKING?

If you are eating until you are comfortably stuffed at every meal, you will not want to snack between meals. That is how you know you are eating enough. But in the beginning, while you are learning to interpret your true hunger cues, a snack here and there may be helpful. A snack could also help you get past a sugar craving. It could be that you need another meal, but you won't know that unless you eat a little something.

So, if you want to have a snack, make it a carnivore snack! Here is a list of yummy carnivore snacks that will help get you through the first month or two:

- Bacon
- Beef sticks
- Biltong
- Butter
- Butter bites
- Carnivore Bars
- Cheese

- Cut-up leftover meats
- Deli meat
- Gardner's Baked Cheese
- Hard-boiled eggs
- Jerky
- Pemmican
- Pork rinds
- Sardines or other canned meats

After you get used to the carnivore way of eating, you will not be snacking much. The only time I snack is when I am on a road trip. If you find yourself mindlessly snacking after a few months on carnivore, you need to eat more food at every meal. You want to give your body time to digest each meal, and that means not eating between meals.

WHAT TO EXPECT IN THE FIRST MONTH

The first month on carnivore is a roller coaster, and it's a bit different for everyone. Some people don't experience any keto flu, but most do. For some, keto flu is a passing annoyance. For others, it's debilitating. I fell into the latter camp. My first month on carnivore was difficult. I experienced severe fatigue and light diarrhea. I couldn't do any exercise other than walking. Looking back, I think my keto flu lasted as long as it did (six weeks) because I was oxalate dumping on top of the carbohydrate withdrawal. I did not know about oxalate dumping when I started carnivore, and if I could go back, I would've followed the gradual carbohydrate reduction protocol that I built for you (see pages 84–87). That being said, I lost 8 pounds in the first month, which was a huge amount of weight for me. That, along with my fifteen- to twenty-point reduction in average blood glucose levels, is what kept me going and convinced me to commit to carnivore for another thirty days.

Other common issues that people encounter in the first month are loss of appetite, undereating, and food aversions. You may find that you can't look at another piece of beef or chicken. Both appetite and food aversions tend to improve after that first month.

While many people report amazing weight loss the first month, there are some who lose only a little, lose none, or even gain weight. If you have been undereating for many years, gaining a little weight is a distinct possibility, and you should not fear it. Sometimes, in order to get healthy, your body needs to recover from years of nutrient starvation. But typically, if you have weight to lose, you will lose some of it in the first month. (If you continue gaining weight on carnivore, turn to chapter 5 for tips on tweaking your carnivore diet.)

Most people begin to see improvements in whatever conditions they are seeking to heal from. The improvements may be drastic, or they may be minor. That's why I advise you to write down everything that is an issue for you before starting the diet and then revisit that list after a month and see what improvements you have made. You may be surprised when something that you did not originally consider to be a problem improves.

On the other hand, conditions sometimes get worse before they get better. Some people get a rash or break out as their body detoxes. Sometimes the body needs more than a month to get used to the higher fat-to-protein ratio and lack of carbohydrates, so your stools may be looser. Some people have low stomach acid, so when they switch to eating meat, they experience heartburn or acid reflux (I talk about how to address those problems in chapter 5).

Some experience keto breath, a phenomenon where you have sweet-smelling breath. That is your body reacting to a new fuel source, and it typically goes away within a few weeks.

But overall, the pros tend to outweigh the cons, even as you're adapting to carnivore. Many people report increases in energy and strength. Blood glucose levels tend to regulate quickly, as does blood pressure. Most people lose some weight. Inflammation levels and joint pain can decrease. It will be interesting to see how you respond!

MONTH 2

You have made it through the first month! I hope you experienced enough positive results that you will commit to another month. I think you need to stay on carnivore for at least ninety days to start seeing serious healing, but committing to it one month at a time makes it seem less daunting. If you continue, here is what you can expect in month 2:

- Keto flu symptoms should have subsided by now.
- Oxalate dumping will continue if you were eating a high-oxalate diet before starting carnivore; you can slow it by consuming one cup of black tea per day this month.
- Your body will become more efficient at using fat as fuel. You will have more energy and stamina, and your strength will improve. If you are tracking ketones, your levels may begin to rise.
- Mental health will improve.
- Inflammation will continue to decline.
- Weight loss will continue.

MONTHS 3 TO 12

The benefits of carnivore compound over time. If you stay carnivore for three to twelve months, here are some things you can expect to see:

- Sugar cravings will begin to decline and eventually disappear. My sugar cravings disappeared after month 4.
- Meal frequency and hunger cues will become settled. You will not be ruled by food anymore. You may begin to incorporate fasting.

- Your body will continue to heal. Inflammation will continue to decline, along with fasting insulin, fasting glucose, A1c, and triglycerides.
- Mental health improvements will continue, allowing you to operate at a much higher baseline.
- Many people begin to recover from chronic illnesses and diseases. Type 2 diabetes responds very well to carnivore and other low-carb diets; some people even go into remission.

New issues may pop up, too. Oxalate dumping can continue for a very long time, sometimes years. You may have no symptoms for a while, and then they will start up again. Weight-loss stalls can happen as well, even on carnivore.

If you are not feeling your best after about six months on strict carnivore, sometimes the solution is not to "carnivore harder" or become even stricter. You may have an underlying condition that is the root cause, and while carnivore is incredible, it cannot address everything. If you are running into issues, chapter 5 will be very helpful for you.

ONE YEAR AND BEYOND

It is entirely possible to follow a carnivore lifestyle for the long haul. Dr. Lisa Weideman, known as the Carnivore Doctor, has been a carnivore for more than sixteen years. Amber O'Hearn, another thought leader in this space, has been a carnivore since 2009. Dr. Shawn Baker started carnivore in 2016, and Dr. Ken Berry started in 2017. Dr. Robert Kiltz has been carnivore since 2011. I have been carnivore since December 2022 and have only seen metabolic health improvements. There are plenty of long-term carnivores out there, and you shouldn't be fearful of eating only animal products for years to come.

As you stay on carnivore for a longer period of time, your food preferences can shift. You may start out preferring chicken and fish and evolve to eating only red meat. You may play around with fat-to-protein ratios depending on your goals. You may evolve into more of a moderator and be able to have a high-carb cheat meal once in a blue moon without spiraling into a three-month sugar binge.

A species-appropriate diet like carnivore can vastly improve your quality of life and your health span. While there is no guarantee that it will extend your life, carnivore can help you reach your goals and live out your Whys while feeling great. Perhaps you will be able to add your name to the list of long-term carnivores! Only time will tell.

But there are other factors besides nutrition that contribute to your metabolic health and well-being. I will discuss those additional factors in the next chapter.

HOW TO KNOW WHEN IT'S TIME TO BE LESS RESTRICTIVE: REINTRODUCING FOODS

You may decide to add plants back into your diet. Ketovore, keto, Paleo, primal, animal-based, and meat-and-fruit diets are also amazing, and staying carnivore forever may not be the right path for you.

When you can reintroduce plant foods depends a lot on your Whys and goals. If you have reached your goals and achieved your Whys, you can think about bringing back plants.

I advise you to start with one food at a time, eating a small amount of it every day for a few days and then waiting a week to see if any symptoms pop up. Keeping a food journal can be helpful. If you notice pain flare-ups, skin issues, declines in energy, general malaise, digestive discomfort, or any other negative symptom, you may not be able to consume that plant at this time. That doesn't mean you can't eat it forever, but you may need to do a bit more healing first. You can try to reintroduce it again in a few months to see if you have a similar reaction.

Some people find that they feel their best when they stay on a strict version of carnivore. But most can start to include some plant material and not experience devastating effects on their health. One caveat is fruit. For some people, the sugar in fruit reactivates their sugar addiction and leads them back to ultra-processed foods. I would also avoid foods that are high in oxalates, lectins, and gluten (such as spinach, tomatoes, or wheat) or eat them only once in a while. I have been carnivore for three years, and I incorporate a keto cheat meal once a month. I have a salad, some Brussels sprouts, and maybe some asparagus along with a ribeye steak. This approach works well for me because while I enjoy vegetables, I feel my best when I stick to beef, butter, bacon, and eggs 90 percent of the time.

While you may be able to reincorporate some plant material eventually, you can never return to eating ultra-processed foods, seed oils, and sugar on a regular basis. Those are not real foods, and if you get back to eating them regularly, your health will decline quickly. Stick to real, whole foods. Test them one at a time to see if you have any reactions. Build a way of eating that works for you in the long term. Your way of eating needs to be a permanent lifestyle shift, not a temporary fix. You will figure out what works best for you.

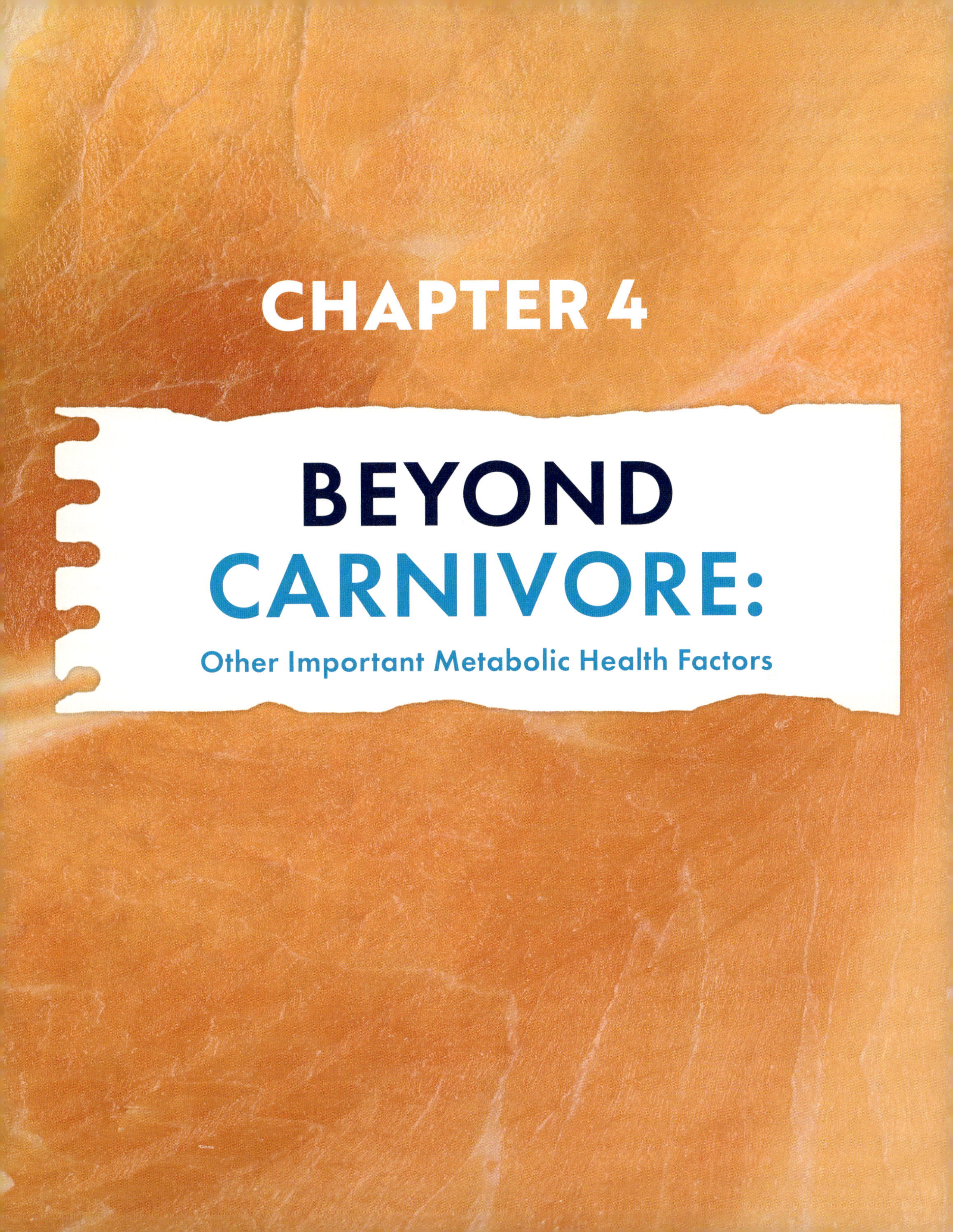

CHAPTER 4

BEYOND CARNIVORE:

Other Important Metabolic Health Factors

While the focus of this book is nutrition, there are many other factors that play a part in your health. Once you have your diet under control, here are some other things you can start to dial in.

THE PILLARS OF HEALTH

Nutrition is one of the four pillars of health. I've already covered that in quite a bit of detail, so I won't rehash it here. The other three pillars are movement, sleep, and stress management. If you can excel at these four pillars, you're going to be operating at a much higher baseline than most of your peers.

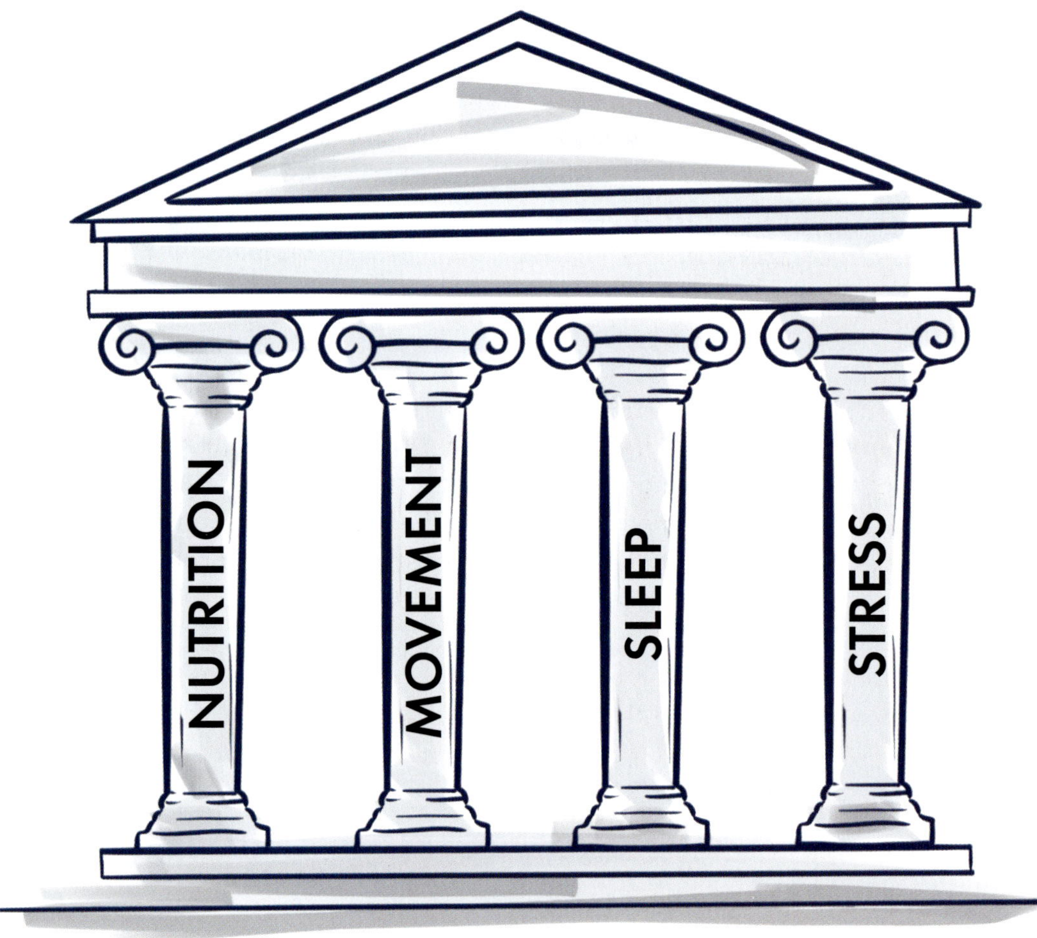

MOVEMENT

Humans are designed for movement. But it doesn't have to be as extreme as competitive bodybuilding or hours of hardcore cardio. Think back to our ancestors, who would do a lot of walking, sprinting, and lifting of heavy things—not "to get some exercise," but because these activities were built into their daily lives. We modern humans must make time for movement.

Going from a sedentary lifestyle to a light activity level is the first step for many people. At the beginning of any exercise program, you want to ensure you don't get injured. Being sedentary can negatively affect your fascia, which is a type of stringy connective tissue surrounding your muscles that provides structure and support. It can become sticky, dry, and tight when you are inactive for even a few weeks, and that is why you may feel some pain even though you aren't moving around much. Stretching helps, as does massage therapy and cupping. Just getting up and moving around more and increasing your hydration levels can do wonders as well.

If you are currently sedentary, then your big goal will be to get up and get moving, be it taking a walk around the block, parking the car farther away from the entrance of the store, or doing stretches with resistance bands in your chair—anything to get the blood flowing and that fascia stretching and loosening. The first few weeks of this transition may be difficult, but just focus on doing a little more every day.

I am a big fan of low-impact forms of exercise that don't overtax your joints: walking, elliptical training, cycling, stair climbing, etc. You don't want to do chronic cardio, where you are working out for hours every day. That is a quick and easy way to burn out your metabolism and raise your cortisol levels. Cortisol is a hormone produced by the adrenal glands that helps regulate metabolism, blood sugar, blood pressure, and the body's response to stress. Chronic cardio is a stressor that can raise it to unhealthy levels.

I also recommend sprinting in whatever form you enjoy: running sprints, going as fast as you can on your bike, swimming a lap as fast as possible, doing one minute on the stair climber at the fastest pace you can, etc. Sprinting is beneficial because it builds muscle, burns fat, and improves cardiovascular health in a short amount of time. It boosts metabolism, enhances insulin sensitivity, and stimulates the release of growth hormone. Sprinting also supports mental resilience and overall athletic performance. Sprinting is a more advanced exercise method, so don't go from sedentary directly to sprinting if you want to avoid injury. Work your way up to sprinting.

I'm a big advocate of strength training, too. Building a solid amount of muscle on your body helps with mobility and flexibility and helps prevent broken bones if you fall. Muscles are repositories for glucose, so the more muscle you have, the more glucose you can store. This can help keep glucose from building up in your bloodstream and keep you insulin sensitive.

The key to any movement regimen is to be consistent with it and constantly challenge yourself. It must also be fun, because you won't keep up with a routine that is boring! Some people really enjoy group fitness, and others thrive when working with a personal trainer. Figure out what works best for you, and if you start getting bored, switch it up!

My Favorite Workouts:

- Walking 3 to 5 miles 3 to 5 days per week
- Strength training 3 or 4 days per week
- Stair climber: glute routine and sprints
- Swimming
- Cycling
- Hiking
- Kayaking

If you are already getting movement and are happy with your regimen, that's great! Staying active is important for longevity and health. My grandmother played tennis until she was ninety-one, and she is still kicking at ninety-seven. She was a physical education teacher and has always been active. In addition to tennis, she walked, handled all her own lawn care, and did light strength training. It really doesn't take much to stay healthy! Just figure out what suits you best.

SLEEP

We all know we need sleep, but getting enough is a struggle. We are surrounded by artificial lights, a barrage of digital content, and endless reasons to delay or avoid sleep. But there is a reason we spend roughly a third of our lives sleeping. Reductions in sleep can increase your appetite. Not getting enough sleep can also ratchet up your stress levels. Night shift work has even been shown to have the same carcinogenic effect as cigarette smoking.[1] Most adults need seven to nine hours of sleep every night, with children and teens needing a bit more and the elderly a bit less.

Sleep timing matters, too. Heading to bed before 10 p.m. helps you take advantage of the natural surge of human growth hormone, which peaks between 10 p.m. and 2 a.m.

Humans are affected by circadian rhythms, just like any other animal. One of the signals that affects our circadian rhythms is light. For millions of years, humans lived by the rising and setting of the sun, and only fairly recently in our evolutionary history did fire begin to be utilized in the evenings. In the 1800s, people began to light up the night even more with kerosene lamps and, later, electric lamps. Nowadays, you could have full illumination twenty-four hours a day, seven days a week, until the grid failed or you didn't pay the electric bill. There is a lot of talk about blue light in particular and how we need to shield our eyes from it in the evenings to avoid disruptions to our sleep and circadian rhythms. But we also need to get as much sunlight into our eyes as possible during the day to keep our circadian rhythm in balance. Especially important is that early morning sunlight. Waking at dawn and immediately going outside to get that sunlight into your eyes and on your skin is a great way to improve your overall health and your sleep.

---

[1] Hogne Vikanes Buchvold et al., "Associations between night work and BMI, alcohol, smoking, caffeine and exercise—a cross-sectional study," *BMC Public Health* 15, no. 1112 (2015), doi:10.1186/s12889-015-2470-2.

Vitamin D synthesis
Early morning light sets your circadian rhythm and primes your skin for UVA/UVB exposure later the day
Low light in the evening triggers melatonin production
NOON
DAWN
DUSK

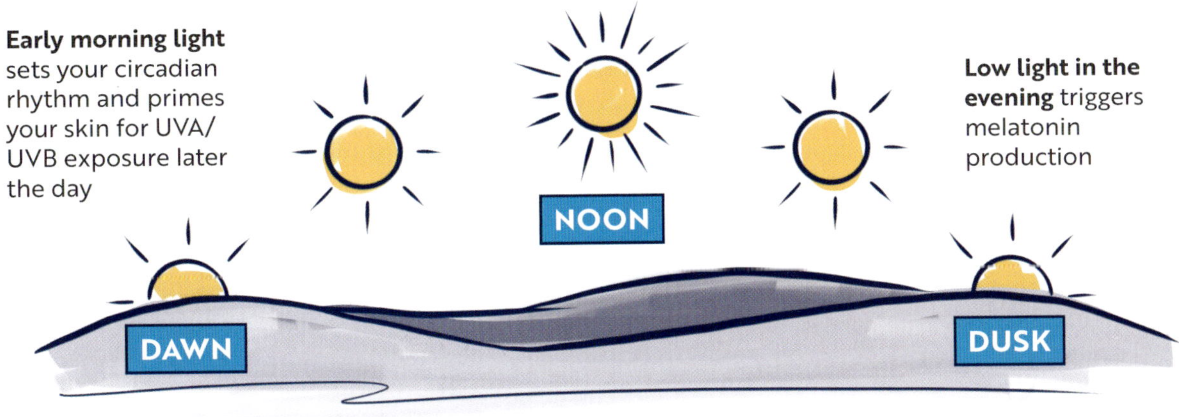

How does your brain know that it is dawn, midday, or dusk? Scientists used to think that only the rods and cones in the eyes could detect light, but another kind of cell, known as a photosensitive retinal ganglion cell (pRGC), senses light levels using a blue-light-sensitive molecule called melanopsin. Because they're especially sensitive to blue light, these cells likely help regulate your circadian rhythms by detecting changes in light at dawn and dusk. Your skin is also full of light-sensitive cells.

But how much will light in the evening trip you up? It's a lot more than you might think. Bottom line: Stop using your phone and other screens within thirty minutes to an hour of bedtime to allow your brain to calm and decompress. You can choose to wear blue-light-blocking glasses as well, but be sure the lenses are orange or red. Clear or light yellow lenses don't work.

This research is part of a wonderful book on sleep and circadian rhythms called *Life Time* by Russell Foster. I suggest reading it if you want the most up-to-date sleep science available. But here are several more ways to improve your sleep, starting well before bedtime.

Sleep Hygiene Tips:

- Get sunlight in the early morning to set your circadian rhythm
- Exercise in the morning or afternoon
- Stop eating at least 3 hours before bedtime
- Stop using screens 30–60 minutes before bedtime
- Build a sleep routine
- Take a hot shower/bath before bed
- Plan the next day
- Read
- Charge your phone on the other side of the room or in another room
- Keep your bedroom between 62°F and 68°F
- Sleep in complete darkness
- Wear an eye mask

STRESS MANAGEMENT

Stress can be a killer, and we deal with so much of it in today's world. While some acute stress can be productive, chronic stress is a cardiovascular risk factor and can cause a plethora of health issues, including weight loss or gain, over- or undereating, sleep disturbances, anxiety, and depression.

Knowing you need to reduce stress is one thing, but actually *doing* it can be a battle. How can you reduce stress when it seems that stressful things are coming at you from every direction?

The first key is recognizing that **time is your greatest asset**. You need to figure out what stuff you absolutely *must do yourself* and what stuff you can *farm out to others*. This starts with prioritization. Sit down and make a list of everything you do in a day. As you move down the list, think about whether this task really needs to be completed today or if it can wait. Focus on the items that absolutely must be done today. For items that can be done later, make a note of the deadline on your calendar and put it on your to-do list closer to when it needs to be completed.

Also, think about whether *you* need to be the person to complete a task, and if not, delegate it. Start a second list with the heading "Delegate" and move any tasks that you can give to someone else over to that column. For example, perhaps you need to be in certain work meetings and calls, but others could be attended by your assistant. There are a lot of AI tools that can be very helpful for lightening your workload.

I always complete the most difficult tasks at the beginning of the day when my brain is fresh so that I don't procrastinate on them.

PRIORITIZATION		DELEGATION	
Daily activities	Needs to be done today	Can someone else do this task?	
1. ______	☐	yes ☐	no ☐
2. ______	☐	yes ☐	no ☐
3. ______	☐	yes ☐	no ☐
4. ______	☐	yes ☐	no ☐
5. ______	☐	yes ☐	no ☐
6. ______	☐	yes ☐	no ☐
7. ______	☐	yes ☐	no ☐
8. ______	☐	yes ☐	no ☐
9. ______	☐	yes ☐	no ☐
10. ______	☐	yes ☐	no ☐
11. ______	☐	yes ☐	no ☐
12. ______	☐	yes ☐	no ☐

Another important stress management skill to cultivate is saying no to unimportant tasks. This circles back to the fact that time is your greatest asset. If you say yes to everything, be it at work, home, or your kid's school, you are going to have sky-high stress levels. Use the same listing method to figure out what are the true priorities, and say no to everything else.

Unfortunately, it's not just tasks, deadlines, and overscheduling that make work life stressful. Sometimes it's a difficult boss or an underperforming coworker, or an unhealthy work environment or corporate culture. In those cases, figure out a way to avoid the toxic person or environment as much as possible (maybe switch to remote work), or perhaps even think about finding a new job. You spend a huge chunk of your time at work, and if it is your main source of stress, you need to reevaluate and decide if it's worth it. Chronic work stress can cause strokes and heart attacks, and you don't want to play Russian roulette with your life.

You can use the same technique of prioritization and delegation at home. If you have kids, a partner, or a roommate, see if you can divvy up the household management and chores. If you have young children, involve them in cooking and other daily chores, and don't tie it to an allowance. Your family is a team, and you don't get paid to do what it takes to run the household. Having the kids help around the house also teaches them how to do so for themselves when they are adults. If you have the budget, hiring a housekeeper or lawn care service is another great way to save time.

There are a ton of activities that can be stress relievers. Many people swear by meditation. Getting a massage can help loosen tight muscles. Dinner and a movie can be a fun way to spend time with your significant other. Scheduling some "you time" if you have a heavy workload is essential. Solo time is super important, especially for busy parents who must wear many hats in their day-to-day lives. For me, managing a sixty-plus-hour workweek, plus twin toddlers, plus a household can be very taxing mentally, and I purposefully schedule "me time" to make sure I fit it in. It can be as simple as taking fifteen minutes to sit with a cup of coffee on the back porch, or an hour and a half to get a massage, or even a full weekend to rest and recuperate. Figure out what you can do and put it on the schedule.

Stress can be difficult to dial in because a lot of it comes from outside sources that you don't have much control over. The trick is to figure out what you *do* have control over and make changes where you can. You always have control over your perception and judgment of a situation, and working on that alone can sometimes be a game changer. I recommend checking out Stoicism. It's an excellent everyman's philosophy that is super easy to understand and has been invaluable to me in shaping my perception of the world. Head to Appendix B for a list of great Stoicism reads to get you started.

Stress Management Tips:

- Exercise
- Meditation
- Prioritization/delegation
- "Me time"
- Scheduled rest
- Therapy
- Sex
- Hobbies
- Reading
- Hot bath
- Hormesis—cold plunge, sauna

OTHER METABOLIC HEALTH FACTORS

The four pillars of health are the backbone of your well-being. Here are some other things that you can work on to get yourself to an optimal baseline. Don't be overwhelmed by this list; just do what you can and figure out what benefits you the most.

SUNLIGHT

The human body evolved to get daily sunlight. When sunlight hits your skin, your body converts cholesterol to vitamin D, an essential nutrient that plays a role in immunity, mental health, inflammation, bone health, muscle function, and glucose metabolism, among other things, and exposure to sunlight is the only way to get it naturally. But most of us are wildly deficient in vitamin D because we spend most of our lives indoors. When we do venture outside, we slather ourselves with sunscreen.

Unfortunately, a lot of the sunscreens on the market today contain toxic chemicals and can cause more damage than the sun[2]—the very thing they are marketed to protect you against! Also, note that the most malignant skin cancer, melanoma, is most likely to start on the trunk of the body, which typically gets the least sun. If you choose to wear sunscreen, be sure to get a mineral-based product. Mineral sunscreens are considered safer because they sit on the skin and reflect UV rays rather than being absorbed like chemical sunscreens. They're less likely to cause irritation or hormone disruption and are also reef-safe. Plus, they provide immediate protection.

As you continue carnivore, you may find that your sensitivity to sunburn improves. One theory is that this is due to cutting seed oils from your diet. Seed oils are high in linoleic acid and omega-6 and can make you more sensitive to sunburns.[3]

Another theory is that improving your circadian biology will reduce your skin's tendency to burn. Circadian training can reduce sunburn risk by syncing sun exposure with your body's natural rhythms. Early morning light boosts skin repair, hormone balance, and builds UV resilience, while late-day exposure increases risk.[4] Gradual morning sun exposure helps your skin adapt and better tolerate UV rays. Training your circadian biology could result in less sunburn over time. I've experienced this firsthand. When I began going outside at dawn, I noticed I could spend more time in the midday sun without burning. To learn more about this topic, check out the work of Zaid Dahhaj and Dr. Jack Kruse.

Geography and genetics play a part in how

---

[2] Sonia Santander and Maria Jose Luesma, "Toxicity of different chemical components in sun cream filters and their impact on human health: a review," *Applied Sciences* 13, no. 2 (2023): 712.

[3] Joseph Mercola and Christopher R. D'Adamo, "Linoleic acid: a narrative review of the effects of increased intake in the standard American diet and associations with chronic disease," *Nutrients* 15, no. 14 (2023): 3129.

[4] Zhi Su et al., "The influence of circadian rhythms on DNA damage repair in skin photoaging," *International Journal of Molecular Sciences* 25, no. 20 (2024): 10926.

much sunlight you need, but in general, it's a good idea to get outside and expose as much of your skin as possible to the sun every day for at least twenty to thirty minutes. I like to stay out until I get a bit pink (I am translucently pale after a long Chicago winter, so this doesn't take long at the beginning of the season), and then I put on clothing to cover myself instead of using sunscreen on my body. I do wear mineral sunscreen on my face every day to prevent wrinkles and brown spots, but that is due to vanity and habit.

You can increase your vitamin D levels by using a supplement, but it's not the same as getting it from the sun. I discuss supplementation at the end of this chapter.

COMMUNITY

Surrounding yourself with a circle of people who care about you is very important for your well-being. There is a reason that safety and security and then love and belonging are just below physiological needs on Maslow's hierarchy. You can't move on to self-actualization until you feel you have stability and support.

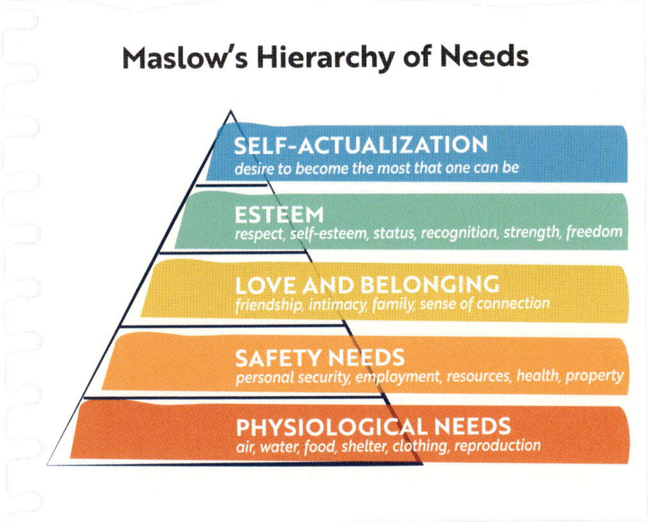

Maslow's Hierarchy of Needs

Having a close circle of friends and family makes a world of difference, especially in difficult situations. Humans are social creatures and need close relationships with others. You may be more of an introvert and not require as much human contact as an extrovert, but no one is an island. We all need some people in our lives. Strong ties to community and high rates of social engagement are among the reasons people in Blue Zones are living longer and healthier lives. Blue Zones are regions of the world where people live significantly longer, healthier lives. These areas share common lifestyle habits like a mostly whole-food diet, regular movement, strong social connections, and low stress (whether their diets are actually a factor is a matter of debate; the food data in that study was not collected in a rigorous way and then was cherry-picked to confirm the researchers' vegetarian biases.)[5] Humans thrive on healthy social interaction.

The quality of the relationship is what's important here. Relationships need to be life-giving, not draining. You know how it is when you are around a toxic person. They tend to suck the energy right out of you. It is essential to clear toxic people from your life. Sometimes doing so is difficult, especially if that person is a family member. But if a relationship is draining you, it's in your best interest to avoid that person as much as possible, define clear boundaries with them, and focus instead on the people in your life who lift you up.

---

[5] Harriet Hall, "Blue zones diet: speculation based on misinformation," *Science-Based Medicine*, October 12, 2021, https://sciencebasedmedicine.org/blue-zones-diet-speculation-based-on-misinformation/.

MENTAL HEALTH

This is a topic that is close to my heart because I used to suffer from extreme anxiety and depression. I self-medicated with drugs and alcohol in my teens and twenties, but now, in my early forties, I no longer suffer from these conditions. I love that we live in a time when we can be more open about our mental health struggles, but more work needs to be done to address this common issue.

The thing about mental health is that it affects your physical health. The brain and body are not separate. Anyone who has experienced depression can tell you that it feels like your shoes are made of cement. You have zero energy and no desire to do any of the things you used to enjoy. Depression can also cause aches and pains, sleep disturbances, digestive issues, and so much more. People with schizophrenia and/or bipolar disorder die from cardiovascular disease at much higher rates than the general population.[6] And mental health struggles affect your quality of life, too. For many people, taking a boatload of meds with their accompanying side effects can make life very unsatisfying.

Addressing trauma is essential. Most people have experienced some kind of trauma, to varying degrees. The more trauma you've faced, the more mental and physical health troubles are going to plague you. And the longer you sweep the trauma under the rug, the more harm it will do. Trust me, I have done loads of therapy, and I wish I had started earlier. While it is scary to shine a light on those skeletons in your closet, it is the best thing you can do for your mental and physical health. I advise finding a trustworthy therapist, counselor, or group that is experienced with this kind of deep, difficult work and getting started as soon as possible. I found cognitive behavioral therapy to be highly effective. Nowadays, you can even find a therapist online! The keys are to find someone you are comfortable with and can trust, and to be consistent with your appointments. If you don't click with the first therapist you find, move on to another until you find a good fit.

Another great practice for mental health is journaling. I started journaling as a young child and have always found it cathartic. It's also nice to be able to go back and read the thoughts of my younger self. Seeing my past thought processes and what I used to think was a big deal can be a bit embarrassing, but it also shows me how far I've come and how much I've grown. I find that to be invaluable. I also love gratitude journaling. It is hard to feel negative emotions when you are thinking about what you're grateful for, and gratitude journaling can be an effective way to shift your mindset over time. A great, quick option is *The Five Minute Journal*. There is more information about this resource in Appendix B.

I mentioned Dr. Ede's book in chapter 2, but it is so good that it deserves to be mentioned again here. *Change Your Diet, Change Your Mind* is a must-read if you suffer from mental health issues. Also, be sure to follow the YouTube channel *Metabolic Mind*, which focuses on using therapeutic ketogenic diets in the treatment of mental health disorders. Another great YouTube channel is *Living Well After Schizophrenia*, where Lauren Kennedy West chronicles her journey of living with schizophrenia, schizoaffective disorder, and mental illness. It is an excellent channel and well worth a watch if you or a family member are dealing with these types of issues.

---

[6] Christoffer Polcwiartek, Kevin O'Gallagher, Daniel J Friedman, et al., "Severe mental illness: cardiovascular risk assessment and management," *European Heart Journal* 45, no. 12 (2024): 987–997.

HYDRATION

Most people do not drink enough water. Dehydration is common. In addition, today's tap water is heavily filtered, which removes a lot of essential minerals. Despite that filtration, tap water can still contain chlorine, lead, pesticides, and bacteria. It is also fluoridated, and I personally don't want to be drinking that halide. So, what to do? I recommend filtering your water and then reintroducing some minerals. I use a countertop water filter that removes fluoride and other chemicals. Adding a bit of Celtic sea salt to your water after filtering is a cheap and easy way to replace essential minerals.

As far as how much water to consume, take your body weight and divide it by 2. If you weigh over 200 pounds, you can divide by 3. Drink that amount of water in ounces per day at a minimum. If you consume caffeinated coffee, you will need to drink more water because coffee is a diuretic (which means it can cause dehydration). For every eight-ounce cup of caffeinated coffee you drink, add twelve ounces of water to your daily intake.

FASTING

Fasting is a commonly underutilized tool to regulate metabolic health that I think deserves a lot more attention. We simply are not supposed to be eating all the time. If you think back to our ancestors, they would have to hunt and gather to eat, and sometimes they would have to go days without eating. Most people couldn't imagine missing even one meal today, but that is because of the carb-heavy diets that most people consume. When you are following a carnivore lifestyle, it becomes much easier to fast because your hunger cues are stable, and your blood sugar is under control. You can more easily tap into the fat stores on your body and use them as fuel.

Fasting is simply not consuming calories, by choice, for a certain amount of time. Technically, anytime you are not eating, you are fasting. But what is the purpose of fasting? For one, it is highly effective at lowering insulin levels, which allows you to burn stored sugar or body fat. If you are constantly eating, you never give your body the opportunity to tap into those stores, and over time, you become overloaded with potential energy. This leads to insulin resistance in the long term. Pairing fasting with a carnivore diet can supercharge your return to metabolic health. Many religions incorporate fasting, and fasting has been used since ancient times as a medical intervention for epilepsy.

There are many different types of fasting that can be deployed for various purposes.

Intermittent fasting involves alternating between periods of eating and not eating. Time-restricted eating, where you eat all your food within a specific feeding window, is a type of intermittent fasting. The 16:8 version is the most common, where you eat for eight hours and then fast for sixteen. Alternate-day fasting is another example of intermittent fasting, where you eat one day and then fast the next, leading to a thirty-six-hour fast.

Water fasting is where you consume nothing but water and perhaps supplements for a certain period. Dry fasting is where you consume no food or liquids. There are also protein-sparing modified fasts, which are low in calories but mostly protein so that you can avoid losing muscle mass during your fast. Sardine fasts are a good example of a protein-sparing modified fast, as long as you eat sardines canned in water. A fat fast, where you consume only fats for a period of time, is yet another variation.

Here is my take: Fasting can be a highly effective strategy after your body has gotten used to carnivore. If you are already an experienced faster, go ahead and continue using it to your heart's content as you embark on the carnivore diet. But if you are new to carnivore and to fasting, please allow your body some time to get used to carnivore first and then work on incorporating fasting. Your body will naturally start relaxing into longer intervals between meals as your blood sugar regulates. Once you can go at least sixteen hours between meals *naturally*, you are ready to play around with extended fasting. By naturally, I mean you don't even notice you haven't eaten for sixteen hours, and when you do notice, it isn't because you are super hungry or suffering. One day, you will just realize that you haven't eaten for sixteen hours, and you will say to yourself, "Huh, I guess I could eat, but I would be fine if I didn't."

I do regular sixteen- to eighteen-hour fasts. I typically eat breakfast with my twins between 8 and 9 a.m. and then have my last meal of the day by 3 or 4 p.m. I also like to throw in twenty-four- to thirty-six-hour fasts occasionally, and I have had some fun playing with sardine fasts and fat fasts.

Fasting can be an excellent strategy for lowering insulin and glucose levels, losing some weight, and gaining energy if used correctly. I highly recommend checking out Dr. Jason Fung's book *The Complete Guide to Fasting*. More info about that book is in Appendix B.

HORMESIS

Hormesis is an adaptive response to a stressor that makes you stronger over time. You can use hormesis to improve your stamina, boost your immune system, and lower inflammation, along with aiding in healthy aging. Fasting, sauna, steam room, cold plunges, exercise, meditation, and brain exercises are all examples of stressors that induce hormesis. I use all of those methods to varying degrees, and I think they are things that you can deploy as you continue your journey to metabolic health.

Examples of Hormesis:

- Sauna
- Steam room
- Cold plunge
- Fasting
- Exercise
- Meditation
- Brain exercises

SUPPLEMENTATION

Supplementation is a hot topic in the carnivore space. Many people feel that you should meet all your vitamin and mineral needs using food, while others think you absolutely need to supplement, regardless of your diet.

For me, the short answer is that you do not *need* to supplement on a carnivore diet, but you can supplement if you want to. I don't see supplements as a bad thing and believe they can bolster an already strong nutritional intervention. There are some exceptions, however:

- People who have had bariatric surgery may need to supplement even on a carnivore diet because they can no longer absorb nutrients in the same way that people with intact digestive systems can.
- People dealing with chronic inflammatory response syndrome (CIRS) may need to supplement and perhaps take some toxin binders to regain their health. A toxin binder is a substance or compound that is intended to help the body eliminate unwanted substances through digestion by "binding" with the toxin and removing it from the body.
- People with hypothyroidism benefit from supplementation to bolster and support their thyroid.
- Anyone with severe nutrient deficiencies may need help getting back to baseline, and supplementation may be the only way to get there.

While carnivore is a nutrient-dense diet, there are some nutrients you may not get enough of. Take iodine, for example. Most people are iodine deficient, and you aren't likely to consume a lot of iodine on any diet. Even the amount in iodized salt is only enough to prevent goiters, not enough to ensure optimal health. Iodine is a supplement that I think most people should be taking, regardless of diet.

Another example is vitamin D. I talked about vitamin D in the "Sunlight" section, but the fact is that most people are deficient. The easiest way to raise vitamin D levels quickly is to supplement. But if you choose to use vitamin D, you need to take K2 and magnesium along with it to ensure that it works effectively.

You should work with your healthcare provider to determine what supplements will work best for you and will not negatively interact with any medication you are taking, but here are some examples of what I think are no-brainer supplements to use with carnivore.

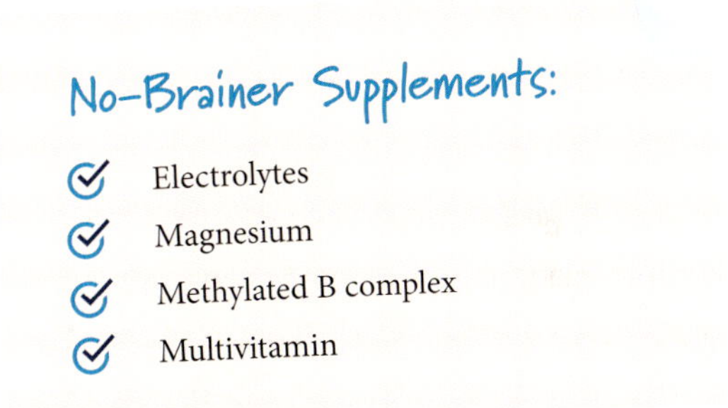

A common concern for people trying carnivore is meeting recommended daily allowances (RDAs) on the diet. RDAs are educated guesses of minimum nutrient needs based on consuming a high-carb, high-grain diet. RDAs are not the amounts of nutrients needed for optimal health in a lot of cases. When you are no longer consuming large quantities of carbohydrates, your needs for certain vitamins may decline. A great example is vitamin C. When carbs are low, glucose competition decreases, oxidative stress is reduced, and vitamin C is used more efficiently—so the body needs less of it to meet its needs. This is part of why people on strict carnivore diets show no signs of scurvy despite getting only minimal amounts of vitamin C from animal foods.

Every person's situation is unique, and you should do what works best for you. I like to test for deficiencies (see chapter 8 for more on what kinds of testing to pursue) and then supplement as needed. Again, working with a knowledgeable health practitioner is advised.

Note that nutritional supplements are not regulated by the FDA, and there are some sketchy products out there. Here are some tips to help you pick the highest-quality supplements:

- Make sure the supplement is in the most absorbable, bioavailable form. For example, when choosing a B12 supplement, go with methylcobalamin, not cyanocobalamin. Always choose folate over folic acid.
- Avoid fillers, colors, flavors, sugars, etc.
- Don't pinch pennies. Higher-quality supplements have undergone more rigorous third-party testing, contain higher-quality ingredients, and are manufactured in cleaner facilities. They will likely cost more.

Bottom line: If you want to supplement, go ahead. But be sure to pay attention to the quality of the supplements you purchase and take only what you truly need.

ENVIRONMENT

Finally, we spend a lot of time worrying about what we eat, but we tend to forget about the environment in which we live! You can clean up your diet, get good exercise, dial in your sleep and stress, and get an appropriate amount of sunlight, but if you are living in a heavily polluted area or in a mold-infested home, that environment is going to affect your health negatively.

If you are still experiencing issues with your health after optimizing all of these other factors, you may be dealing with another root cause. Getting your home checked for mold is a great first step. Having the air quality checked in and around your home and neighborhood could give you another data point. A high-quality commercial-grade air filter, like a Jaspr, could be helpful in controlling the quality of the air inside your home.

Microplastics and forever chemicals are something that we all must deal with in today's world. Minimizing exposure to microplastics and forever chemicals is important because they can disrupt hormones, cause inflammation, and build up in the body. They also persist in the environment, contaminate the food chain, and harm wildlife. Reducing exposure supports both your health and the planet. You can minimize your exposure by avoiding detergent pods, choosing natural fibers over synthetic ones, opting for glass storage containers and glass or metal water bottles and drinkware, avoiding nonstick cookware with Teflon coatings, minimizing shellfish consumption, avoiding ultra-processed foods (which you will already be doing on carnivore), and filtering your water.

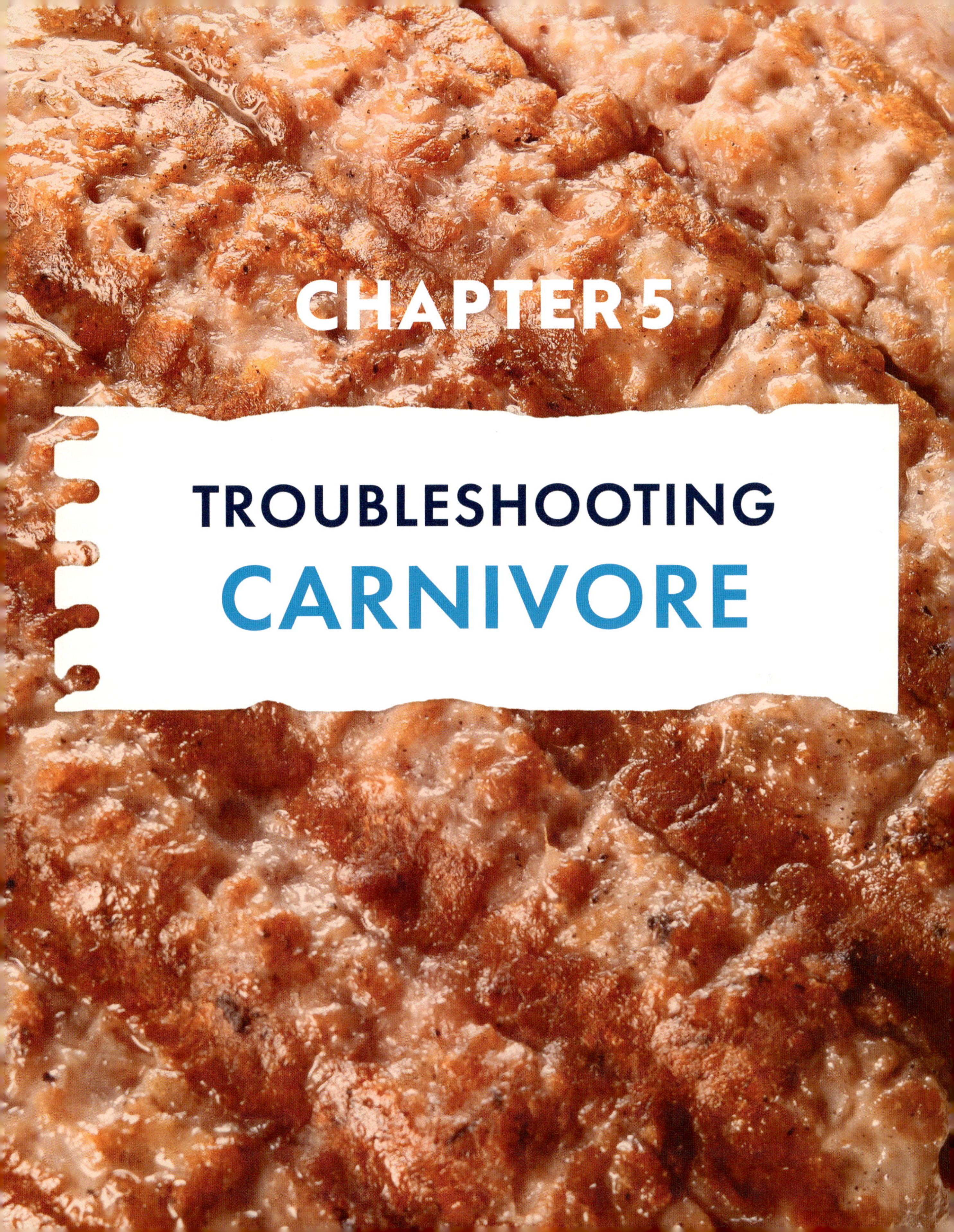

CHAPTER 5

TROUBLESHOOTING CARNIVORE

Unfortunately, it's not always smooth sailing on the carnivore diet. You may run into some issues. In this chapter, I hope to address all of the problems you could encounter and give you actionable steps to deal with each one.

THE FIVE MOST COMMON MISTAKES NEW CARNIVORES MAKE

Do you feel that your carnivore diet is not going as well as it should be? Let's start by tackling the most common mistakes that new carnivores make.

NOT EATING ENOUGH

The first mistake is not eating enough food. This can be exacerbated by loss of appetite and food aversions, but after the first month or so on carnivore, things should even out. If you don't eat enough for a long enough period of time, your metabolism will slow down and adjust to the level of energy you are consuming. So be sure to consume enough food, referring to the minimum consumption guidelines on pages 89 to 95.

Some people go carnivore and do not see their appetite improve after the initial adaptation period, when appetite sometimes drops temporarily. They cannot seem to eat enough fat, protein, or food in general. If that is the case for you, I recommend going off how you feel. If you are feeling energetic and healthy, keep doing what you're doing. If you start feeling sick or getting negative test results, you will need to address the lack of appetite. You may need to schedule two or three mealtimes per day and eat something at each meal. Some people find a lot of success using a high-quality protein powder to reach their protein goals.

But sometimes it's time to try something new. Carnivore isn't for everyone, and you shouldn't stay on it if you are not thriving. I think whole-food, low-carb diets free from ultra-processed foods, added sugars, and seed oils are great in general, and perhaps it is time for you to start incorporating some variety. You can always return to carnivore down the road.

EXPECTING EXTREME RESULTS

The second most common mistake is expecting extreme results in a short time. Some people think they can do carnivore for two weeks and see miraculous drops in weight and drastic improvements in metabolic health. But remember, you didn't get to where you are today in a couple of weeks. You are likely dealing with years of metabolic dysfunction and weight gain. Results are not going to occur overnight. That being said, a lot of people do lose large amounts of weight during the first ninety days. Many see significant improvements in blood pressure, glucose levels, and overall health. But I don't want you to feel discouraged if you are not one of those people. You will get there eventually with time and consistency.

EATING TOO MUCH FAT

The third mistake is adding too much extra fat when you still have a lot of weight to lose. Animal fats are healthy and should be part of your diet, but if you're insulin resistant and pile on butter or cream, you may end up gaining instead of losing. For now, stick to the fat that naturally comes with your meat. Think of the fat on your body like sticks of butter—you want to burn that first. If you keep eating extra fat, your body won't tap into its own stores. As you lose weight and get closer to your goal, you'll need to increase fat since you'll have less on your body to use.

NEGLECTING HYDRATION

The fourth most common mistake is neglecting hydration levels. Simply drinking enough water will take care of a lot of the issues you may be encountering, from headaches to constipation.

NOT GETTING MORNING ELECTROLYTES

Finally, the fifth mistake that new carnivores often make is not drinking electrolytes first thing in the morning. I don't think you need to take electrolytes forever, but you will almost certainly need them in the beginning. Your electrolyte balance can get out of whack, and it is essential to replace them while your body gets used to this way of eating. Simply stirring a powdered electrolyte mix into your water can mitigate the worst keto flu symptoms.

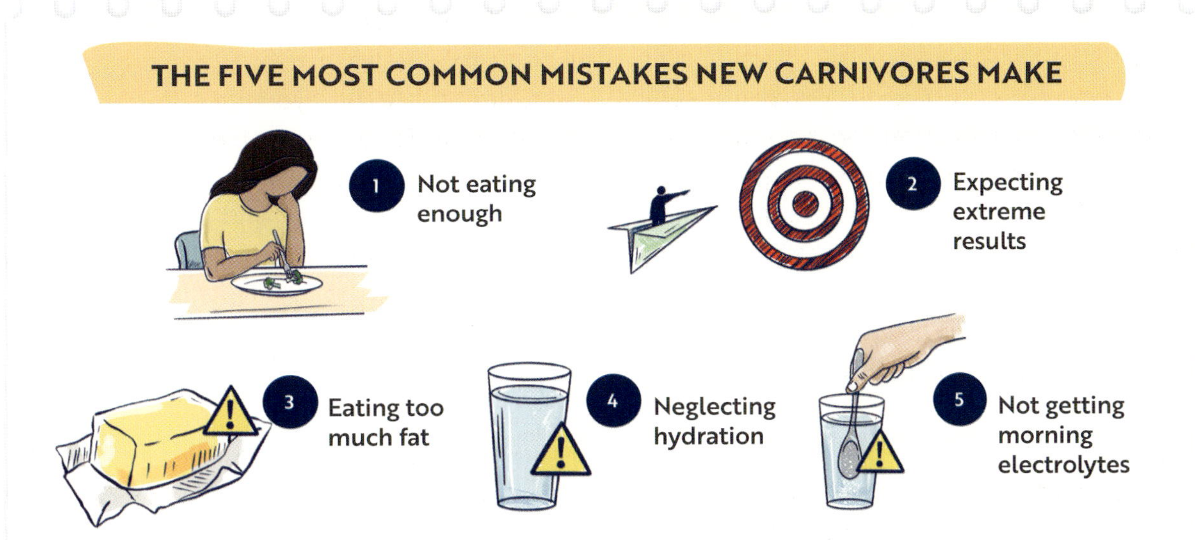

Now that we've covered the most common mistakes, let's dive into the troubleshooting.

WEIGHT-LOSS STALLS

You can hit stalls on carnivore, even if you are doing everything "right." But what is a true weight-loss stall? I think that once you have stayed around the same weight for at least two months and you still have weight to lose, you've officially hit a stall. It is normal to not lose weight for a few weeks. That's why I want you to take measurements, DEXA scans, blood work, and more (refer to chapter 8). There may be improvements in that data that don't show up on the scale.

If you have hit a weight-loss stall, there are a few tweaks you can make to get the scale moving again. Let's address the most common reasons people experience stalls and some easy-to-implement solutions for each.

CIRS/Mold

Long-term exposure to mold can wreak havoc on your metabolic health. Chronic inflammatory response syndrome, or CIRS, is most often triggered by mold exposure and has a myriad of symptoms including fatigue, brain fog, headaches, and chronic sinus congestion. If you suspect CIRS is an issue for you, the first thing you can do before diving into expensive blood work is an inexpensive online vision test. If you fail that test, you can explore other options for determining whether CIRS is your root cause issue. Here are some places to start your exploration:

- **www.survivingmold.com:** You can take the CIRS vision test here and get tons of information on next steps.
- ***Nutrition with Judy* YouTube channel:** Judy Cho is a nutritionist with a thriving practice who works with lots of CIRS clients. Her YouTube channel has a wealth of information on CIRS and is a great place to learn more.

Note: If, after taking the following measures, you still are not seeing the results you would like, I recommend looking to your environment for mold, air or water pollution, and the like. If you have developed chronic inflammatory response syndrome (CIRS) or if you have Lyme disease, your body may be hanging on to extra fat to protect itself.

SWITCH IT UP

When you hit a weight-loss stall, the key is to switch things up so your body doesn't get too comfortable with the routine. If you eat the same meals at the same times with the same exercise regimen for months, your body will adapt and create a new baseline. One of the easiest changes is to adjust your macros—try lowering the extra fat you add to meals and swapping a fatty cut like ribeye for a leaner one such as sirloin or chicken breast at least once a day. This encourages your body to burn stored fat instead of relying on dietary fat. At the same time, raise your protein a bit so you don't undereat. Playing with meal timing can help, too: Intermittent fasting (like 16/8), finishing meals earlier in the day, or even doing an occasional 24-to-48-hour fast can help you break through a plateau. The idea is to keep your body guessing. Small adjustments in fat intake, protein balance, and/or fasting windows can get fat loss moving again.

CUT INFLAMMATORY FOODS

Are you consuming dairy in your version of the carnivore diet? That is the first thing I ask my coaching clients and YouTube commenters. A lot of people don't realize that they have a dairy intolerance until they cut it from their diet for at least thirty days. If you are still eating dairy and have hit a weight-loss stall, omit the dairy for a month and see what happens.

After this thirty-day period, I recommend reintroducing one dairy product at a time to see which ones, if any, make you feel achy, give you indigestion or bloating, or cause you to feel a little sad. If you feel any of those things, I would exclude that dairy food from your diet. (There is an argument that raw dairy doesn't cause the inflammatory effects that conventional dairy does, so perhaps you could experiment with raw dairy and see if you still have an issue.) If you don't feel any of those things, perhaps you can reincorporate that dairy food in reasonable amounts. But remember, dairy is easy to overeat, so be sure to portion it out. Also remember that when I refer to dairy, I am not including butter or ghee, only liquid dairy and cheese.

The next inflammatory food item to look out for is eggs. Try omitting them for thirty days, and then reintroduce whole eggs and see what happens. If you have a reaction, cut out eggs for another couple of weeks, and then reintroduce just the yolks. A lot of people who have reactions to eggs are only sensitive to the whites.

Finally, if you have been having high-carb, standard American diet (SAD) cheat meals or cheat days, you must stop. Every time you eat like that, you will get inflamed, and not just for one day; sometimes the inflammation can last for weeks. The longer you eat a species-appropriate diet such as carnivore, the more your body will not tolerate poisons such as ultra-processed foods. This happened to me after my husband and I shared a pizza while we were in Chicago. I was achy and bloated for a week and suffered mental health symptoms for two weeks afterward. It was not worth it. So, if you need a treat, consider a keto cheat meal instead of a SAD cheat meal. I like to eat a keto cheat meal once a month that includes a salad and some smothered Brussels sprouts (see page 323 for the recipe) alongside my normal ribeye steak. When I eat this instead of a high-carb, ultra-processed cheat meal, I don't suffer negative consequences and don't lose any of the progress I've made.

EAT MORE

Calorie restriction only works to a point. I discussed minimum calorie and protein goals in chapter 3, but if you have stuck to your minimums for months, you are physically active and you haven't upped your caloric intake, or you have no appetite and you have been eating only once a day or once every couple of days, your weight loss will eventually slow to a halt. It may take a while to get to that point, but it will happen. You simply must get enough food and nutrients consistently, or your body will go into conservation mode.

Here is what I recommend in this situation: First, if you are not already tracking your food, start tracking. Log your food for a week so you can get an accurate estimate of calories, protein, and fat. Then figure out your total daily energy expenditure (TDEE). There are plenty of free online calculators out there—just search for "TDEE calculator" and a bunch will pop up. You input your gender, age, height, weight, and activity levels, and the calculator outputs the number of calories you should be consuming to maintain your current weight. For example, based on my info, I get 2,132 calories per day.

Next, compare your maintenance calories to what you are currently consuming. If you are a few hundred calories or more below maintenance, I recommend upping your calories to at least maintenance for one to two months. I would prefer you to be at least a few hundred calories *over* maintenance for this time period, which will allow your body to soak in all of the nutrition it needs and has been denied. It will also let your body know that there is not a famine. You may gain a couple of pounds, but don't worry too much about that. This technique is called reverse dieting or refeeding.

After one to two months of reverse dieting, you can start to think about cutting the calories a bit, but in a tactical way. I recommend cutting your daily caloric intake to only 100 to 200 less than your TDEE maintenance number. Here's why: Your metabolism is going to adjust to whatever amount of energy you are giving it. If you are chronically undereating, your metabolism is going to slow down so that you stay alive in this underfed state. This effect is amplified if you are also very physically active, and it can have disastrous long-term effects on your metabolism. Once you start feeding yourself enough energy, your metabolism will slowly adjust up to that level of energy. Then, once you cut calories again, you will start to lose weight again because your metabolism is now used to burning the higher amount of energy, but you will be feeding it slightly less.

Now, this is going to take some experimentation to see what works best for you. You could even do it in cycles: Reverse diet for one month and then cut your calories to 200 below maintenance for one month. Then repeat the cycle. This will allow your body to maintain a higher metabolism, never allowing it to slow down because you are not restricting calories for longer periods of time.

Check out page 127 for more on reverse dieting and priming.

One more thing about undereating in general: I think we have been brainwashed to believe that 1,200 calories per day is enough for an adult to thrive on. I also believe we live in a toxic culture that is obsessed with doing whatever it takes to lose weight, even if it means sacrificing our health. But you do not have to stay on that hamster wheel. You simply must eat enough food, or it will be harder to lose weight in the long term. I know that sounds counterintuitive, but it is the truth. Feed your body enough of the right foods, and it will eventually get to a healthy, optimal baseline.

EAT LESS

Another reason you may not be losing weight on carnivore is that you're eating way too much. I know this one will be unpopular because there are people out there who think calories don't matter and that we can eat endless amounts of carnivore foods and not gain weight. I do think it is nuanced and complicated, and the standard information about calories out there is garbage (refer to page 92). But the simple truth is that it is entirely possible to eat too much on carnivore and slow or stop your weight loss.

Here are the situations I see the most often:

- **Overeating dairy products:** 3 tablespoons of heavy cream and butter in coffee, bricks of cheese, dairy products at every meal
- **Snacking:** Instead of focusing on one to three meals per day, constantly snacking or grazing, even if those foods are carnivore
- **Overeating carnivore foods:** Eating very high fat, high calorie for an extended period of time, never allowing the body to tap into its own fat stores

You may not realize you are eating too much. This is where tracking for a week can come in handy. Just eat the way you've been eating, track your food, and see what you come up with. If you're consuming more than 500 calories over your TDEE maintenance calories, consider ramping down by a few hundred calories per week and see if it makes a difference.

ADDRESS THYROID ISSUES

Thyroid issues are super common, especially in women. Hypothyroidism, or a slowdown in thyroid hormone production, is most prevalent. Symptoms include extreme fatigue, hair loss, feeling cold all the time, irregular menstrual cycles, infertility, and inability to lose weight or even weight gain. If you are experiencing any of these symptoms, it is worth it to get a full thyroid panel from a practitioner who is experienced in thyroid health. Unfortunately, conventional doctors are trained to check only thyroid-stimulating hormone (TSH), so most of them have no idea how to evaluate a full thyroid panel. If your doctor won't test anything except TSH and maybe T4, it's time to find a doctor who will. You can also order all of these blood tests online in most states. Head to page 171 for a list of tests to order and some values to look for. It is worth getting this panel done just to eliminate a thyroid issue as a possibility for why your weight loss has stalled.

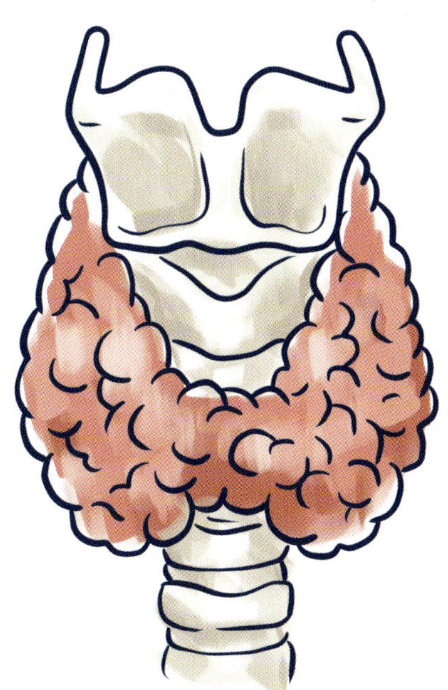

TRY FASTING

If you are experiencing a very stubborn weight-loss stall, incorporating some fasting may be helpful for you. I know it was helpful for me. I had been stuck between 152 and 158 pounds (69-71.7 kg) for about six months, so finally I did a seven-day sardine fast and dropped to 148 pounds (67 kg). While fasting for weight loss should be used sparingly by people at a healthy weight, aggressive fasting is recommended for those with insulin resistance (see the next section for more details). I do a three- to seven-day sardine fast (see below) once a month, and I do occasional twenty-four- to thirty-six-hour water fasts as well. I also intermittent fast every day, typically 16:8 (sixteen hours of fasting followed by an eight-hour feeding window). I recommend reading the book *The Complete Guide to Fasting* by Dr. Jason Fung, which has a ton of info about how to fast safely and effectively. I also recommend working with a medical professional who has experience with fasting that can help guide you through the process.

Here are a few fasting protocols you can try to get the scale moving again:

- **24 to 72 hours:** Shorter fasts are a great introduction to fasting. Some people eat every other day, incorporating a thirty-six-hour fast several times a week. I like to fast for this length of time on travel days. One of these shorter fasts can be a great experiment once your body is used to daily intermittent fasting.
- **3 days on, 4 days off:** This intermediate-level fasting regimen can be effective for lowering insulin, glucose, and weight. I recommend doing at least three cycles in a row to see maximum benefits.
- **5 days on, 2 days off:** This more aggressive weekly fasting regimen might be warranted if your insulin resistance is not responding quickly to three days on, four days off.
- **Extended fasting:** Seven-plus straight days of no food. The longest fast on record is 382-plus days, by a morbidly obese man named Angus Barbieri. He consumed only liquids, vitamins, and electrolytes during this time and lost 276 pounds (125.2 kg). I do not recommend trying to fast for that long, but I mention it because people get freaked out about not eating for extended periods. If you have a ton of extra fat on your body, you will not starve to death. You do need to pay attention to your hydration levels, but that is easily managed.
- **Sardine fasting:** On a sardine fast, you consume only sardines for a certain amount of time. Sardine fasts are effective because they combine natural calorie restriction, high satiety, zero carbs, and dense nutrients that support fat burning, hormone balance, and metabolic reset. Typical sardine fasts last three to fourteen days, with one person I am aware of going for 120-plus days consuming only sardines. I personally have done three-, seven-, ten-, and fourteen-day sardine fasts with great success. I now do a sardine fast at least once a month.

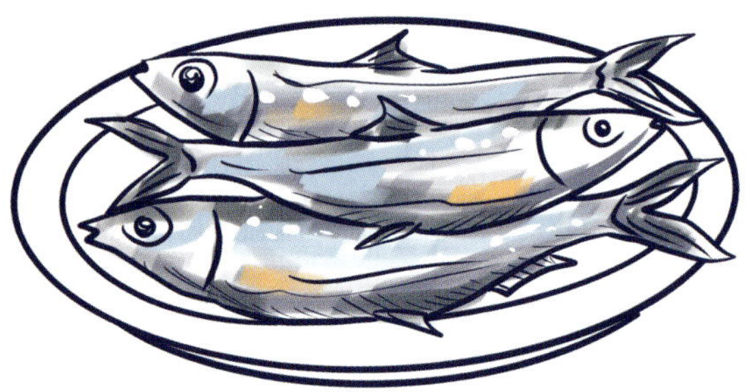

- **PSMF:** On a protein-sparing modified fast, you consume just enough protein to "spare" your lean mass while fasting. This allows your body to tap into your fat stores while maintaining muscle mass. Typically, you would throw in a couple of protein-sparing modified fasting days per week in place of your normal diet. There are many PSMF calculators online that you can use to calculate your macros for those days. A hypothetical meal plan would include egg whites and grilled chicken breast for breakfast, 99 percent lean ground turkey for lunch, and sirloin steak for dinner. If you would like more information on this style of fasting, Maria and Craig Emmerich have a great book on the topic that is listed in Appendix B.

If you're struggling with insulin resistance or excess weight, morning glucose and ketone readings can help you decide whether to eat or fast. If your blood glucose is 100 mg/dL (5.6 mmol/L) or higher, it's best to fast until it drops below 99 mg/dL (5.5 mmol/L). Ketones offer another clue: If they're below 0.5 mmol/L, keep fasting; if they're above 0.5 mmol/L, it's fine to eat. This simple method, used by Dr. Annette Bozworth (Dr. Boz) in her clinic, is an easy way to tell whether your body needs more food—or more fasting. See chapter 8 for more on these readings.

How to Practice Religious Fasting on a Carnivore Diet

Many religious traditions incorporate fasting, and it is possible to stay close to a carnivore approach while honoring these practices. In Orthodox Christianity, fasting excludes meat, dairy, and eggs, but fish and seafood are permitted. Leaning on salmon, sardines, shrimp, and mussels provides protein and fat while respecting the guidelines and keeping meals simple. In the Catholic tradition, fasting during Lent and on Fridays requires abstaining from meat but allows fish, making seafood the best carnivore-friendly option. On other days, meat, eggs, and dairy can be eaten within the traditional fasting meal structure. During Ramadan, the restriction is on timing rather than food, with no eating or drinking from sunrise to sunset. Here, nutrient-dense proteins and fats at suhoor (such as eggs, beef, or lamb) help sustain energy, while breaking the fast at iftar with broth, eggs, or fish before a larger meat-based meal supports digestion and recovery.

In all cases, planning around the rules of each tradition makes it possible to keep meals simple, nourishing, and aligned with both spiritual practice and a carnivore lifestyle.

NOT LOSING WEIGHT AND METABOLIC HEALTH DECLINING

Perhaps you haven't run into a weight-loss stall; maybe the problem is that the scale didn't move much in the first place, and your biomarkers weren't improving, either. If you have been doing carnivore for at least ninety days without cheating and haven't lost much or any weight, *and* you're not seeing improvements in your blood glucose, triglycerides, HDL, fasting insulin, and blood pressure levels, you will need to take a different approach temporarily.

When most people go ultra-low carb, they see improvements in their metabolic health along with significant weight loss. But a small percentage of people do not lose any weight, or maybe even gain, and they see declines in their metabolic health.

My husband was one of these people. We went carnivore at around the same time, and while I lost a ton of weight, he lost none. His fasting glucose continued to average in the low 100s mg/dL (5.56 mmol/L), and he would have an early-morning ("dawn effect") rise to 130 mg/dL (7.22 mmol/L). His triglycerides were still elevated at 200 mg/dL (2.26 mmol/L), his HDL wouldn't go higher than 35 mg/dL (0.91 mmol/L), his fasting insulin remained elevated at 18 uIU/mL (125 pmol/L), and his blood pressure was hovering between 140/90 mmHg and 155/100 mmHg. We were at a loss as to why this was happening until we learned that high glucose, triglycerides, insulin, and blood pressure and low HDL are just symptoms—indicators of metabolic dysfunction.

What my husband was experiencing is called lipotoxicity, which can happen when you have reached your personal fat threshold and your body cannot store excess fat in your fat cells anymore. Your body will begin to deposit this fat internally, on and around your organs. This fat is called visceral fat, and it drives persistent insulin resistance.

What causes lipotoxicity? Years and years of high carbohydrate consumption. Your body simply gets to a point where it can no longer deal with the elevated glucose levels that are the consequence of eating so many carbs. Your insulin remains high because your glucose is constantly elevated, so you eventually build up a resistance to it, hence the term *insulin resistance*.

Insulin is a fat storage hormone (among other things), so if it's always high, you are always in storage mode. Your fat cells become packed to the brim, and eventually they cannot store any more fat without becoming diseased and inflamed. This is lipotoxicity. It doesn't necessarily mean that you are overweight. Genetics play a role in how much fat your fat cells can hold, and some people can be thin and still have reached their personal fat threshold. This is why there are so many thin type 2 diabetics.

Back to my husband. After we saw that his biomarkers were so dysfunctional, we got him a body composition DEXA scan and discovered that 9 of the 70 pounds (4 of the 31.75 kg) he had left to lose were visceral fat, which is a clear indicator of insulin resistance. It is like a feedback loop: The more visceral fat you have, the more insulin you produce, which leads to more visceral fat storage.

My husband was still very insulin resistant, despite having been carnivore for over a year at that point. We were puzzled because most of the recommendations in the carnivore space were to increase the fat and "carnivore harder." It wasn't until I spoke with Dr. Nadir Ali, an interventional cardiologist out of Houston, Texas, that we connected all of the pieces and figured out that Goran was experiencing lipotoxicity. For him, a high-fat carnivore diet wasn't going to work; in fact, it could have made his health worse, at least until he could empty his fat cells and resolve his metabolic dysfunction. Thankfully, there is a threefold treatment that is relatively quick and easy to implement and can reverse lipotoxicity. In just ten months (as of June 2025), Goran has been able to reduce his weight from 270 to 214 pounds (122.5 to 97 kg) and improve all his biomarkers using the methods that follow.

But before you start implementing this protocol, you need to determine if you are truly experiencing lipotoxicity. Make sure you have been consistently carnivore or ultra-low carb for at least ninety days, and then test for the following biomarkers. (It is ideal if you have some "before carnivore" numbers to compare these updated tests to so you can see if your health is improving or declining.) Fast for twelve to fourteen hours before the test—no more, no less. Drink only water in this period, no coffee.

- **Elevated triglycerides:** 100 mg/dL (1.13 mmol/L) or higher
- **Elevated fasting insulin:** In the double digits (69.45 pmol/L or higher)
- **Elevated fasting glucose:** 95 mg/dL (5.28 mmol/L) or higher
- **Low HDL:** Below 50 mg/dL (1.29 mmol/L)
- **Low adiponectin:** Single digits to low teens (below 333 nmol/L)
- **TG/HDL ratio:** Above 2 (above 1 in international units)
- **HOMA-IR:** Above 1.3
- **Visceral fat accumulation** (as measured through a body composition DEXA scan or MRI, not a body composition scale or InBody scan): Above 2 pounds (1 kg)

If only a few of the above criteria match yours, you most likely are not lipotoxic; something else is going on. If most or all of your tests match these criteria, then you likely are lipotoxic. In that case, I recommend that you implement the following interventions:

- **First, temporarily adjust your macros to be low to moderate fat, low carb, and high protein.** This will allow your body to tap into its own fat stores more effectively. For example, if you ate 200 grams of protein, you could do 75 grams of fat and up to 50 grams of carbs. It's not zero fat, just lower fat. Eat leaner cuts of meat, don't top your steak with butter, and you should be fine.
- **Next, throw in some zone 2 exercise.** Zone 2 exercise is low-to-moderate intensity cardio that keeps your heart rate within a range where you can still hold a conversation—usually 65 to 75 percent of your max heart rate. You can estimate your max heart rate by subtracting your age from 220. Exercising at this level of intensity is great for burning fat and emptying out your fat cells.
- **Finally, add in some fasting.** This can be as simple as doing some intermittent fasting every day, or you can go up to more

aggressive water fasting of three days or more. You can tailor your fasting to your personal preferences and abilities, but know that the more fasting you do, the quicker you can resolve the lipotoxicity. I listed several fasting protocols earlier in this chapter.

After following this protocol for three months, rerun the blood tests and do another DEXA scan. Again, fast for twelve to fourteen hours only and drink only water before the test. You will know that the lipotoxicity has resolved when you experience the following improvements:

- **Triglycerides:** 100 mg/dL (1.129 mmol/L) or less
- **Fasting insulin:** In the single digits, ideally 2–6 uIU/mL (13.89–41.67 pmol/L)
- **Fasting glucose:** 95 mg/dL (5.27 mmol/L) or less
- **HDL:** Above 50 mg/dL (1.29 mmol/L)
- **Adiponectin:** 20+ (667 nmol/L+) for men, 25+ (833 nmol/L+) for women
- **TG/HDL ratio:** Below 2 (below 1 in international units)
- **HOMA-IR:** Below 1.3
- **Visceral fat accumulation:** Under 2 pounds (1 kg), ideally 1 pound (0.5 kg) or less
- **Overall weight loss**

Once everything is moving in the right direction again, you can begin to raise your fat intake. But be sure to keep an eye on your biomarkers by testing every three to six months for at least a year afterward.

Only a small subset of people will run into the issue of lipotoxicity. Again, most people who follow a carnivore diet experience health improvements and weight loss. But I wanted to share my husband's story with you to illustrate that there is no one-size-fits-all dietary intervention, and it is important to get blood work periodically to look under the hood, so to speak. The fact that lipotoxicity happens to certain individuals doesn't make the carnivore diet "bad." It just means that some people need to do a couple of extra things to get their metabolism working correctly again. Lipotoxicity doesn't occur in metabolically healthy people! Without the blood testing and DEXA scan, we would have had no idea that something was going wrong with Goran, and that could have led to disaster. Please take this to heart and keep an eye on your biomarkers!

If you would like to learn more on this topic, I have several videos on lipotoxicity on my YouTube channel. You will also want to dive into Dr. Nadir Ali's channels, as he treats patients experiencing lipotoxicity on a daily basis and has a lot of great content on this topic.

PRIMING/REVERSE DIETING

If you are coming from a place of nutrient deficiency or calorie restriction, it is important to rebuild your nutrient stores and show your body that you are not experiencing a famine. There are several ways to do so. The first, called priming, was created/popularized by "Steak and Butter Gal" Bella Ma and one of her coaches, Raymond Nazon. Priming is a technique where you basically refill your body with nutrients for two weeks. Here's what you do:

In week one, you eat three carnivore meals per day, plus snacks. Some people eat upwards of 6,000 calories during this time. In week two, you eat three meals per day, no snacks. By the end of this priming period, you should feel full and no longer want to eat three meals per day. Then you can return to your normal carnivore meal frequency.

Priming is just a regimented form of reverse dieting, which is another way to boost your metabolism after an extended period of calorie restriction. Reverse dieting is just that: Instead of calorie restriction, you aim for calorie abundance. Here is how I use reverse dieting: I like to eat a ton of carnivore foods for a few weeks, typically between 2,500 and 3,500 calories per day, with a fat-to-protein ratio of at least 70/30, but typically higher fat, like 75/25 to 85/15. Then I cut my calories down to 2,000 to 2,300 for a few weeks while lowering my fat intake and increasing my protein. I also do some reverse dieting after a long fasting protocol. So, if I did a seven-day sardine fast, I eat high-fat, high-calorie carnivore for a few days afterward. By doing so, my body never has time to think it is going into famine mode. It always has the nutrients it needs, and that allows me to shed extra pounds in the long run. I cycle back and forth between reverse dieting, "normal" food consumption, and fasting. Play around with reverse dieting and see how you can make it work for you.

PHYSICAL SYMPTOMS

LOW ENERGY

Many people experience low energy in the beginning stages of carnivore, but if it extends past ninety days, it's time to take a closer look. You should be feeling full of energy most of the time.

First, look at your protein intake. If you are not eating enough protein, you can start to experience fatigue. Same with fat intake. Remember the In-Depth Guide: Proteins are the building blocks for your vehicle, and fat is the fuel. If you are not getting enough of either or both, your vehicle will begin to run inefficiently. Also remember that if you are not eating enough food for an extended period, you may begin to experience low energy levels. Sometimes just eating more food in general can do the job.

Low energy could also be the result of an electrolyte imbalance. Try consuming some salt or other electrolytes and see if that does the trick. Simple dehydration could also be the issue, so be sure to pay attention to your hydration levels.

I discussed this next issue in the "Weight-Loss Stalls" section, but it needs to be mentioned again because low energy is one of the most common symptoms of a thyroid disorder. If your fatigue levels are high and you are eating clean, getting enough sleep, and feeling generally healthy otherwise, it's time to get your thyroid checked. Head over to chapter 8 for a list of the tests to get done.

Low energy could also be related to something completely separate from your diet. Look into your environment and see if there are any issues such as mold, pollution, or air or water contamination. It would also be worth it to do a genetic test to see if you have the MTHFR mutation, because if you do, you will need to supplement with methylated B vitamins, and that could be a reason your energy is low. More info on that in chapter 8.

MUSCLE CRAMPING

Muscle cramping is another common complaint on carnivore. Unfortunately, there is not a clear answer as to why it happens, and different interventions work for different people. Here are some things you can try.

First, make sure your hydration levels are adequate. I know I keep going back to that, but it is a common cause of so many issues.

Next, check your electrolyte levels. Not getting enough sodium, potassium, and/or magnesium can cause muscle cramping. Taking some magnesium supplements can be helpful, specifically magnesium glycinate. On the flip side, maybe you are taking too many electrolytes, and ramping down could be helpful. If a potassium deficiency is causing your cramping, taking too much magnesium can make that imbalance worse. Some people find that taking a teaspoon to a tablespoon of apple cider vinegar with a large glass of water lessens the cramping. Another thing that sounds crazy but really helps is yellow mustard. If you are getting muscle cramps, eating a teaspoon of plain yellow mustard will help instantaneously. My grandma shared that tip with me years ago, and I still use it occasionally. I've also heard that a shot of pickle juice has the same effect.

Kelly Hogan tells me that mouth taping can be helpful for cramping because it improves oxygen saturation. Dr. Ken Berry has an entire video on medications that can cause leg cramping.

HEART PALPITATIONS, RACING HEART, AND ANXIETY

Some people experience heart palpitations, racing heart, and/or anxiety in the beginning stages of carnivore. This is a common keto flu or carbohydrate withdrawal symptom that typically does not persist beyond the first month. Make sure you stay hydrated and pay attention to your electrolyte levels. If the symptoms become unbearable, eat some low-sugar fruits or vegetables. Eating some carbohydrates may stop the withdrawal symptoms in their tracks.

If these symptoms are extending past the first month or two on carnivore, it is time to look at non-carnivore root causes. How is your sleep? How are your stress levels? How is your work/life balance? Have you had blood work done lately? What's your environment like? I recommend starting a journal to see if you can identify common triggers for your racing heart. Perhaps it's every time you meet with a specific person. Or maybe it happens after you've had three cups of strong coffee. Maybe you have an undiagnosed thyroid condition or mold infestation in your home. Simply keeping a journal for a couple of weeks could give you some insight on what changes need to be made.

DIARRHEA OR LOOSE STOOLS

Diarrhea is a common complaint, especially in the beginning of carnivore. When your body is adjusting to a new fuel source, it can react in all sorts of ways. Be sure to stay hydrated and keep up with your electrolytes first and foremost. Next, try reducing your fat intake a bit, especially hot, rendered fats like melted butter and the fat from ground beef. Stick to cold or room-temperature fats like cold butter and pemmican (Carnivore Bars are an excellent option). Also, the fat on your meat that retains its structure after cooking won't run through you like hot, rendered fats will.

If you have loose stools after more than ninety days on carnivore and lowering your fat consumption isn't helping, it is time to look for a different root cause. You could have some kind of intestinal bacteria, infection, or parasite that you were unaware of. Something in your environment could be affecting your body. Maybe you have a sensitivity to something you are eating, like dairy or eggs. It could also be a histamine issue. Unfortunately, carnivore is not a magic bullet and cannot cure every ailment. You may need to dig deeper.

CONSTIPATION

On the other hand, perhaps you are feeling a bit constipated, or maybe you are not going number two as frequently as you were when you were consuming carbohydrates. If you are truly constipated, with the accompanying bloated and uncomfortable feeling, simply increasing your fat consumption can get things "flowing" again. If your bowel movements are hard and/or pellet-like, increasing the fats can help stool come out more easily. You want your bowel movements to be sausage shaped, easy to pass, and with either a cracked or smooth surface. Refer to the Bristol Stool Chart below for more information.

Bristol Stool Chart

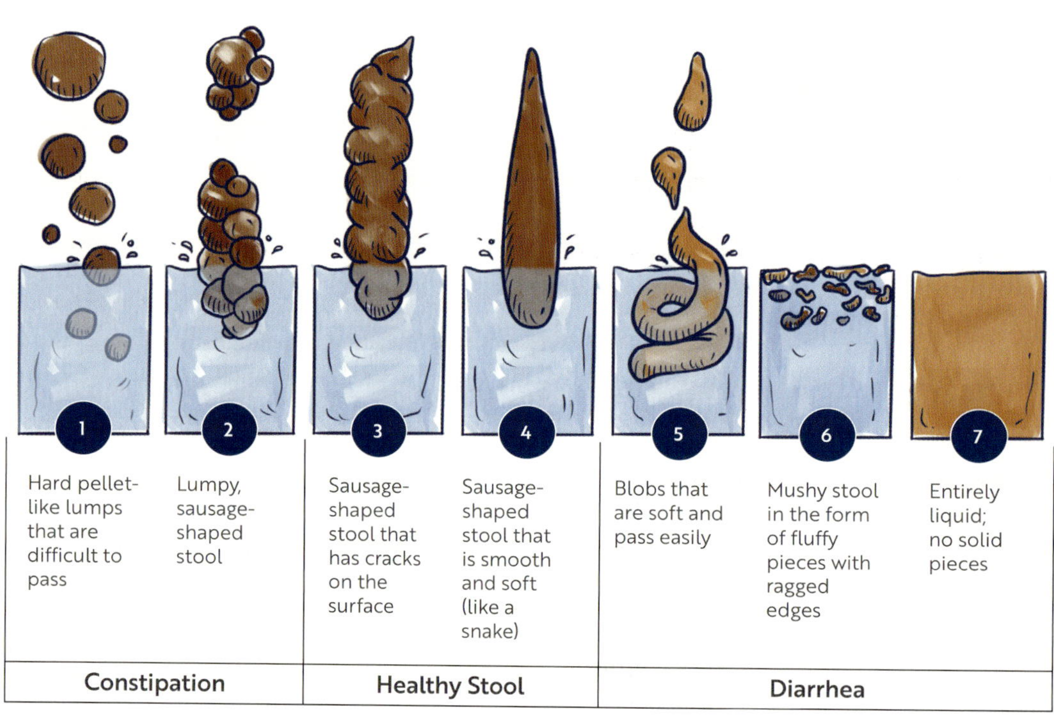

Another thing to note is that you may not be creating as much fecal matter as you were when you were consuming carbohydrates. Your body utilizes most of the animal fats and proteins you consume, so there is not a lot of waste material left behind. You may not be constipated; you may just not have to poop as often.

ACID REFLUX

Acid reflux typically goes away after the first few months on carnivore. But what if you are still experiencing it after ninety-plus days? Acid reflux or heartburn is not a problem of too much stomach acid; it is a valve problem. There is a little valve that prevents your stomach acid from going up your esophagus. If that valve is open when it shouldn't be, you experience heartburn. But the solution is not to lower your stomach acid. What keeps that valve shut is the high acidity levels in your stomach. If you lower it with an antacid, you will be keeping that valve open when it should be closed.

How can you address this issue? First, you need to *increase* the amount of acid in your stomach. You can do so with a betaine HCL supplement or even apple cider vinegar. If you experience a burning sensation in your gut, you may be experiencing gastritis or a stomach ulcer, which means you cannot add more acid until you heal that issue. Adding some fermented foods like sauerkraut and kimchi could be helpful. Another recommendation from a few low-carb practitioners is to begin supplementing with vitamin B1 (thiamine), magnesium, and zinc.

Next, look at what you are eating. If you have not been strict carnivore, you need to address that. Alcohol, seed oils, and refined carbohydrates must go. Of course, if you smoke, that must stop as well. If you are still drinking coffee or tea, those beverages can be a common trigger. Certain medications could also be giving you issues, so you may need to work with your doctor to reduce or eliminate them. Chronic stress can also be a root cause of acid reflux.

SYMPTOMS GETTING WORSE BEFORE THEY GET BETTER

Sometimes, symptoms get worse before they get better. If you aren't prepared for this possibility, your gut reaction will be, "Oh well, carnivore didn't work for me," when in reality, you just need to make some tweaks.

Let's touch on oxalates first. Most people have no idea what oxalate is or how it can affect metabolic health. Oxalates are natural compounds found in many plant foods. If you consume oxalates daily and then suddenly stop eating them, you might experience something called oxalate dumping, which can be highly unpleasant. I touched on oxalate dumping in previous chapters (see pages 61 and 85), but just know that it is a real thing that can have serious health consequences. When you stop consuming oxalates, your body will think it is time to purge all of the stored oxalates from your system. This can lead to gout flare-ups and/or kidney stones, among other things, especially if you have experienced them in the past. A lot of people think that carnivore gave them a gout flare-up or a kidney stone when in fact it's not carnivore but oxalate dumping. If you have had gout or kidney stones, it is highly advisable for you to ease into carnivore. Please use the carb reduction guide beginning on page 84 to get started and take it slowly. You can also slow oxalate dumping by keeping some oxalate in your diet for a time. Simply drinking one cup of black or green tea a day can slow oxalate dumping and allow your body to rid itself of oxalate slowly.

Gallstones are another possibility, especially if you have had them before. Here's why they happen: Carnivore is a typically a high-fat, moderate-protein style of eating. Your gallbladder holds a reservoir of bile that is used to emulsify the fats you consume. If you have been eating a low-fat diet for a long time, your gallbladder may be out of practice. You need to give it time to start working correctly again. If you go cold turkey into carnivore, your gallbladder may have issues accommodating all that fat at first. A gallstone is just a hardened deposit of digestive fluids. If you suddenly up the need for digestive fluids, there could be some kinks in the system. This is why it is so important to slowly ramp up the fat consumption if you have had gallstones in the past. You need to give your body time to build up its supply of bile, and the simple act of consuming higher levels of fat and protein will allow your gallbladder to fully drain and refill itself more often, which will "clear the pipes," so to speak. I talk about what to do if you don't have a gallbladder later in this chapter.

Skin conditions such as psoriasis, acne, and rosacea can also flare up before they improve. Sometimes this is just your body doing some elimination and detoxing itself. Insulin resistance can be a driver of some skin conditions and food sensitivities. So, if you have been doing carnivore for ninety days and are still experiencing issues with your skin, the next step is to eliminate common allergens such as eggs and dairy. If you are still experiencing some insulin resistance, doing some fasting in addition to eating a carnivore diet could be an effective solution.

MEAT AVERSIONS OR FOOD BOREDOM

Meat aversions and food boredom are common among new carnivores. This happened for me at around week three. I could not stand to look at another steak. By week five, the aversions went away.

If you have hit this point, find something different to eat. There are eighty recipes in this book that you can incorporate into your weekly meal plans. There are even more recipes on YouTube. Just a few of my favorite sources for creative carnivore recipes are Courtney Luna, "Ketogenic Woman" Anita Breeze, and Chris Cooking Nashville. Sometimes you just need a bit of variety! I like to throw in some chicken or go out for tuna sashimi. Figure out what works best for you.

SPECIAL HEALTH OR DIETARY ISSUES

HOW TO GAIN WEIGHT ON CARNIVORE

To intentionally gain weight on a carnivore diet, the key is to eat in a caloric surplus by increasing both protein and fat intake. Prioritize fatty cuts of meat like ribeye, short ribs, brisket, and lamb, along with additions like butter, tallow, and bone marrow to boost calorie density. Eating more frequently—such as three main meals plus a snack of eggs, cheese (if tolerated), or fatty fish—can help push calories higher without feeling overly stuffed. Dairy, particularly cream and cheese, can also be useful for adding extra calories if it works for your digestion. By consistently eating beyond maintenance and focusing on rich, nutrient-dense animal foods, weight gain on Carnivore becomes both intentional and sustainable.

AUTOIMMUNITY

Leaky gut is linked to many autoimmune issues, so supporting gut health is crucial. A great resource is *Gut and Physiology Syndrome* by Dr. Natasha Campbell-McBride (see Appendix B). To help heal the gut lining, consume collagen-rich meat stock made from cartilage-heavy cuts like pig's feet or pork shanks (1 to 2 cups daily, cooked for 3 to 5 hours without skimming the fat). You can also add collagen to your morning drinks and use targeted supplements: L-glutamine (10 to 12 grams daily, unless you have a history of cancer, increasing slowly), inulin (a prebiotic fiber), and quality probiotics to restore healthy gut bacteria.

NO GALLBLADDER

You can do carnivore if you don't have a gallbladder, but you may need to make some minor adjustments. First off, your body is still making bile; you just don't have a large bolus of it available at one time. That is all the gallbladder is: a reservoir for digestive fluids. So, if you suddenly increase the amount of fat you are consuming, you may develop loose stools and/or intestinal distress because you don't have a reservoir of bile to emulsify those fats. But once your body recognizes that you are now consuming a fat-heavy diet, it will increase bile output. It just needs some time to get used to the change in dietary composition.

If you are running into a lot of digestive and bowel-related issues in the beginning, perhaps you need to ramp the carbs down slowly while gradually increasing your intake of fats and proteins to allow your body time to adjust. Some people in this situation utilize digestive enzymes or ox bile to aid in breaking down fats. You will have to experiment to see what works best for you.

HISTAMINE ISSUES

As discussed in chapter 1, you can do carnivore even if you are experiencing histamine issues. Avoiding processed meats, aged cheeses, and bone broth is a highly effective strategy. Also, freezing any meat soon after you purchase it will stop the aging process and keep the meat as low in histamines as possible. Freezing the meat close to the time of slaughter will minimize histamines. Try working with a local farmer to see if they can accommodate your needs. Some highly sensitive people find that avoiding meat from single-chamber-stomached animals, such as pork and chicken, and consuming only ruminant meats, such as beef, lamb, mutton, venison, and elk, can be helpful. A wonderful supplier of low-histamine meats is BillyDoe Meats. They freeze their meat immediately after slaughter. You can find a discount code for BillyDoe at JennyMitich.com.

Mold is a common trigger for histamine issues; see page 118 for more information. Many people who experience histamine reactions also have leaky guts, and doing a strict version of carnivore allows their digestive systems to heal. There is hope. If you can address the root cause of your histamine issue, you can experience healing and perhaps return to a less restrictive way of eating.

BARIATRIC SURGERY

I went over these tips in chapter 2, but I wanted to put them here as well for easy reference. If you have had bariatric surgery, you may run into some roadblocks when starting a carnivore diet. You can still succeed on carnivore if you have had bariatric surgery, but you will want to use the following tips:

- Ease into carnivore instead of going cold turkey.
- Consume three to six or more smaller meals in an eight- to ten-hour feeding window.
- Stay away from liquid fats and hot, rendered fats like melted butter.
- Chew your food slowly and thoroughly.
- A sip or two of water during each meal may help with digestion.
- You may need to use HCL supplements, ox bile, or other digestive aids.
- Your protein minimum is the same as everyone else's, but you may have a tough time reaching it. Protein powder added to shakes works for some but runs right through others. You could incorporate protein powder into eggs, pancakes, meatloaf, etc. to increase the amount of protein you are consuming without increasing the volume of food. Powdered dehydrated meats can work as well.
- Vitamin and nutrient deficiencies are a real concern for you. Continue taking your supplements and/or getting vitamin infusions as needed. Get regular blood work to test your vitamin and mineral levels.

I have several videos on this topic on my YouTube channel, so feel free to check those out if you would like more information for your unique circumstances.

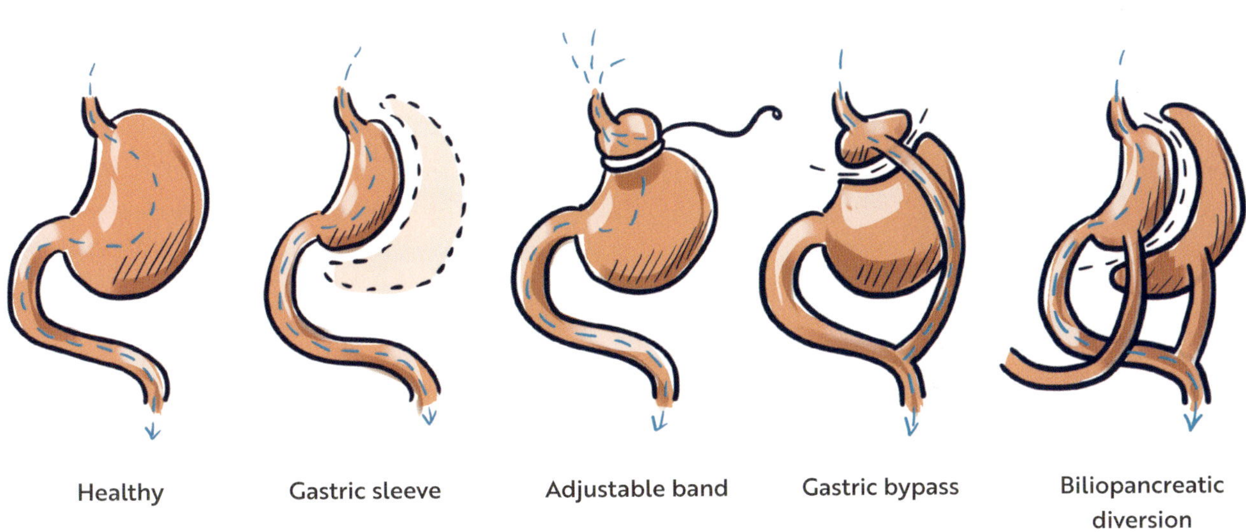

TALKING TO OTHERS ABOUT YOUR NEW LIFESTYLE

When you decide to go carnivore, you must also decide if you are going to share your new lifestyle with others, especially early on. We all have naysayers, pushers, and Debbie Downers in our lives, so let's talk about some ways to broach the topic of carnivore with your family and friends.

Your first option is to say nothing at all. You may think that people are watching your every move, but most are so wrapped up in their own thoughts that they aren't paying much attention. If, down the road, people start noticing changes and ask about what you are doing, then you can tell them more. But only if you want to. Don't feel like you must share everything going on in your life with every person you encounter.

Your next option is to reference it only vaguely by saying you are doing a low-carb elimination diet. This is a good option if you don't really feel like getting into the details. There are a ton of different "low-carb" diets out there, and most people don't really know the difference. You could also say that you have some food sensitivities, and you are trying to figure out what is causing them.

Another option is to tell people outright that you are doing carnivore when they ask. I advise waiting to do that until you have been carnivore for at least sixty days so that people don't think it is a passing phase. You will be surprised by how many people are aware of carnivore or know someone who is trying it. It's not as niche as it was a few years ago.

Here's how I look at it: I'm a lighthouse, not a tugboat. I don't randomly bring up my diet, but if someone asks me a question, I answer it. I will steer people in the right direction if they are curious, but I am not going to force it down their throats. Carnivore is just one small part of my life. I live by the philosophy of "watch their feet." I pay more attention to people's actions than their words, and I try to let my own actions lead the way. People can see the benefits of my lifestyle through the fruits it produces: a healthy weight, glowing skin, a positive and upbeat demeanor, and a thriving work and home life. If they see all that and ask what I'm doing, I tell them. Otherwise, I just live my life and don't worry too much about what others think, especially about what I'm eating.

HOLIDAYS

Over the holidays, you are going to encounter lots of opportunities to partake in high-carb cheat meals. Holidays are not going to sneak up on you; you can prepare for the occasion. If you're headed to a family gathering, one thing you could do is bring a few carnivore dishes to ensure you will have something to eat. Another tactic is to eat before you go so that you won't succumb to temptation when you are there.

Still another option is to actively designate this holiday celebration as a cheat meal. This is what I do for Thanksgiving and Christmas. Most of the time I don't go off the rails with super-high-carb, sugary items, but I do partake in vegetables, cranberry sauce, and other standard holiday fare. If I have a piece of pie, I don't eat the crust. I also pick only one of the several celebrations we attend to partake in a cheat meal. I don't cheat at every get-together over the holiday season.

If you are starting your carnivore journey during the holiday season, you may still be dealing with sugar cravings. In that case, I think avoiding high-carb, high-sugar cheat meals is best. If you are dealing with insulin resistance, avoid a high-carb cheat meal until you are in better health. A keto cheat meal could be a good alternative for you. Bottom line: Plan what you are going to do for each of the holiday events you attend and stick to the plan. If you fall off the wagon, that's okay! Just get right back on the next day and release any guilt or shame you feel. Those feelings don't serve you in any way and could prevent you from getting back to carnivore.

WORK-RELATED ACTIVITIES

You may work in an office where there are always goodies in the breakroom. You may have a regular midday slump that leads you to reach for a snack. Maybe there is a time of day that you gather with coworkers over coffee and chat. Whatever it is, you can still manage these things on carnivore; you just have to adapt. If saying no to the goodies in the breakroom is difficult for you, avoid the breakroom. Pack yourself some carnivore snacks for your midday munchies. Drink coffee and munch on a couple of pieces of bacon while you gossip with your coworkers. You can make this lifestyle work in just about any environment.

If you travel or drive a vehicle for work, eating before or after work can be helpful. For over-the-road truckers, packing carnivore meals in your fridge or lunchbox is essential. Hitting fast-food restaurants and ordering burger patties à la carte is also a viable strategy. I have talked to a few truckers who have run into issues with reheating the food that they pack. Every truck stop I've been to has a few microwaves, so take advantage of that option. I bring an air fryer with me when I'm driving long distances so I can fry up a steak on the go. Camping stoves are also a great option. Be creative! You can make this lifestyle work regardless of your work travel schedule.

"PUSHERS"

A "pusher" is someone who is always trying to force food or drinks on you (of course, what they're pushing could be something more nefarious, but let's focus on food and drinks for the moment). These people typically mean well, but their efforts can get overwhelming if you are trying to avoid carbs or experiencing sugar cravings.

You will need to practice a few good responses to extricate yourself from the grasp of a pusher. My first excuse is the elimination diet: "Sorry, I can't have the delicious cake you made right now because my doctor has me on an elimination diet." My second go-to is the food allergy or reaction excuse: "I've been having some weird food reactions, and we are trying to figure out what is causing them, so I can't eat that today." My final go-to is a simple hard no. Now that I have been on carnivore for a long time, everyone around me knows that I don't eat carbs or drink alcohol very often. Just saying "No thank you" is effective with most of the pushers I encounter. But for the ones who are persistent, I go into detail about how eating carbs, sugar, or gluten makes me feel crummy, or I talk about how I won't be able to function as an effective parent for a few days if I eat or drink whatever they are offering. If you say no often enough, they will eventually stop asking.

Remember that *you* are the only person who is going to look out for your metabolic health. You have to live in the body you were gifted with, and you are the only person who is 100 percent invested in its care. When you encounter a pusher, it's good to have made up your mind ahead of time that you are sticking to carnivore. That is half the battle. The other half is having those responses at the ready. Come prepared with a few lines of your own the next time you know you will be around a pusher!

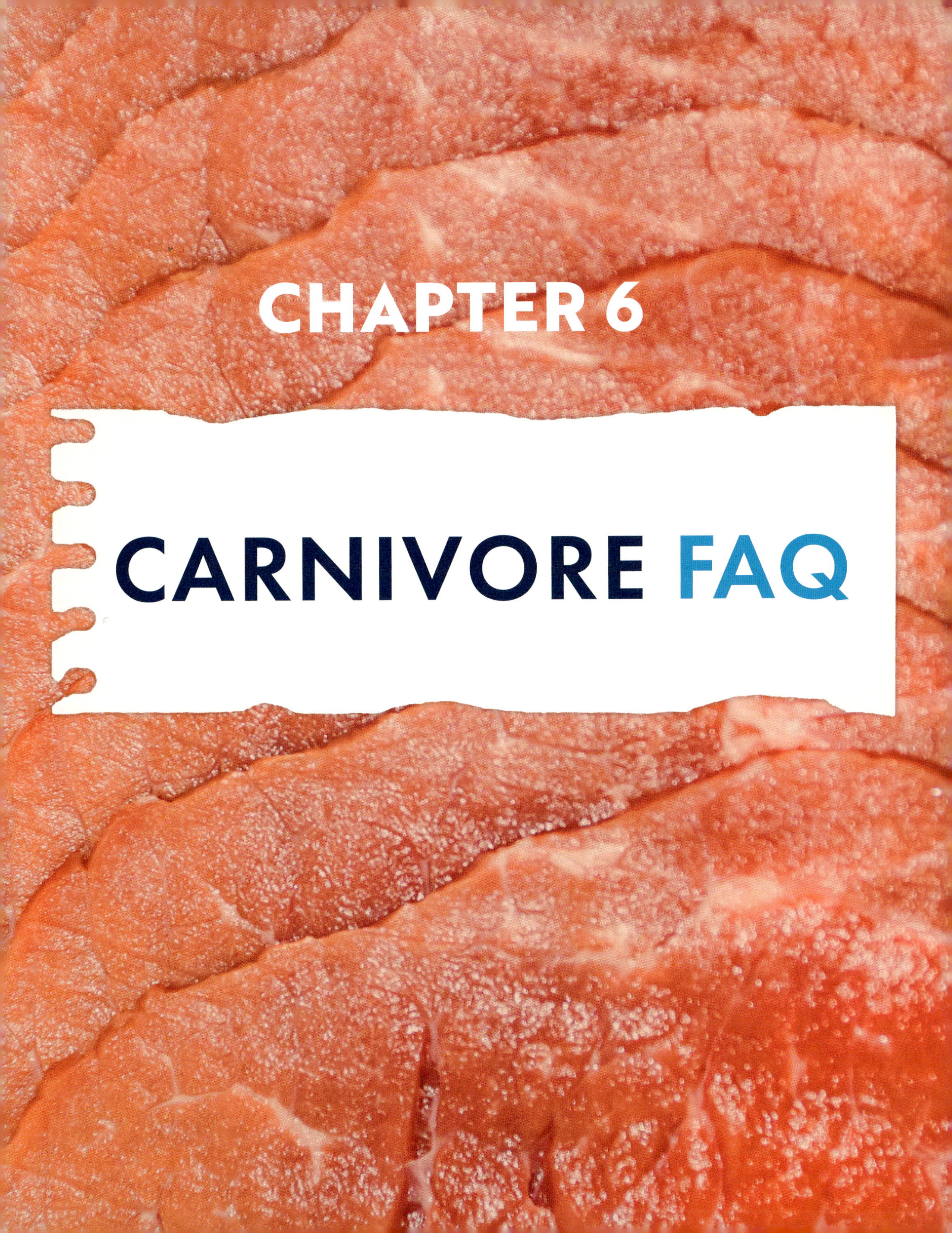

CHAPTER 6

CARNIVORE FAQ

By this point in the book, I hope that you have found the answers to most of your questions related to the carnivore diet. Maybe you saw this chapter listed in the table of contents as you were browsing in a bookstore and flipped to this page to see if your question is covered. However you got here, welcome!

This chapter is split into three sections: food and drink, metabolic health, and miscellaneous. Some of these questions have been answered in other chapters, but I wanted to collect them all in one place so you can quickly refer to them as needed. Chapter 7 addresses common myths about carnivore, so if the answer you are looking for isn't here, perhaps it is there.

FOOD AND DRINK–RELATED QUESTIONS

CAN I DO CARNIVORE ON A BUDGET?

Yes, it is entirely possible to do the carnivore diet on a strict budget. First, try some smart shopping strategies to save money on the meat you buy. Head to your local grocery store early in the morning to get first pick of the discounted meat. Every day, the meat manager must mark down the meat that needs to be sold by that day, and I find discounts of 30 to 50 percent. Next, start paying attention to the meat deals commonly available in your area. I live in the Chicagoland region, and one of our main grocery stores is Jewel. They have weekly deals that can be out of this world, so I always shop those deals and freeze the meat that I am not going to use immediately. Cheaper cuts of meat include pork and chicken, along with skirt steak, higher-fat ground beef, and organ meats.

Another great way to save money on meat is to buy it in bulk, either from a big box store like Costco or from a local farm or ranch. Investing in a deep freezer and purchasing half a cow can be a huge money saver and feed your family for months.

Finally, you will be saving money in lots of ways when you switch to carnivore. You won't be eating as often, and the food you will be eating is the most nutrient-dense food you can get for your money. You will no longer be purchasing side dishes, fruits and vegetables that will go bad in your fridge, sodas, snacks, and packaged foods. My family is actually saving money on grocery bills on carnivore.

DO I HAVE TO BUY GRASS-FED MEATS TO REAP THE BENEFITS OF CARNIVORE?

There are conflicting opinions on this topic. Nutritionally, there are some advantages to grass-fed beef over grain-fed beef. Grass-fed beef has a slightly better omega-6 to omega-3 ratio and a slightly better nutrient and phytonutrient profile. A major difference is that grass-fed beef typically has less fat than grain-fed beef, and cooking a grass-fed steak requires a bit of practice. Grass-fed beef also has a slightly different flavor that can take some getting used to. Environmentally, raising grass-fed cows on a regenerative farm can be a carbon sink, meaning they lock up carbon from the atmosphere over time. But here's the thing: All cows are fed mostly grass for most of their lives. Conventionally raised cattle are only fed grain for the last few weeks to few months of their lives to fatten them up before slaughter. Lots of ethically raised cows eat grass and then are finished with grain to improve their fat profile.

Here's my opinion: Get what you prefer and can afford. I eat conventionally raised beef most of the time. I buy a whole ribeye from Costco every four to six weeks and then pick up any half-price ribeyes I find at my local grocery store. I do purchase American Wagyu ground beef from a ranch in Minnesota because the taste is out of this world. And I get a delivery of grass-fed, grass-finished beef from ButcherBox once a month. But the bottom line is that all beef, whether grass or grain fed, is nutrient dense, and you need to include as much of it as you can afford on the carnivore diet.

CAN I EAT PROCESSED MEATS ON CARNIVORE?

This is another highly contentious topic in the carnivore world. In my opinion, yes, you can include processed meats (including bacon, sausage, pepperoni, lunch meats, etc.), but with some caveats. First, you need to read the ingredient label, just as you would with spices and seasonings. Avoid dextrose, corn syrup and other added sugars, and seed oils such as canola, soybean, and sunflower. I look for the shortest ingredient list. I also try to avoid anything with carbs, but if that isn't possible, I like to keep it to 2 grams of carbs or less per serving. Some people claim that nitrates in processed meats are bad because they can form cancer-causing nitrosamines in the body, which have been linked to increased cancer risk in some studies. But I think those concerns are overblown, and I don't worry too much about some nitrates in processed meats.

Would you want to make processed meats the focus of your carnivore diet? No. But if you want to include some, I think that's fine. If processed meat is all you can afford, then get processed meat! It is still infinitely better than ultra-processed carbs, seed oils, and sugar.

My twins and I eat breakfast sausage and thick-cut bacon every morning. I include some deli meats on a charcuterie board a couple of times a month. I also use some deli meats in recipes. Making your own sausages and deli meats is going to be your best bet if you have the time because then you can control the ingredients. Purchasing from a local farm or butcher is another great option because they typically don't use a ton of added ingredients.

DO I NEED TO EAT ORGAN MEATS?

Some people swear by organ meats, while others avoid them completely. I used to think they weren't necessary, but over time I've come to see their value on a carnivore diet. Certain nutrients—like those in beef liver—are hard to get anywhere else. If the taste is tough for you, desiccated organ supplements or even organ-based seasonings (like Pluck) are a great option. I recommend experimenting to find a way to work some organ meats into your routine.

IS CHARRED MEAT BAD FOR YOU?

While I advise against overcooking meat in general—you don't want to be consuming a hockey puck for dinner—a little bit of blackened char on meat isn't the end of the world. The key here is that you don't want to destroy the nutrients. So, in general, stick to medium-rare or medium for your steaks and burgers.

TO SALT OR NOT TO SALT?

There are varying schools of thought on salt use while eating carnivore. Old-school carnivores from the Zeroing In On Health forum of the late 1990s and early 2000s used little if any salt on their meat. Cut to the present, and most carnivore influencers are talking about the importance of salt. Here is my take: Electrolytes are essential in the beginning of carnivore (to help mitigate the worst keto flu symptoms), and salt is an electrolyte. But, as your body adapts to the diet, your need for salt may decline. I think you should do some experimenting with varying amounts of salt in your version of carnivore. Like some people on ultra-low-carb diets, you may find you feel best with as much as 3 to 7 grams of salt per day, or you may feel best on the other end of the spectrum with zero salt. Figure out what works for you.

CAN I USE SEASONINGS AND SAUCES?

Some purists argue that if you include any kind of plant material in your diet, you are no longer doing carnivore, but I disagree. Plenty of carnivores add some spices to their meats or use some sauces. In my opinion, it's only when you are chewing plant materials that you are no longer technically eating carnivore. A little bit of garlic powder isn't the end of the world for most people.

There are some exceptions, though. If your Why is to address a severe autoimmune condition, food allergies you can't seem to pin down, or another health condition that is severely impacting the quality of your life, I suggest avoiding all seasonings except for salt for the first ninety days of carnivore. You may be highly sensitive to some or all plant materials, and you will have to reintroduce them one at a time down the road (I go over the reintroduction process on page 100).

When it comes to seasonings, there are a few things to watch out for. In general, I always spring for organic and avoid anything with anti-caking agents (which are typically labeled as such), dextrose or other sugars, or any kind of filler. I choose organic because there tends to be a lighter pesticide load in these spices along with less heavy metals. But spices can be pricey, so get what works best for your budget. You are only going to be using a little bit here and there, so it's okay if you can't get the highest-quality spices.

Typically, mustard, avocado oil–based buffalo sauce, and vinegars are okay on carnivore. Some people also use sugar-free ketchup and BBQ sauce sparingly. Just don't drown your meat in sauce. Keep it to a tablespoon or two, and if you start to crave sweets or carbs, cut out the sauce. I avoid anything containing seed oils or added sugar.

CAN I USE ARTIFICIAL SWEETENERS OR SUGAR SUBSTITUTES?

This is yet another topic that has a lot of opinions floating around about it in the carnivore world. Here's the thing: Plenty of long-term carnivores use artificial or natural sugar substitutes and have success with it. And then there are others who can't touch the stuff because it triggers a previous sugar addiction or gives them gastrointestinal distress. You are going to figure out what works best for you, but I have some tips to get you started.

I advise you to avoid all sugar substitutes, natural or artificial, for at least the first ninety days on carnivore. After that, you can reintroduce them one at a time to see if they give you any sugar cravings or gastrointestinal distress. If you are addicted to sugar or carbs, you may need to avoid all sweeteners in the long term because they may reactivate that addiction. Personally, I do not use many sugar substitutes, artificial or natural. Occasionally, I use an electrolytes packet that is sweetened with stevia. If I am making an egg pudding or carnivore cheesecake around the holidays, I use allulose to sweeten them. But in general, I avoid sugar substitutes. You figure out what works best for you the longer you are on carnivore.

DO I HAVE TO EAT STICKS OF BUTTER?

You've probably seen carnivore influencers biting into sticks of butter, but you don't need to copy that unless you truly want to. The point they're making is that butter isn't harmful and that high-fat diets can be healthy. Many of them are already at their goal weight and actually need the extra fat since they don't have much stored on their bodies. When I first started carnivore, I tried eating butter straight from the stick and thought it was strange. A couple of years in, I found myself occasionally craving frozen butter and enjoying it—but that was much later. If you're still carrying extra weight, you don't need to pile on added fat, because your body already has plenty in reserve. Listen to your body and find what works best for you.

CAN I HAVE PROTEIN POWDER?

Yes, although I prefer that you get your protein from whole-food sources. But sometimes it's hard to consume that much food. Some people, especially those with compromised digestive systems due to bariatric surgery, find it difficult to reach their daily protein goal. In that case, incorporating a high-quality protein powder may be appropriate. Protein powder also may be recommended for bodybuilders. Read the ingredient label and avoid any protein powder that contains seed oils, added sugars, or other harmful ingredients. Also, keep in mind that pulverized protein can have a large glucose impact if you are insulin resistant.

WHAT CAN I DRINK ON CARNIVORE?

In general, water is going to be your main beverage. Sparkling water is good, too. Sugar-free electrolyte drink mixes are allowed. But what about tea, coffee, diet soda, and sugar-free energy drinks? Can you still drink that stuff on carnivore? This is the subject of many arguments in the carnivore space. In general, I think coffee is fine. Some carnivores can drink diet soda or other sugar-free beverages without triggering sugar cravings. I would steer clear of tea because of the high oxalates (see page 78), but a cup here and there won't kill you. I would definitely stay away from energy drinks because there are way too many ingredients in them. I think you will discover that you no longer need heavily caffeinated drinks because your energy levels are going to go up on carnivore.

CAN I HAVE ALCOHOL ON CARNIVORE?

Alcohol is not carnivore, and I do not recommend drinking during your first ninety days on the diet. First, whenever you consume alcohol, your body must stop what it is doing to detox itself. It must process the alcohol first, before whatever food you just ate. Second, alcohol can trigger sugar and carb cravings. Third, if you include alcohol, you will not reap the full benefits of the diet, such as mental health improvements, inflammation reduction, and abundant energy. So, for the first three months at least, do your best to not drink any alcohol.

If that is not workable for you, or if you are in a social situation where drinking is unavoidable, keep it to one drink and pick something very low in carbs, like a vodka soda or a whiskey on the rocks. If you want to feel included but not drink, ask the bartender to make you a sparkling water in a lowball glass with a lime. No one will notice that you aren't imbibing.

If you continue carnivore long term, having a drink once in a while is a possibility. As an established carnivore, I enjoy a drink or two every few months. I typically keep it low carb, but I will admit to having a couple of beers in the summertime or a margarita at a Mexican restaurant. You will figure out what works best for you.

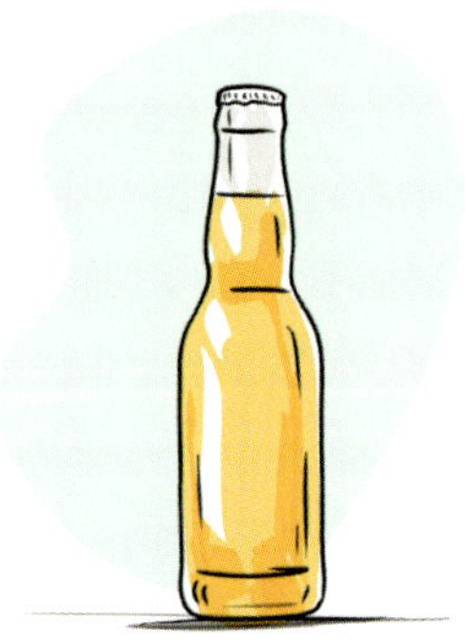

CAN OR SHOULD I EAT RAW MEAT?

Some carnivore doctors and influencers claim eating raw meat is the best way to preserve nutrients. Personally, I'll enjoy a black-and-blue steak, tuna sashimi, or the occasional steak tartare—but that's where I draw the line. I've known people who became very sick from raw ground beef, and I would never risk eating raw chicken. If you do choose to include raw meat, use discretion, handle it carefully, and always wash your hands and any surfaces it touches.

CAN I FRY FOOD ON CARNIVORE?

Sure, you can fry foods, but only use animal fats to do so. Ground pork rinds and Parmesan cheese make excellent carnivore breading for deep-frying.

ARE NONSTICK COATINGS OKAY?

If you are trying to eliminate toxins from your diet, why would you cook with a typical non-stick pan? Nonstick coatings are notorious for leaching toxic chemicals into food. To prevent this from happening, invest in a high-quality set of ceramic-coated or stainless-steel pots and pans, and choose an air fryer with a ceramic-coated or glass cooking vessel.

HOW DO I STAY CARNIVORE WHILE TRAVELING?

With a little practice, staying carnivore while traveling isn't difficult. Most restaurants serve meat. You can ask for no seasoning, breading, or oils—only butter. Many fast-food restaurants will serve meat patties à la carte. Grilled chicken or "naked" nuggets are also an option. Some places offer egg bites or protein bowls. You can even build a meat-only salad at a salad bar with whatever protein options are available.

When you are away from home, you may have to consume something with seed oil or some other questionable ingredient in it. Remember, a little bit of ultra-processed stuff once in a blue moon isn't going to kill you; it's chronic use of these items that affects your metabolic health. But if it makes you feel like crap, avoid it. Your body will let you know if it doesn't like a particular item.

Here are some travel tips: If you are staying in a hotel, try to get one with a kitchenette or at least a refrigerator. That way, you can go to a grocery store and pick up some carnivore foods. If I am going to be away from home for more than a few days, I get an Airbnb so I can cook carnivore meals. Hard-boiled eggs and jerky are great carnivore options that travel well.

WHAT HAPPENS IF I GO OFF THE RAILS WITH CHEATS?

It depends on how long you keep eating the offending foods and how insulin resistant you are. It also depends on how much of a carb or sugar addict you were in the past. Some people can have a piece of cake and not think of it at all the next day. For others, that same piece of cake will send them spiraling off on a monthlong carb binge. You know yourself. If you fall into the latter category, avoid high-carb cheat meals.

But the question here is what happens *if* you go off the rails. Well, a few things. First, your blood glucose may be elevated for a few days to a few weeks. Your blood ketones may be low to nonexistent for the same amount of time. Your fasting insulin and triglycerides can rise, while your HDL cholesterol can drop. In addition, you may feel crummy. I get super inflamed and achy after a high-carb cheat meal. My mental health goes down the tubes, and I feel a bit bogged down. You will have a unique response depending on your current metabolic health.

There are a few ways to get back on the wagon after a cheat meal. Most importantly, get back to carnivore foods as quickly as possible, and don't eat any more of the offending food. Next, you can hit the sauna and do some exercise to lower inflammation and burn off some of the excess glucose. You can go into a short fast of twenty-four to thirty-six hours to jump-start ketosis again. You can also use exogenous ketones to get back into ketosis faster. Bottom line: Get back on the wagon and don't beat yourself up about cheating. Just move on and go back to carnivore foods.

HOW DO I STAY CARNIVORE WHILE IN THE HOSPITAL OR CARING FOR SOMEBODY IN THE HOSPITAL?

This one can be difficult, but it's not impossible. I spent one month as a caregiver for a family member in the hospital, and we were able to keep them carnivore/keto for the duration of their stay. Typically, you can special-order a patient's meals every day; you don't have to eat whatever they send up. You may need to work with a nurse to bypass some of the defaults that are in place with the hospital's food-ordering software, such as only allowing one or two burger patties to be ordered at a time. At the hospital we were at, their software required a minimum of 60 grams of carbohydrates to be on each meal tray, even if you didn't order any carbs. All that extra food went straight into the garbage because once it is on the tray, it cannot be reused. Such an incredible waste. It's no wonder the healthcare system makes up 8.5 percent of America's annual greenhouse gas emissions.[1]

I also brought food in that I cooked and purchased from local grocery stores and restaurants. Unfortunately, hospital food is dictated by the Dietary Guidelines for Americans, and we all know how tragic those are. Until ketogenic diets are recognized as healthy, it will be difficult to change the menu at any facility that depends in part on federal funding. Sticking to carnivore/keto while in the hospital can be very helpful for overall recovery and lowering inflammation. Carnivore is also excellent for accelerating wound healing.

[1] Shanoor Seervai et al., "How the U.S. health care system contributes to climate change," The Commonwealth Fund, April 19, 2022, https://www.commonwealthfund.org/publications/explainer/2022/apr/how-us-health-care-system-contributes-climate-change.

METABOLIC HEALTH QUESTIONS

CAN I GET ALL OF THE VITAMINS AND MINERALS I NEED WHILE EATING ONLY MEAT AND ANIMAL PRODUCTS?

I discuss this topic in chapter 1, but yes, you can get all of the required vitamins and minerals by consuming only meat and animal products. Meat is the most nutrient-dense food on Earth. I would be more worried about a vegan diet, which lacks essential vitamins and minerals such as B12, EPA, and DHA, along with heme iron and much more.

WILL MY CHOLESTEROL GO UP ON CARNIVORE?

This is one of the main questions I get about a carnivore diet, and I think a little bit of clarification is needed. When most people say they have high cholesterol, they are referring to total cholesterol or maybe LDL cholesterol. But when I look at a lipid panel, I start with triglycerides, and then check the HDL level. I don't even look at total cholesterol, and I barely glance at LDL. This is because total and LDL cholesterol aren't great biomarkers to measure metabolic health. Triglycerides and HDL, on the other hand, are excellent indicators.

Typically on a carnivore diet, you will see your triglycerides decline and your HDL increase. Total cholesterol and LDL could stay the same, go down, or go up. In general, you want your triglycerides (TG) to be less than 100 mg/dL (1.129 mmol/L), your HDL cholesterol to be greater than 50 mg/dL (1.29 mmol/L), and your TG/HDL ratio to be under 2 (1 IU). These are your goalposts regardless of the diet you follow. You will find more information on blood work and how to track your biomarkers in chapter 8.

As described earlier in this book, some people are lean mass hyper responders, and they have very low levels of triglycerides paired with very high HDL cholesterol levels and very high LDL cholesterol levels. This "LMHR triad" is only seen when these people are consuming a ketogenic or very low-carb diet. It is a rare phenotype, so don't expect to exhibit these characteristics.

ISN'T FIBER REQUIRED FOR A HEALTHY GUT?

Contrary to popular belief, fiber is not required for a healthy gut or microbiome. You can be perfectly healthy without consuming fiber. Some negatives of fiber consumption include digestive discomfort (like bloating, gas, and constipation), interference with mineral absorption (such as iron and zinc), and, in some cases, worsening symptoms for people with certain gut conditions, like irritable bowel syndrome (IBS) and small intestinal bacterial overgrowth (SIBO).

CAN THE KIDNEYS HANDLE THE AMOUNT OF PROTEIN CONSUMED ON A CARNIVORE DIET?

A lot of people assume that meat or protein is bad for the kidneys, but this couldn't be further from the truth. What is harmful to the kidneys is eating too much sugar-containing food or excess carbohydrates. Our kidneys are built to handle large amounts of animal fats and proteins. What they can't handle is the amounts of sugar and ultra-processed foods that are so common in the standard American diet. The shift to high-sugar and ultra-processed foods over the last thirty to fifty years is one of the reasons the rate of kidney disease has jumped significantly.

In addition, it is a common misconception that carnivore is a high-protein diet. It is typically a high-fat, *moderate*-protein diet, and the amount of protein most people consume on carnivore is well within the healthy range, even for people with compromised kidney function.

Many conventional doctors see chronic kidney disease (CKD) as an incurable condition, but with the use of a therapeutic ketogenic diet, kidney function might improve. Among the best things a person with CKD can do are to clear their diet of ultra-processed foods, seed oils, and sugar and then focus on a therapeutic ketogenic diet. I recommend finding a low-carb-friendly healthcare practitioner to guide you through the process, though, as each case is unique.

WILL I HAVE NORMAL BOWEL MOVEMENTS ON CARNIVORE?

This is one of the most frequently asked questions I get on YouTube. Many people assume they will either be super constipated or have explosive diarrhea and won't be able to leave the house. The first month or so of carnivore is when most bowel-related issues occur. Once your body adjusts to the new fuel source and you become fat adapted, your bowel movements should regulate. If you are experiencing diarrhea, be sure to take electrolytes and drink lots of water to stay hydrated. You can also lower your fat intake a little bit, especially hot, rendered fats like melted butter or the fat from browned ground beef. If diarrhea persists after the first few months, look for a possible infection. If you are constipated or have hard stools, increase both your hydration and your fat intake to help get things "moving" again.

WILL CARNIVORE GIVE ME GAS?

I do not have gas on carnivore. Lack of gas was one of the unexpected benefits of this lifestyle. This makes sense, because a lot of gas production is related to plant consumption. When I eat my monthly keto cheat meal, I sometimes have gas for the next couple of days. But in general, carnivores are not walking gas machines. On the contrary, it is typically vegans or vegetarians who have issues with gas and farting.

WILL CARNIVORE GIVE ME BAD BREATH?

In the beginning of carnivore, keto breath can occur. Keto breath is temporary and smells a bit fruity and sweet, or like nail polish remover. Basically, you are exhaling ketones. This usually clears up in a few weeks. Oral health also tends to improve on carnivore—another unexpected benefit that I encountered early on. I used to use breath mints every day, and since switching to carnivore, I haven't needed to. My gum health has improved, and I don't have as much plaque buildup at my twice-yearly dentist visits.

WILL CARNIVORE GIVE ME BODY ODOR?

It always blows me away what some people will leave as comments on posts by a person they don't even know. But people have commented that eating only meat makes you smelly. I have not experienced that problem, nor do I know of any carnivores who have had increases in body odor after going carnivore. If this occurs, I think it would be limited to the very beginning of the new diet when your body is eliminating toxins. But I don't think it is a common occurrence.

HOW CAN I AVOID HAIR LOSS ON CARNIVORE?

Occasionally, people experience hair loss when doing carnivore. This can be due to many factors. One is telogen effluvium, which is when you shed hair after a life stressor, such as divorce, surgery, childbirth, extreme weight loss, or extreme diet change. For telogen effluvium, there isn't much you can do once the hair starts falling out. It typically falls out for a couple of months and then starts growing back. Another reason you may lose hair is not eating enough protein. Be sure to eat at least 1 gram of protein per pound of ideal body weight to prevent hair loss. I experienced hair loss between months 4 and 6 of carnivore and thought it might be telogen effluvium, but later I discovered that it was likely due to Hashimoto's thyroiditis. If your hair is falling out unexpectedly and in large amounts, I would have a full thyroid panel run to see if hypothyroidism is the cause. Details on what you should get tested are in chapter 8.

HOW LONG UNTIL I'M TRULY FAT ADAPTED?

Typically, it takes two to three weeks to become fat adapted, or able to use fat efficiently as a fuel source. It can take up to a few months for some people. But once you are fully fat adapted, your body can switch between burning glucose and burning ketones very efficiently. Your body is built to burn both fuels; you just have to let it "remember" how to do so.

CAN I STAY CARNIVORE WHILE SICK?

Some people on carnivore worry about taking common cold medications when they are sick because they don't want to spike their blood sugar or take anything with questionable ingredients, and I empathize with that. But if you are sick and want to feel better, taking cold medicine is fine. I use sugar-free cough drops as needed, along with several popular cough syrups or pills. There are sugar-free cough syrups that won't spike your blood sugar. Bone broth, hot water with lemon and a bit of honey, and crushed garlic are other remedies that can be helpful. Just read the ingredient labels of the various medications out there and find what works best for you. It's not like you will be taking this stuff forever; it's only temporary.

As far as what to eat when you are sick, I think sticking with meat and animal products is the way to go. You want to keep inflammation low and not make it worse by consuming high-carb, high-sugar foods.

MISCELLANEOUS HEALTH QUESTIONS

WHAT IS THE MINIMUM AMOUNT OF TIME IT TAKES TO SEE THE TRUE BENEFITS OF A CARNIVORE DIET?

Start with thirty days of strict carnivore. That will give you a good idea as to how it will work for you. But to see the true benefits, I think a minimum of ninety days is required. Think of it this way: How long did it take you to get to where you are today...decades? It's going to take more than a few weeks to undo years of eating a standard American diet.

DOESN'T EATING ONLY MEAT GET BORING?

Honestly, yes, it does get a bit boring from time to time. But less often than you might think. I think food boredom is more prevalent in the beginning of carnivore, when you are only weeks separated from a more varied diet. There are plenty of carnivore recipes that you can use to mix up your weekly routine (eighty of which are in this book!). But if I find myself getting bored with the status quo, I go out for some tuna sashimi or Korean barbecue. I am okay with a little less variety overall when I am feeling great, losing weight, and have boatloads of energy. It is a trade-off I am willing to make.

DO I HAVE TO EAT THIS WAY FOREVER?

I think the answer to this question boils down to your Whys. Why are you doing carnivore in the first place? If it is to help manage a severe medical condition, you may need to stay carnivore for the long term. But most people doing carnivore can start to incorporate some plant material again after they do some healing. You can never return to a standard American diet, however. That junk is not real food, and your health will decline again quickly if you go down that path.

SHOULD I STACK HABIT CHANGES OR JUST FOCUS ON CARNIVORE FIRST?

A lot of people ask if they should quit other things when they are going carnivore. Here is my experience with that: If not being able to drink coffee or diet soda is going to stop you from starting carnivore, then keep drinking the coffee or diet soda. In the grand scheme of things, it's not as important as getting your nutrition in order. Perhaps down the line, after you have gotten used to carnivore and seen weight loss and health improvements, you will want to quit other things. But for now, give yourself a break and focus on the lowest-hanging fruit: nutrition.

I will say that if you are still smoking cigarettes and drinking large amounts of alcohol, I advise you to quit as soon as possible. Both cigarettes and alcohol are highly oxidative to your body and cause a lot of damage.

CAN ATHLETES DO CARNIVORE?

Not only can athletes do carnivore, but they can *thrive* on carnivore. Carbohydrates are not necessary once you are fat adapted. If you are an athlete, I suggest starting carnivore on a break from heavy training or during the off-season so that you can give your body time to adjust to a new fuel source and deal with any keto flu symptoms. According to Dr. Anthony Chaffee, a leading carnivore expert and athlete, it typically takes only two to three weeks to become fully fat adapted. I recommend checking out his YouTube channel for more information on this topic.

CAN KIDS DO CARNIVORE?

Yes. Meat is necessary for kids, and they should eat as much of it as possible. I've talked in passing about the safety of carnivore for children, but let's dive into a few references and studies.

In an interesting two-year study out of Kenya, a researcher divided a class of kids into four groups. In addition to their normal diet, one group received two spoonfuls of minced beef per day. The next group received a glass of milk, the third received an equivalent number of calories in the form of vegetable oil, and a control group received no food supplement. The children who ate two spoonfuls of beef outperformed their peers physically, cognitively, and developmentally.[2]

In another article, early beef consumption was linked to better mental and physical health outcomes in young children.[3] Yet another article discusses the importance of iron and zinc. Infants are born with a six-month supply of iron in their bodies, but after that, they need to consume it, and the best sources of iron are red meats. Even a 1- to 2-ounce serving of high-quality meat, such as beef, per day is more than sufficient to meet the vitamin and mineral needs of children aged six months to three years.[4]

Not only is eating meat safe for children, but it's the optimal food for them. Meat is the most nutrient-dense food on the planet, so it just makes sense. Do kids need to go full carnivore to see the benefits? Not necessarily. My kids, who are four, eat meat, fruit, milk, and a bit of organic grains from time to time. As they get older, I will let them decide if they would like to go more carnivore. We will never have ultra-processed foods in the house (mostly because I have zero self-control), but if the boys want to eat some plants, I am not opposed. Carnivore, keto, and low-carb diets are all on the spectrum of healthy eating and represent, as Dr. Ken Berry says, a Proper Human Diet.

DO I STILL NEED TO WEAR SUNSCREEN?

A sunburn is often a sign that your body is out of circadian alignment. The good news: It's simple to fix. Start by getting outside at dawn for about 20 minutes, letting that early light hit your eyes and skin. This primes your body to handle the stronger midday sun. When sunbathing later in the day, build up gradually, and then cover up with clothing once you've had enough. In the evening, mimic nature by dimming the lights in your home, wearing blue blockers after sunset, and limiting screens. Over time, this will help you tolerate more sun without burning. For me, just under a month of following this approach made a huge difference. If you use sunscreen, choose a mineral-based one, which creates a physical barrier against UVA and UVB rays. Keep in mind that sunscreen blocks vitamin D production—so your skin needs some natural, unfiltered sunlight to get what it needs.

---

[2] Michael Hopkin, "Meat diet boosts kids' growth," *Nature* (2005): published online.

[3] Victoria C. Wilk et al., "Early life beef consumption patterns are related to cognitive outcomes at 1–5 years of age: An exploratory study," *Nutrients* 14, no. 21 (2022): 4497.

[4] Keli M. Hawthorne et al., "Meat helps make every bite count: an ideal first food for infants," *Nutrition Today* 57, no. 1 (2022): 8–13.

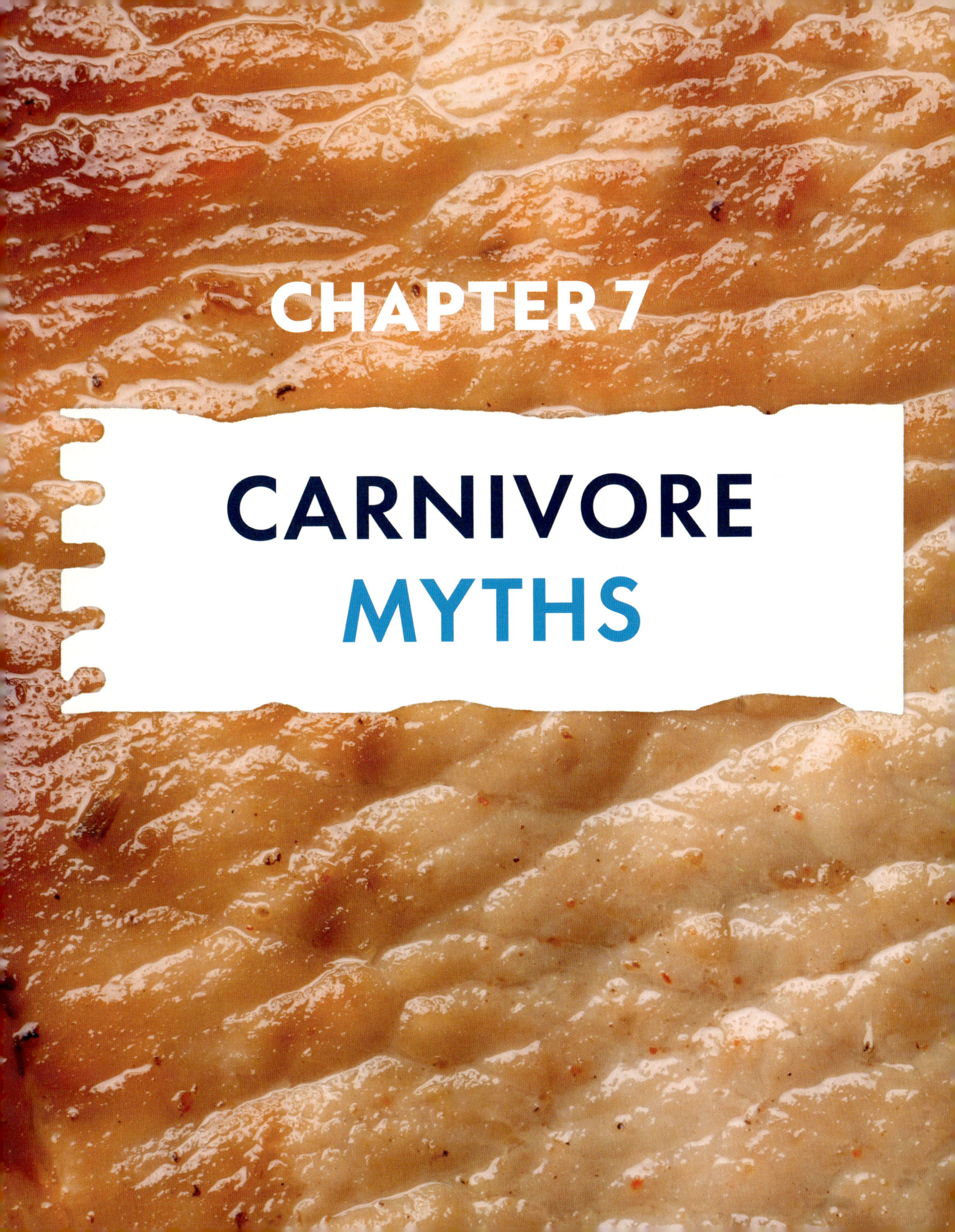
CHAPTER 7
CARNIVORE
MYTHS

It's inevitable: When people hear that you are doing carnivore, you're going to get hit with a barrage of myths. Popular media has done an excellent job of demonizing meat for decades, and now a lot of people assume that these myths are true. This chapter will help clarify what is accurate and what is false and give you some resources for learning more.

MYTH: CARNIVORE IS UNSAFE

You've read the headlines: "Red Meat Causes Cancer!" "Red Meat Kills!" We've been told for the past sixty or so years that animal products are a danger to our health and that we must limit our consumption of them. Well, we've tried that, and our health has suffered. It's simply not true. How could a whole food like meat—which humans have been eating for hundreds of thousands, if not millions, of years—suddenly start killing us?

Most of these sensational news articles reference a study. But if you dig deeper and look at the study itself, it is almost always based on weak observational or epidemiological evidence that cannot be used to prove something *caused* something else to happen. Correlation or association does not mean causation. These types of studies should only be used to identify possible patterns and then to form a hypothesis that can be tested in a more rigorous way, like with a randomized controlled trial. These news articles pop up every day, and to the untrained eye, they are scary! No one wants to die because they eat two eggs a week or consume red meat. But by and large, these articles are misleading at best and egregious at worst.

To combat misinformation, you need to educate yourself. With a bit of training and practice, you can become adept at reading a scientific paper and knowing whether to take it seriously. This is a skill I fostered early on, and now, in less than thirty seconds, I can evaluate an abstract (a short summary at the beginning of a paper that gives the gist of what the paper is about) and decide if this paper is worth getting worried over. Appendix A includes a quick and easy overview of what to look for so that you can develop this skill for yourself.

MYTH: CARNIVORE IS BAD FOR THE ENVIRONMENT

For decades, it has been argued that eating meat—especially beef—is a major cause of climate change. This argument has shifted the pro-vegetarian stance of the plant-based movement from health to environmental activism, but blaming livestock (especially cow burps) oversimplifies the issue of climate change and distracts from the real drivers of greenhouse gas emissions, like transportation, industry, and energy production.

Religious and corporate interests have played a significant role in promoting plant-based diets. The Seventh-day Adventist Church, for example, is a major global educator with deep roots in vegetarian advocacy and has influenced the training of dietitians and nutritionists for decades. Figures like Dr. John Harvey Kellogg developed cereal and bland plant-based diets based on religious beliefs, and over time, the Adventist argument against meat evolved from moral to health-based and now environmental arguments.

Meanwhile, corporations have embraced the plant-based trend because it's profitable. Heavily subsidized ingredients like corn and soy are used to produce ultra-processed vegan foods with high profit margins, marketed as eco-friendly alternatives despite their environmental costs. Regenerative animal agriculture, by contrast, can actually improve soil health and sequester carbon—making a well-managed carnivore approach potentially more sustainable than industrial plant-based alternatives. For a deeper dive, check out *The Great Plant-Based Con* by Jayne Buxton.

MYTH: YOU NEED CARBOHYDRATES TO SURVIVE

There are three macronutrients: protein, fat, and carbohydrates. Only protein and fat are vital for survival. You do not need to consume carbohydrates to survive and thrive. Your body can produce all of the glucose it needs from protein and fat.

MYTH: FIBER IS REQUIRED FOR HEALTH

The myth that we need fiber has become "common knowledge" only because of the clever marketing of cereal companies and the fact that it has been repeated over and over. I just established that you do not need to consume carbohydrates to survive and thrive. Fiber = plant = carbohydrate, which means fiber is not required for health. In fact, fiber can cause many pesky digestive problems. Fiber cannot be broken down by the human digestive tract, so it just passes through. This can result in constipation, gastrointestinal distress, and rectal bleeding.

Your body is intelligent. When you eat something, your body is going to use what it needs and dispose of the rest. Fiber is not used; it is discarded. Why eat something your body isn't going to use? You do not need to consume it to be healthy.

Also, contrary to what you may have heard, fiber is not needed for healthy bowel movements. Once your body is adapted to a carnivore diet, your bowel movements will be regular and daily.

MYTH: EATING RED MEAT CAUSES DIABETES

Quite the opposite. Eating an ultra-low-carb diet such as carnivore, which typically includes plenty of red meat, can put type 2 diabetes into remission.[1] This is another one of those sensational headlines that is based on weak epidemiological studies. Animal-based diets used to be used to manage type 1 and type 2 diabetes before exogenous insulin was available. People with type 1 diabetes can have normal blood glucose and A1c levels and reduce the amount of insulin they need to take by using an ultra-low-carb diet like carnivore. The public is finally rediscovering the knowledge that removing carbohydrates from your diet can normalize blood sugar numbers. The American Diabetes Association considers a diet with as much as 130 grams of carbs per day "low carb." That is way too many carbs for a person with type 1 or 2 diabetes. Go as low carb as possible to get your diabetes under control.

---

[1] Amy L. McKenzie et al., "5-year effects of a novel continuous remote care model with carbohydrate-restricted nutrition therapy including nutritional ketosis in type 2 diabetes: An extension study." *Diabetes Research and Clinical Practice* 217 (2024): 111898.

MYTH: EATING RED MEAT CAUSES CANCER

There is no good evidence that red meat causes cancer. You will see a ton of epidemiological evidence trying to demonize red meat, but again, association is not causation. On the contrary, many people are using therapeutic ketogenic diets for cancer management. Cancer cells love glucose-rich environments, so the theory is that keeping glucose low and ketones high can inhibit tumor growth. Lowering or eliminating carbohydrates from your diet creates a hostile environment for cancer cells. While I cannot say that carnivore can cure cancer, studies have shown that it can help the body deal with cancer treatment and perhaps inhibit tumor growth.[2] Many oncologists in the low-carb space are using therapeutic ketogenic diets to help their patients manage the condition and heal during cancer treatment.

MYTH: EATING MEAT IS BAD FOR YOUR KIDNEYS

A lot of people assume that meat or protein in general is bad for the kidneys. This couldn't be further from the truth. What is harmful to the kidneys is "overnutrition leading to hyperglycemia, insulin resistance and diabetes mellitus."[3] It is a common misconception that carnivore is a high-protein diet. It is typically a high-fat, moderate-protein diet, and the amount of protein consumed daily is well within range of what is required for optimal health. Many conventional doctors see chronic kidney disease (CKD) as an incurable condition, but when using a therapeutic ketogenic diet, it is possible to see improvements in kidney function. One of the best things a person with CKD can do is clear their diet of ultra-processed foods, vegetable seed oils, and sugar and then focus on a therapeutic ketogenic diet. I recommend finding a low-carb-friendly practitioner to guide you through the process, as each case is unique.

MYTH: HIGH LDL CHOLESTEROL CAUSES HEART DISEASE

It is a common misconception that your LDL cholesterol will go up when you eat a low-carbohydrate diet. It is different for every individual, but it might go up, stay the same, or even decline. Many factors influence your LDL levels. But even if it does go up, should you be concerned? Should you worry about LDL cholesterol itself, or are there other, more important biomarkers that you should pay attention to first?

First, understand that LDL cholesterol on its own is *not causal in heart disease*, meaning its existence is not why plaque builds up in arteries. Excluding rare genetic abnormalities such as familial hypercholesterolemia (which causes very high levels of LDL cholesterol in the blood,

---

[2] Bryan G. Allen et al., "Ketogenic diets as an adjuvant cancer therapy: history and potential mechanism," *Redox Biology* vol. 2 (2014): 963–70.

[3] Thomas Weimbs, Jessianna Saville, and Kamyar Kalantar-Zadeh, "Ketogenic metabolic therapy for chronic kidney disease—the pro part," *Clinical Kidney Journal* 17, no. 1 (2024): sfad273.

increasing the risk of early heart disease), only the patients[4] who have increased fibrinogen or other coagulation factors will see increased risk of heart disease.[5] There must be damage to the lining of the arteries before plaque can accumulate. A blood clot forms to cover the damaged area, and then endothelial progenitor cells cover the clot, eventually drawing it into the arterial wall. Think of the way a scab forms when you skin your knee. Eventually, new skin grows over the wound. That same process is happening in your arteries.

Next, macrophages come and clean up the remanent blood clot, and then the healing process is complete—if you are healthy. Plaque will only start to grow if there is something pathological occurring in your system, like continuous damage, if the blood clot formed is abnormally large or hard to break down, or if your repair system is not working correctly.[6]

LDL cholesterol on its own is not causing that damage. It is just one component of the system that comes in to heal the damage after the fact so you don't bleed to death. What's actually *causing* the damage to the arteries can be many things:[7]

- Smoking/Environmental toxins
- Diabetes or insulin resistance
- High uric acid
- High blood pressure
- Severe mental illness
- Stress
- Infections, both bacterial and viral
- Sickle cell anemia
- History of migraines
- And so much more

For the arterial walls to be damaged, the glycocalyx first needs to be damaged. You may not remember the anatomical structure of an artery from high school anatomy class (honestly, it probably wasn't even covered; this may be college-level anatomy), but the insides of your arteries are not smooth. They are covered by a hairlike layer called the glycocalyx that protects the endothelium, or "skin cells" of your arteries, and acts as a gatekeeper of sorts. It's like a nonstick surface for the insides of arteries. A healthy glycocalyx will not allow LDL particles (or much of anything) to stick to or pass through it. For LDL particles to pass into or through the artery wall, the glycocalyx must be damaged.[8]

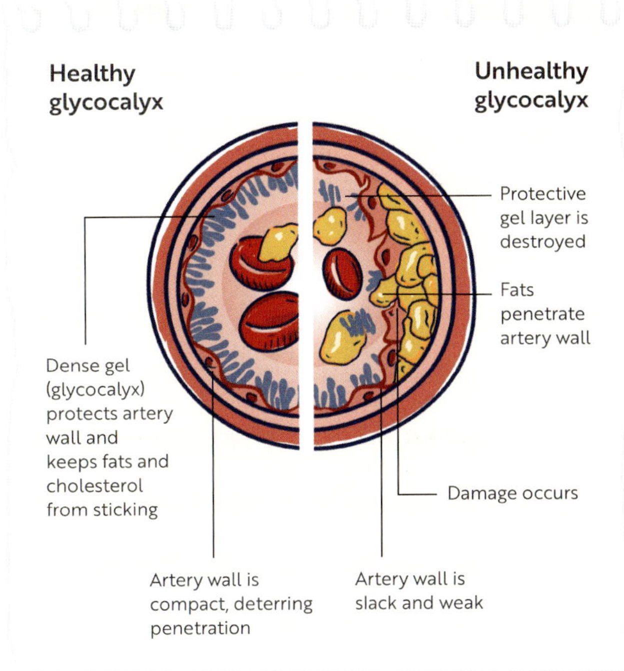

[4] Uffe Ravnskov et al., "Serious flaws in targeting LDL-C reduction in the management of cardiovascular disease in familial hypercholesterolemia," *Expert Review of Clinical Pharmacology* 14, no. 3 (2021): 405–406.

[5] Uffe Ravnskov et al., "Inborn coagulation factors are more important cardiovascular risk factors than high HDL-cholesterol in familial hypercholesterolemia," *Medical Hypotheses* 121 (2018): 60–63.

[6] Dr. Malcolm Kendrick, *The Clot Thickens: The Enduring Mystery of Heart Disease* (Columbia Publishing Ltd., 2014), 103.

[7] Kendrick, *The Clot Thickens*, 109.

[8] Kendrick, *The Clot Thickens*, 88–91.

Next, it is a common misconception that arterial plaque is made up of only cholesterol. Plaques are composed of many substances, including red and white blood cells, platelets, foam cells, bacteria, calcium, and fibrin.[9]

In reality, the causes of heart disease are still being debated, and this is not settled science. But LDL has been unjustly demonized because it is an easy target, and there is a class of drugs that exists to lower it (statins), which makes Big Pharma boatloads of money. In Appendix B, I have listed several books on this topic that are must-reads if heart disease is of interest to you.

MYTH: CARNIVORE CAUSES SCURVY

Scurvy is an extreme degree of vitamin C deficiency. Symptoms start with fatigue, weakness, irritability, and sadness and then move into muscle and joint pain, swollen and bleeding gums, tooth loss, red or blue spots on the skin, and bruising. When most people think of scurvy, they think of sailors or pirates. Yes, sailors were susceptible to scurvy, but only because they were not eating fresh meat; they ate dried meats, along with other preserved foods, plus they smoked and drank alcohol, which is associated with vitamin C deficiency. It is a well-known fact that simply eating fresh meat will quickly reverse scurvy.[10]

A modern carnivore diet is not remotely like what sailors were eating, and scurvy does not occur with a well-formulated carnivore diet. Also, you don't need as much vitamin C when you're not consuming carbohydrates. Vitamin C and glucose fight for the same receptors in your body, so if you don't have as much glucose floating around, your body isn't going to hang on to a bunch of vitamin C. Your body is a highly efficient machine, and it will get rid of anything that it's not using.

Even if you eat a carb-heavy diet, your body only needs 10 milligrams of vitamin C per day to prevent scurvy—a very small amount. Bottom line: If people were regularly getting scurvy on carnivore, nobody would continue eating this way.

---

[9] Marc Sirol, "Atherosclerosis plaque imaging and characterization using magnetic resonance imaging," *US Cardiology Review*, https://www.uscjournal.com/articles/atherosclerosis-plaque-imaging-and-characterization-using-magnetic-resonance-imaging, accessed July 2, 2025.

[10] David L. Harrowfield and Bill Alp, "The diet and incidence of scurvy and adopted preventative measures in the two branches of Shackleton's Imperial Trans-Antarctic Expedition 1914–1917," *Polar Record* 55, no. 2 (2019): 82–92.

ADDITIONAL MYTHS THAT EVEN SOME CARNIVORES BELIEVE

Now that I have covered the most common myths *against* the carnivore diet, let's touch on some myths that some carnivores believe. Overall, I like to think that the carnivore community is less dogmatic than the vegan or vegetarian community, but sometimes I field comments that make me question that position.

MYTH: CARNIVORE IS THE ONLY HEALTHY WAY TO EAT

I do not think carnivore is the only healthy way to eat; I think it is one of a handful of good dietary approaches. If you are eating a whole, real-food diet that is meat heavy and low in carbohydrates, you will be in good shape. Every person must determine the volume of carbohydrates their body can handle. Some people can eat 100 grams per day and maintain an ideal weight and excellent metabolic health. Others can only handle 25 grams, or maybe even zero.

MYTH: FRUIT AND VEGGIES ARE BAD FOR YOUR HEALTH

This myth piggybacks on the previous one. If you think that carnivore is the only healthy way to eat, then it follows that you think all plant foods are bad. I don't think fruits and vegetables are bad for you in the grand scheme of things, but I do think that paying attention to seasonality is important. Also remember that the fruits and vegetables that exist today are not what our ancient or even more recent ancestors would have consumed. We have hybridized and grafted our way to monstrous produce. For example, wild bananas are full of seeds and nowhere near as sweet as the bananas you and I would recognize. Watermelons used to have a lot more rind and many more seeds. Wild strawberries are small and bitter. Our ancestors did not chow down on fruits and veggies like people do today. And again, avoiding plants that are high in oxalates, gluten, lectins, and other toxins is important, as is focusing on organic and pesticide-free options when available.

I think the key here is figuring out which foods make you feel good and energetic and which foods do the opposite. If that means eliminating all plants for the long term, so be it. But plants are not inherently bad; what matters is what does and does not work *for you*.

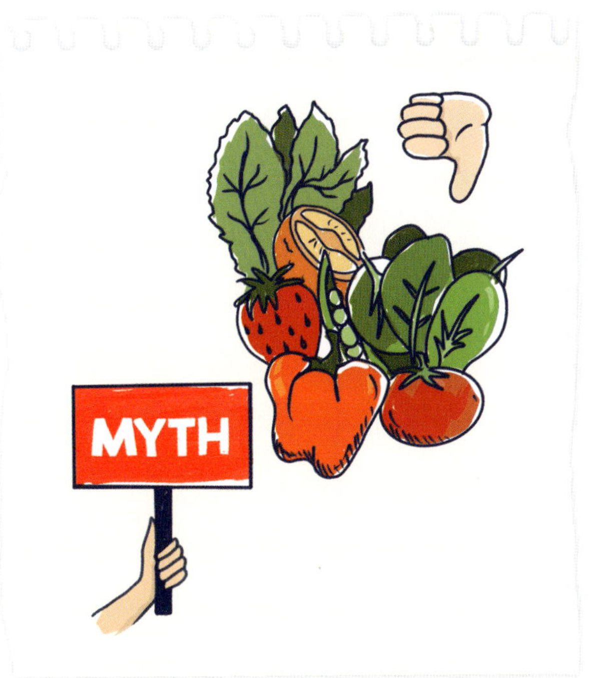

MYTH: YOU ARE AUTOMATICALLY IN KETOSIS IF YOU ARE EATING CARNIVORE

A lot of people think that if they are eating zero carbs, they are automatically in nutritional ketosis. That is not necessarily the case. It depends a lot on your metabolic health and how insulin resistant you are. I've run several fun N-of-1 or N-of-2 experiments on my YouTube channel where I eat a cheat meal and then measure how long it takes for my glucose to return to normal and for my ketones to get back up to at least 0.5 mmol/L (the lowest level required to be in ketosis), and I've found that it can take up to a week. For my husband, it can take even longer—up to a few weeks. Goran and I have different health profiles, so the same cheat meal affects us differently.

Don't assume you are in nutritional ketosis if you are not eating carbohydrates. Measure your blood ketone levels with a continuous ketone meter or a manual ketone/glucose meter so you know what's going on and can adjust as needed. I talk more about ketone measurement in chapter 8.

MYTH: CARNIVORE IS A MAGIC BULLET THAT WILL SOLVE EVERY ISSUE

While carnivore is an excellent dietary philosophy, it's not going to fix everything. You can still get sick. You can still experience negative health symptoms. Your body might start to heal and then begin releasing all of the toxins you've accumulated, making you feel worse before you feel better. Some people's jobs require them to deal with toxic chemicals that impair their health. Some people live in homes infested with mold, and no amount of carnivore eating can make the mold go away. Chronic stress in any form is going to slow your progress, even if you are eating carnivore.

My point is that carnivore can help with a lot, but it can't fix everything. You may need to take additional steps to get to where you want to go.

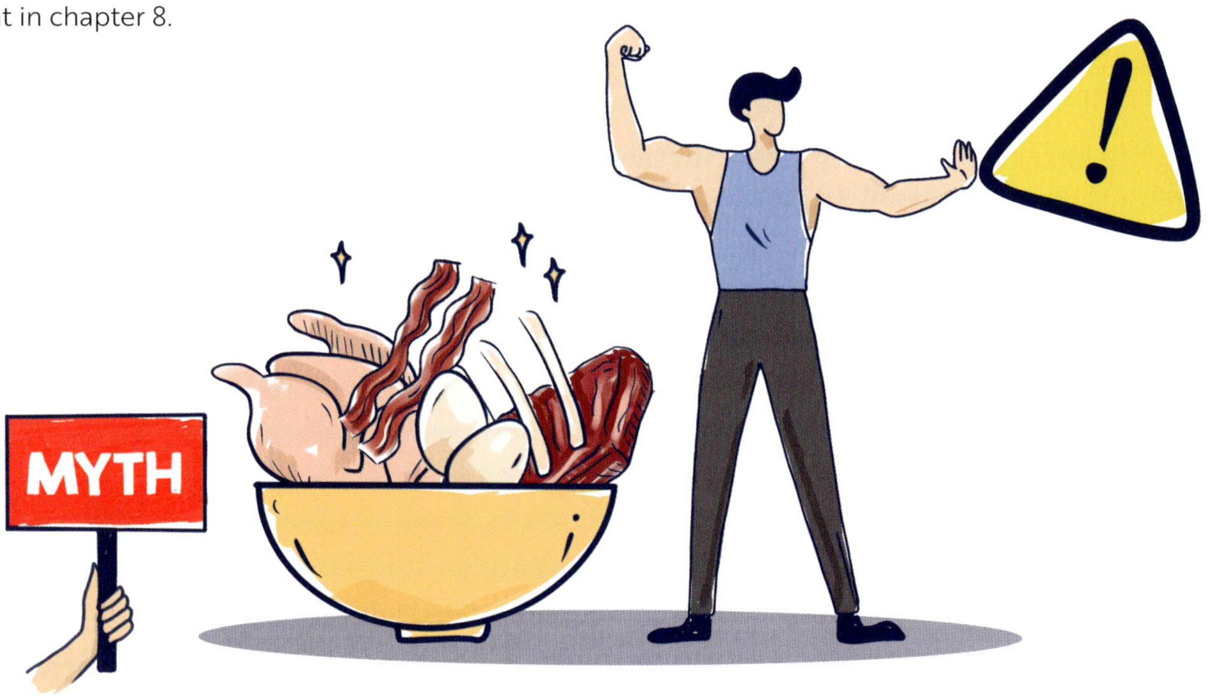

CHAPTER 8

MONITORING YOUR PROGRESS

When working toward a goal, it is essential to have a way to measure your progress. There are plenty of options at different price points, and in this chapter, I share some of my favorites. While I am not a doctor and this is not personal medical advice, consider this chapter a helpful resource to empower you and clarify which targets you might want to aim for. I have compiled this information to save you time, as it took me a lot of effort to figure it all out on my own.

The simplest way to track your progress on carnivore is through body weight and measurements, which is covered in detail in chapter 2. Here, I dive into the analytical side of things and share insights from my personal experiments. If you are a data enthusiast like me, you will find this chapter especially exciting!

BLOOD WORK

Blood testing is my favorite way to monitor my progress on carnivore. It is one of the quickest and easiest ways to measure change, especially if you are trying to improve your metabolic health. I personally get blood work done once or twice per month for the N-of-1 (N=1) experiments I run for my YouTube channel, but I think that everyone should know their own numbers and get tested at least once a year, or more often if you are working toward a goal like improving your metabolic health or losing weight. The tests I am getting done are very common and include lipids, blood sugar, and inflammation markers. By the time you are done with this section, you will know how to read your own blood work results and feel confident in interpreting them.

ORDERING BLOOD WORK

In most US states, you can order your own blood work online without a doctor's referral. The two main labs in the US are Quest and Labcorp, and then there are various other websites from which you can order tests. These sites are typically self-pay and do not take insurance. Here are my top choices:

- Own Your Labs (ownyourlabs.com)
- Ulta Lab Tests (ultalabtests.com)
- Walk-In Lab (walkinlab.com)

You can also ask your doctor to order these tests, and a lot of them will be covered by insurance.

If you do not live in a state where you're allowed to order your own blood work, or if you live outside the US, you will have to get your doctor to order these tests for you. In that case, it's best to approach them in a friendly way; you don't want to turn them off by seeming combative. But be prepared for a bit of push-back on some tests, especially in the realm of thyroid health. Most of this pushback is simply because the doctor doesn't know what these tests are or how to interpret them, and once they run them, they are legally responsible for the results and your care. Keeping this in mind, I have suggested a couple of sentences for each test that explain why it is important so you will have an answer if your doctor asks why you want that test.

If possible, I recommend that you get the following blood tests run before starting carnivore and then retest three months to a year later. It is important to give your body time to get used to the carnivore diet because some of these markers can get out of whack temporarily. There are endless blood tests you can get done, but I think this list is a good place to start; it will give you a lot of data that you can use to track your progress on carnivore. If you want to get hormone testing done, find a knowledgeable practitioner who can help interpret those tests for you.

Basic tests:

- **Lipid panel** includes total cholesterol, HDL cholesterol, LDL cholesterol, and triglycerides. This inexpensive test can tell you a lot about your metabolic health. Doctors will almost always order this common test for you.
- **Comprehensive metabolic panel** includes fasting glucose, kidney and liver function, electrolytes, and protein levels. It's another inexpensive, common test that gives you a lot of good information about your overall health.
- **A1c** measures your average glucose levels over the past three months, though it's skewed toward the most recent month. This test gives you more data than fasting glucose alone.
- **Fasting insulin**, if elevated, is a much earlier indicator of insulin resistance than A1c or fasting glucose. Insulin can be elevated for years before glucose levels start to become pathological. It is arguably one of the more important blood tests to get and is inexpensive, but doctors don't often order it.
- **hs-CRP** (high-sensitivity C-reactive protein) measures systemic inflammation.
- **Vitamin D 25** measures levels of vitamin D, which is vital for immunity and cell, bone, and blood health, among many other things. Most people are deficient in D, so it is important to see where you stand so you can supplement if needed.

If you want even more data, here are a few more tests you can get done:

- **Homocysteine:** An inflammation marker that can indicate B vitamin deficiency
- **Ferritin:** An inflammation marker
- **Uric acid, serum:** An inflammation marker
- **B12 and folate:** Vitamins
- **GGT:** A liver function marker
- **OmegaCheck:** Looks at the levels of omega-3 and omega-6 fatty acids in your blood
- **NMR LipoProfile:** An advanced lipid panel that includes a standard lipid panel in addition to lipoprotein particle number (LDL-P), particle concentration and size (HDL-P, small LDL-P, LDL size, large VLDL-P, large HDL-P, HDL size), and insulin resistance score (LP-IR), as well as a graph of reported results

Extreme fatigue, hair loss, weight gain, and stubborn weight-loss stalls are common symptoms of thyroid dysfunction. If you are experiencing any of these symptoms, I recommend that you get a full thyroid panel run. This panel includes the following:

- **TSH** measures how much thyroid-stimulating hormone the pituitary gland is releasing to regulate thyroid function.
- **Free T4** measures the level of unbound thyroxine hormone available to enter cells and regulate metabolism.
- **Free T3** measures the level of triiodothyronine (T3), the active thyroid hormone, that is unbound and available for use by the body's cells.
- **Reverse T3** measures the level of an inactive form of T3 that blocks active T3 from binding to receptors, often reflecting the body's response to stress, illness, or low calorie intake.
- **TPO antibodies** measures the level of immune proteins targeting thyroid peroxidase, an enzyme essential for thyroid hormone production, often indicating autoimmune thyroid conditions like Hashimoto's thyroiditis.
- **Thyroglobulin antibodies** measures immune activity against thyroglobulin, indicating possible autoimmune thyroid disease.

Unfortunately, most conventional doctors are not trained to look past TSH and maybe T4. But without the rest of this data, you won't know the true state of your thyroid health. Here is what you can say to your doctor if you get pushback: "TSH and T4 can be normal, but if my reverse T3 is elevated and my free T3 is low, that's an indication of a hypothyroid condition, and if I have any thyroid antibodies, that is an indication of Hashimoto's, so I need to have all those markers run so that I can rule out thyroid issues." It also may be time to find a knowledgeable thyroid practitioner who knows how to interpret these labs and what to do when they are off.

PREPARING FOR BLOOD WORK

Let's go over some important things to remember when going in for blood work. First, avoid eating anything for twelve to fourteen hours beforehand. Any more or any less time than that can skew the results. Next, drink only water during that time. Coffee, even black coffee, can skew triglyceride readings in about 30 percent of the population. Stop taking any vitamins, supplements, or electrolytes at least two days before any blood tests. If you are measuring B12, folate, or fasting insulin, discontinue any biotin supplements for at least seventy-two hours before the test.

In the case of thyroid testing, stop taking any medications containing T3 or T4 twenty-four hours beforehand. Resume taking your medications after the test.

Fasting Etiquette

- No food for 12 to 14 hours
- Only drink water, no coffee or tea
- Stop taking all vitamins, supplements, and electrolytes at least 2 days before
- Stop biotin at least 72 hours before
- For thyroid tests, stop intake of medication containing T3 and T4 24 hours beforehand

Finally, don't do any strenuous exercise for at least one day before a blood test. Exercise can temporarily raise your glucose levels, among other things, so save the workout for after your test. The exception is walking, which is generally okay.

REVIEWING THE OPTIMAL RANGES

Now that we've covered which tests to get done and how to prepare for them, let's go over the optimal ranges you're looking for. These are the ranges that doctors in the low-carb/keto/carnivore space recommend, and they may differ a bit from the reference ranges you see on the results themselves. Keep in mind that those reference ranges are based on what is normal for the population getting blood work done, and a lot (if not most) of those people are in poor health. Also, remember that conventional reference ranges are often used to put people on medications, so sometimes that plays a role in why a reference range is as it is. For example, the usual target for LDL cholesterol nowadays is 100 mg/dL (2.6 mmol/L) or less. That maximum has been lowered in recent decades, one consequence of which is that more people qualify for statins. Instead of going for the standard reference ranges, which are based on an unhealthy population, I want you to work toward the functional medicine ranges, which aim for optimal metabolic health. I have included both US and international units of measure for each marker where applicable.

LIPID PANEL

When reviewing a standard lipid panel like the one shown below, I look at triglycerides and HDL first. Elevated triglycerides and low HDL are strong indicators of insulin resistance. LDL can go up, down, or stay the same on carnivore, and total cholesterol is mostly arbitrary because LDL cholesterol is estimated, not directly measured like HDL cholesterol and triglycerides. A more important number than total cholesterol is the triglyceride-to-HDL ratio. These two markers and one ratio are what to look for on a lipid panel:

- **Triglycerides (TG):** Under 100 mg/dL (1.13 mmol/L)
- **HDL:** Above 50 mg/dL (1.3 mmol/L)
- **TG/HDL ratio:** Under 2

Test	Current Result and Flag		Previous Result	Units	Reference Interval
Cholesterol, Total	285	High	325	mg/dL	100–199
Triglycerides	49		68	mg/dL	0–149
HDL Cholesterol	88		87	mg/dL	> 39
VLDL Cholesterol Cal	7		9	mg/dL	5–40
LDL Cholesterol Calc (NIH)	190	High	229	mg/dL	0–99

Caveats to Cholesterol Tests

There are a few things you need to understand when looking at a lipid panel. First, your cholesterol numbers are not static. They rise and fall throughout the day and are influenced by many factors. A lipid panel is just a snapshot in time. Thinking your numbers will stay the same from one yearly test to the next is a common misconception.

Next, there is no such thing as good or bad cholesterol. The cholesterol in an LDL particle is the exact same as the cholesterol in an HDL particle. LDL, which is often called bad cholesterol, is a lipoprotein that carries cholesterol, among other things. Dr. Zoe Harcombe describes the LDL particle beautifully as a "carrier of fresh cholesterol (going out to cells to do vital work)." She goes on to explain that HDL particles are just "carriers of unused cholesterol (going back to the liver for recycling)."[1] Both LDL and HDL particles carry the exact same cholesterol, along with triglycerides, proteins, and phospholipids.

Lastly, a lipid panel is not an exact measurement of each marker. An equation is used to determine LDL cholesterol, most often the Friedewald equation. Here are the equations:

- **For countries using mg/dL (US):** total cholesterol in mg/dL = LDL-C + HDL-C + (triglycerides / 5)
- **For countries using mmol/L (UK, Australia):** total cholesterol in mmol/L = LDL-C + HDL-C + (triglycerides / 2.2)

However, these equations fail when people have extremely high triglycerides. They don't work well for people with type III hyperlipidemia. Even people with normal triglyceride levels can see high levels of variation.

I tell you all this because lipid panels are used as a gold standard for prescribing statins when they do not even measure the exact amount of LDL in your blood. It is just an estimate. And because there is no such thing as good and bad cholesterol, why are we even worried about this?

That being said, I still find lipid panels to be valuable. They give you a picture of your overall metabolic health and tell you if something is out of whack. But you need to realize that you will see a range of values if you are measuring often enough. For example, from month to month, I see a range of 65 to 100 mg/dL (1.7 to 2.6 mmol/L) for HDL, 175 to 265 mg/dL (4.5 to 6.5 mmol/L) for LDL, and 40 to 70 mg/dL (0.5 to 0.8 mmol/L) for triglycerides. I do not freak out if my triglycerides "go up" from 43 to 60 mg/dL (0.5 to 0.7 mmol/L). Those numbers are well within the normal range for me. If my triglycerides suddenly shot up to 150 mg/dL (1.7 mmol/L), however, that would be concerning. When looking at cholesterol markers, a change of less than 19 percent is not significant.[2]

Because testing errors can occur, I retest if a marker is out of whack. If the second test came back with a similar number, only then would I begin to put some thought into what is going on.

---

[1] Zoe Harcombe, PhD, "How Accurate Is Your Cholesterol Test?" weekly newsletter, December 9, 2024.

[2] "Interpreting laboratory results," *British Medical Journal* 298 (1989): 1659.

BLOOD SUGAR MARKERS

Next, I look at blood sugar–related markers:

- **Fasting glucose (typically part of a comprehensive metabolic panel):** On carnivore, 70 to 95 mg/dL (3.9 to 5.3 mmol/L)
- **A1c:** On carnivore, 5.4 percent or less; in general, under 5.6 percent. Sometimes carnivores see slightly elevated A1c. It is theorized that red blood cells are living longer and thus have more time to accumulate glucose molecules, but that hasn't been proven yet. I have seen my A1c as high as 5.7 percent on carnivore, while my glucose level averages 85 mg/dL (4.7 mmol/L), so do not be alarmed if your A1c is slightly high. I will talk about some practical interventions to address elevated A1c in the next section.
- **Fasting insulin:** On carnivore, between 2 and 6 uIU/mL (13.9 and 41.7 pmol/L); in general, in the single digits

	Estimated Average Glucose (eAG)	
A1c (%)	**mg/dL**	**mmol/L**
5	97 (76–120)	5.4 (4.2–6.7)
6	126 (100–152)	7.0 (5.5–8.5)
7	154 (123–185)	8.6 (6.8–10.3)
8	183 (147–217)	10.2 (8.1–12.1)
9	212 (170–249)	11.8 (9.4–13.9)
10	240 (193–282)	13.4 (10.7–15.7)
11	269 (217–314)	14.9 (12.0–17.5)
12	298 (240–347)	16.5 (13.3–19.3)

KIDNEY AND LIVER FUNCTION

Then I look at kidney and liver function:

- **Comprehensive metabolic panel** (see the example on the following page):
  - **eGFR:** As high as possible, but at a minimum above 59 mL/min/1.73. This is just an estimate, though, and not something to be too concerned about.
  - **AST and ALT:** As low as possible, ideally under 40 IU/L
  - **BUN/Creatinine ratio:** Within the conventional reference range of 10:1 to 20:1, but a slight elevation isn't a big deal
- **GGT:** Single digits IU/L

[3] American Diabetes Association Professional Practice Committee, "Glycemic targets: standards of medical care in diabetes—2022," *Diabetes Care* 45, Suppl. 1 (2022): S83–S96.

Test	Current Result and Flag	Previous Result	Units	Reference Interval
Glucose	86	80	mg/dL	70–99
BUN	11	11	mg/dL	6–24
Creatinine	0.63	0.66	mg/dL	0.57–1.00
eGFR	115	114	mL/min/1.73	> 59
BUN/Creatinine Ratio	17	17	mg/dL	9–23
Sodium	138	136	mg/dL	134–144
Potassium	4.4	4.3	mg/dL	3.5–5.2
Chloride	103	99	mg/dL	96–106
Carbon Dioxide, Total	20	20	mg/dL	20–29
Calcium	9.0	9.7	mg/dL	8.7–10.2
Protein, Total	6.6	7.1	mg/dL	6.0–8.5
Albumin	4.4	4.7	mg/dL	3.9–4.9
Globulin, Total	2.2	2.4	mg/dL	1.5–4.5
Bilirubin, Total	0.4	0.3	mg/dL	0–1.2
Alkaline Phosphatase	51	52	mg/dL	44–121
AST (SGOT)	19	14	mg/dL	0–40
ALT (SGPT)	21	15	mg/dL	0–32

OTHER MARKERS

Then I look at inflammation markers, vitamins, and minerals:

- **hs-CRP:** Ideally under 1.0 mg/L (9.52 nmol/L)
- **Homocysteine:** Ideally in the single digits µmol/L
- **Ferritin:** 300 ng/mL (674.1 pmol/L) or less
- **Uric acid, serum:** 3 to 5 mg/dL (178 to 297 µmol/L)
- **Vitamin D 25:** Ideally 60 ng/mL (150 nmol/L) or higher, but at a minimum above 40 ng/mL (100 nmol/L)
- **B12 and folate:** At the high end of the conventional reference ranges of 190 to 950 pg/mL (140 to 701 pmol/L) and 2 to 20 ng/mL (4.5 to 45.3 nmol/L), respectively

The next tests are a bit more advanced.

OMEGACHECK

The OmegaCheck (see the example on the next page) looks at omega-3s, omega-6s, and various ratios. When looking at this test, start with the Omega-3 Index, which is EPA + DHA as percent of total RBC fatty acids. Your goal is to be greater than 6 to 8 percent, with higher than 8 percent being optimal. As far as the omega-6 to omega-3 ratio is concerned, you want that to be less than 4:1. For the omega-6s, you want them to be on the lower end of normal or at least in balance with your omega-3s. In general, you want higher omega-3s (EPA, DPA, and DHA) and lower omega-6s (arachidonic acid and linoleic acid).

Test	Current Result and Flag		Previous Result	Units	Reference Interval
OmegaCheck(TM)	8.6		**3.3**	% by wt	>5.4
	Relative Risk: LOW Increasing blood levels of long-chain n-3 fatty acids are associated with a lower risk of sudden cardiac death (1). Based on the top (75th percentile) and bottom (25th percentile) quartiles of the CHL reference population, the following risk categories were established for OmegaCheck: A cutoff of >5.5% by wt defines a population at moderate relative risk, and <=3.7% by wt defines a population at high relative risk of sudden cardiac death. The totality of the scientific evidence demonstrates that when consumption of fish oils is limited to 3g/day or less of EPA and DHA, there is no significant risk for increased bleeding time beyond the normal range. A daily dosage of 1g of EPA and DHA lowers the circulating triglycerides by about 7–10% within 2 to 3 weeks. (Reference: 1-Albert et al. *NEJM*. 2002; 346: 1113–1118).				
Arachidonic Acid/EPA Ratio	4.9		**57.3**		3.7–40.7
Omega-6/Omega-3 Ratio	4.3		13.3		3.7–14.4
Omega-3 Total	8.6		3.3	% by wt	
EPA	**2.8**	**High**	0.3	% by wt	0.2–2.3
DPA	0.9		0.9	% by wt	0.8–1.8
DHA	4.9		2.2	% by wt	1.4–5.1
Omega-6 Total	37.1		44.3	% by wt	
Arachidonic Acid	13.8		15.5	% by wt	8.6–15.6
Linoleic Acid	21.4		26.0	% by wt	18.6–29.5

NMR LIPOPROFILE

This advanced lipid panel provides a lot of information, but I look at only a few things. First, I look for an A pattern. If you have an A pattern, you know that your LDL particles (LDL-P) are generally large, buoyant, and healthy and that only a tiny fraction of them are small and dense. A B pattern tells you that some sort of metabolic dysfunction, typically insulin resistance, is damaging your LDL particles, causing you to have an abundance of small, dense LDL-P and an overall small LDL size, which is not what you want.

I am not as concerned with the particle number (LDL-P), which can depend on many factors. For example, if you were to eat extremely high-fat and high-calorie carnivore for three days before taking this test, you would see a dramatic reduction in your LDL-P number. If you were to do a ten-day sardine fast before taking this test, you would see a dramatic rise in your LDL-P number. Instead of focusing on how many particles there are, focus on the health of the particles. With an A pattern, you know your particles are functioning as they should.

The NMR LipoProfile also generates an LP-IR score, which estimates your level of insulin resistance. You want this marker to be as low as possible. Here is one of my NMR LipoProfiles to give you an idea of what the report looks like:

PARTICLE CONCENTRATION AND SIZE

Lower CVD Risk ← Higher CVD Risk

Percentile in Reference Population

LDL AND HDL PARTICLES

		High	75th	50th	25th	Low
HDL-P Total	39.6 µmol/L		34.9	30.5	26.7	
		Low	25th	50th	75th	High
Small LDL-P	< 90 nmol/L		117	527	839	
LDL Size	22.1 nm	23.0 Large (Pattern A) 20.6			20.5 Small (Pattern B) 19.0	

Small LDL-P and LDL Size are associated with CVD risk, but not after LDL-P is taken into account.

Insulin Sensitive ← Insulin Resistant

Percentile in Reference Population

LIPOPROTEIN MARKERS ASSOCIATED WITH INSULIN RESISTANCE & DIABETES RISK

		Low	25th	50th	75th	High
Large VLDL-P	0.9 nmol/L		0.9	2.7	6.9	
		Low	25th	50th	75th	High
Small LDL-P	< 90 nmol/L		117	527	839	
		High	75th	50th	25th	Low
Large HDL-P	15.5 µmol/L		7.3	4.8	3.1	
VLDL Size	*** nm	VLDL levels not sufficient for VLDL size determination.				
		Large	75th	50th	25th	Small
LDL Size	22.1 nm		21.2	20.8	20.4	
		Large	75th	50th	25th	Small
HDL Size	10.1 nm		9.6	9.2	8.9	

INSULIN RESISTANCE SCORE

		Insulin Sensitive	25th	50th	75th	Insulin Resistant
LP-IR Score	< 25 /100		27	45	63	

THYROID MARKERS

Here are the optimal ranges for thyroid health:

- **TSH:** 2 uIU/mL or less
- **Free T4:** 1 to 1.5 ng/dL (12.9 to 19.3 pmol/L)
- **Free T3:** In the upper quadrant of the reference range (this will be different for each lab, but aim to be in the upper quadrant of the range)
- **Reverse T3:** If free T3 is good, 15 ng/dL (150 pg/mL) or less; ideally 12 ng/dL (120 pg/mL) or less
- **TPO:** Zero
- **Thyroglobulin antibody:** Zero

If you think you might be dealing with thyroid issues, I strongly recommend finding an experienced thyroid practitioner to work with. As stated earlier, conventional doctors are not trained to look past TSH and maybe T4. It is imperative that you address any thyroid issues sooner rather than later because they can severely damage your metabolic health over time.

Carnivore is an excellent dietary intervention, but sometimes it is not enough, and medication and/or supplementation is needed. It can be frustrating to find the right practitioner, but do not give up. With persistence, you will find one. Here are some resources to get started:

- Dr. David Brownstein, www.centerforholisticmedicine.com
- Dr. Amie Hornaman, www.betterlifedoctor.com
- Dr. Isabella Wentz, www.thyroidpharmacist.com

I also strongly recommend working with a knowledgeable practitioner for any kind of hormone replacement therapy. Bioidentical hormones are essential for many people, especially women coming into middle age. The key is to find a practitioner who knows what they are talking about, what to look for, and how to treat these issues. Don't just go to a med spa and get hormone injections; this process needs to be closely monitored.

IMPROVING YOUR MARKERS

Now that you know the optimal ranges you should be aiming for, let's go over some ways you can improve each marker if it is out of range. Remember that improvements in metabolic health can take time, so practice patience if the improvements come more slowly than you expect.

LIPIDS

In general, a low-carbohydrate, high-fat diet will do most of the work when it comes to blood lipids. Over time, you may see a reduction in triglycerides and a rise in HDL cholesterol as you become more insulin sensitive. Your LDL cholesterol could go up, down, or stay the same. Total cholesterol is not something to worry about unless you have a genetic anomaly like familial hypercholesterolemia (marked by high levels of LDL; a genetic test is needed to confirm). As you are losing weight, you might see a slight elevation in your triglycerides, but they will stabilize. This happens because when you are losing fat, your body breaks up your fat stores into components it can use, including triglycerides. If your triglycerides do not improve on carnivore, check out the section on lipotoxicity in chapter 5.

Another excellent way to improve cholesterol markers is to get enough sunlight. Our bodies use sunlight to synthesize vitamin D out of cholesterol, so the more sunlight you get, the better.

BLOOD SUGAR–RELATED MARKERS

In general, eating a low-carbohydrate, high-fat diet should be enough to normalize your glucose levels and lower your A1c and fasting insulin. If your A1c remains elevated on carnivore, throw in a high-quality berberine supplement to help bring it down. It has been theorized that red blood cells live longer in people who are carnivore, and that could be a reason why your A1c is slightly elevated even if your glucose levels are great. This theory hasn't been proven, but berberine is an effective way to lower A1c. I experienced this phenomenon with an average glucose level of 85 mg/dL (4.7 mmol/L) and A1c of between 5.4 and 5.7 percent (36.3 and 39.9 mmol/mol). Since I started taking berberine, my A1c has been declining (down to 5.0 percent, or 31.9 mmol/mol).

Another fantastic way to clear excess glucose is regular exercise. Make sure you break a sweat; don't just do light exercise. Muscles are like a storage facility for glucose, and a good workout depletes your muscles' glucose supply. Then the glucose in your bloodstream can refill those muscle stores, leaving less glucose in your blood.

If your fasting insulin and glucose remain elevated after three to six months on carnivore, it's time to start throwing in some fasting and lower your fat intake a bit. I recommend getting a DEXA scan (discussed in the next section) to determine your level of visceral fat and see how aggressive you will need to be with the fasting. For more information on fasting, head to chapter 5, where I have laid out a complete fasting protocol for you.

KIDNEY AND LIVER MARKERS

In general, kidney and liver markers will improve as you continue a low-carbohydrate, high-fat diet. The kidneys are especially sensitive to high blood sugar levels, so normalizing blood sugar is the best way to improve your kidney health. Exercise and staying hydrated are also important.

hs-CRP

You should see improvements in your hs-CRP levels on a long-term low-carbohydrate diet. Losing weight, exercising, fasting, and getting enough vitamin D can help as well. It can take time for this marker to improve, though. For example, my husband's hs-CRP was as high as 6 mg/L, but once we addressed his lipotoxicity, we got it down to 1 mg/L. That took ten months of work, but we got there, and I am very pleased with his progress.

Homocysteine

If your homocysteine is in the double digits, I recommend supplementing with a high-quality methylated B vitamin complex and retesting in a month. *Methylated* is the key word here; don't take just any B vitamin. Methylated B vitamins are better because they are in their active form, allowing for better absorption and utilization. I also recommend a genetic test for MTHFR and other gene mutations that impair your ability to methylate B vitamins. You may need to supplement with B vitamins for the rest of your life if you have any of those mutations. I have information on genetic testing at the end of this chapter.

Ferritin

If your ferritin is elevated (above 300 ng/mL or µg/L), there are a couple of things you can do. One of the most effective solutions is donating blood. Doing so will drop your ferritin levels quickly and efficiently. Some people naturally accumulate ferritin and don't clear it very well. For them, blood donation is the best solution. My husband has this issue, so he does a whole blood donation every two months.

Rigorous exercise has also been shown to lower ferritin levels. If your ferritin levels remain high after these interventions, have your doctor run some additional tests to see if they are elevated due to an underlying condition. Overall systemic inflammation can cause elevated levels. Figuring out the root cause of your inflammation and addressing it can lower your ferritin levels quickly.

Uric acid

Typically, uric acid is not an issue unless you have gout. In that case, losing weight by eating a low-carbohydrate diet will be extremely helpful. Getting your blood sugar markers under control goes hand in hand with losing weight. If you are a gout patient, I think easing into carnivore is the way to go because it gives your body time to get used to this way of eating and allows for improvements in your metabolic health. It also gives your body time to expel the uric acid crystals from your joints back into your bloodstream so that they can be cleared from your body through your urine. If you need help with this process, I have a full guide to slowly reducing carbohydrate consumption in chapter 3. Pay special attention to the oxalate portion of the guide and do not cut oxalate-rich foods all at once. If you have gout, it is imperative that you remove all alcohol, sugar-containing products, and anything with corn syrup in it from your diet because these are the main culprits in uric acid overproduction.

If you do not have gout, you may see a temporary rise in uric acid levels after consuming sardines or other high-purine foods, but levels typically normalize after a few days to weeks without causing any issues. It takes years of having uric acid levels over 10 to 15 mg/dL (868.6 to 1,300 µmol/L) to cause gout.

VITAMIN D

The best way to maintain high vitamin D levels is to get plenty of sun on your skin. To avoid sunburn and support circadian alignment, try this approach: Start your day with about 20 minutes outside at dawn, letting the early light reach your eyes and skin—this primes your body for stronger midday sun. When sunbathing later, increase exposure gradually and cover up once you've had enough. In the evening, follow nature's cues by dimming indoor lights, wearing blue blockers after sunset, and minimizing screen time. Over time, this method will help you tolerate more sun without burning—I noticed a big difference in under a month. Remember, sunscreen blocks vitamin D production, so some natural, unfiltered sunlight on your skin is essential.

Supplementing with a high-quality D3 supplement, specifically cholecalciferol, is another excellent way to boost vitamin D levels. Be sure to supplement with vitamin K2 as well because the two work together. D3 helps your body absorb calcium, and K2 helps your body transport the calcium to your bones rather than letting it sit in your arteries and other soft tissues.

If you are interested in circadian biology and vitamin D, be sure to follow Zaid Dahhaj on Instagram.

B12 AND FOLATE

If you are eating a carnivore diet, your B12 and folate levels should be great. But if they are not, I recommend supplementing with a high-quality methylated B vitamin complex and retesting after a month. Like with elevated homocysteine, I also recommend a genetic test for MTHFR or other gene mutations that impair your ability to methylate B vitamins. If you do this and your B levels continue to be low, I would next look at leaky gut and/or compromised nutrient absorption.

THYROID MARKERS

If you have a thyroid condition, it is imperative that you cut gluten, liquid dairy, and cheese from your diet if you have not done so already. These foods can be highly inflammatory for anyone with thyroid issues, especially Hashimoto's thyroiditis. Carnivore is one of the best dietary interventions for people suffering from thyroid conditions because it eliminates so many inflammatory foods, so you will have a leg up on most other people if you are already eating this way. But again, collaborating with a knowledgeable practitioner who has experience treating thyroid conditions is important. As far as supplements, a regimen of selenium, a high-quality methylated B vitamin complex, and iodine is a good place to start. A skilled thyroid practitioner will be able to provide guidance on dosages.

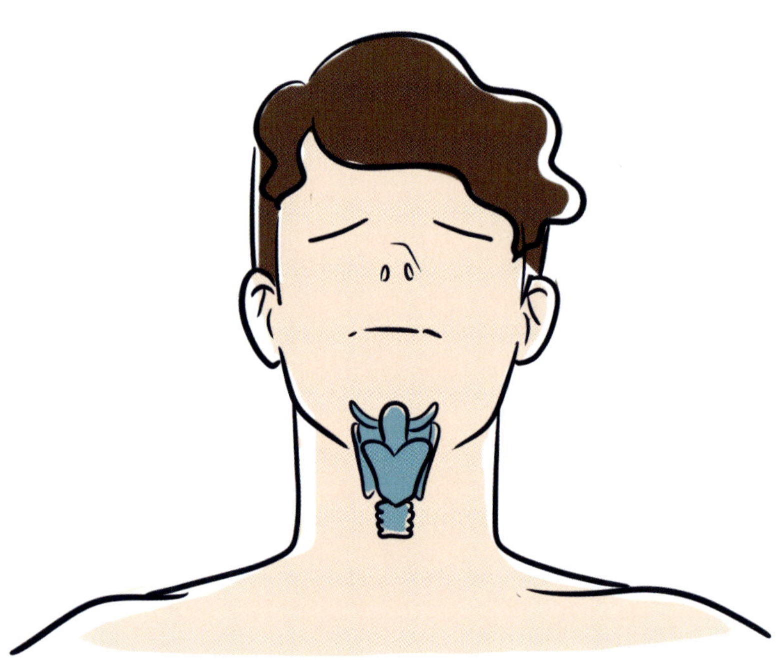

DEXA

DEXA scans are my favorite body composition measurement tool. They measure the amount of fat, muscle, bone, and water in your body. This data can help you make informed decisions about exercise and nutrition. I love the visceral fat measurement, as visceral fat levels are an important metabolic health indicator. Visceral fat is the fat that accumulates inside your abdominal cavity, around your organs. You don't want much of it; less than a pound is optimal. It's also cool to see how much progress you've made and if the weight you've lost is fat or lean mass.

WHAT IS A DEXA SCAN?

DEXA stands for dual-energy X-ray absorptiometry. There are a couple of versions of DEXA: One is used for diagnosing osteoporosis, and the other is used for measuring body composition. The main differences between them are the purpose of the scan and the areas of the body being examined. The DEXA scan that you want is the one that measures body composition.

WHERE CAN I FIND ONE, AND HOW MUCH DOES IT COST?

Head to the search engine of your choice and search for "DEXA scans in my area." Dexascan.com has an impressive "Find a Testing Location" page where you can find providers in the United States, Europe, Asia, and Australia. DEXA scans typically cost less than $200, making them a reasonably affordable option for measuring body composition. The types of businesses that typically provide body composition DEXA scans are gyms, wellness centers, and weight-loss clinics.

WHAT ABOUT RADIATION LEVELS?

The amount of radiation delivered in a body composition DEXA scan is very small, so it's nothing to worry about. According to an article in the journal *Bone*, "The effective radiation dose from a single whole body DEXA (< 10 microSieverts) is similar to the normal background radiation received over one day at sea level."[4]

HOW OFTEN SHOULD I GET A DEXA SCAN?

If you are trying to lose weight or improve your body composition, I recommend getting a DEXA scan every one to three months. Once you have hit your target weight and/or body composition goals, once every six to twelve months is sufficient.

WHAT DO I NEED TO DO TO PREPARE FOR A DEXA SCAN?

Fasting for several hours before a DEXA scan is ideal, but eating a little something is okay. Also, make sure you are hydrated. If you plan

[4] John Shepherd, Bennett Ng, Markus Sommer, and Steven B. Heymsfield, "Body composition by DXA," *Bone* 104 (2017): 101–105.

on getting DEXAs often, I advise eating and drinking the same things before each scan and getting the scan done around the same time of day every time. I also prefer getting scanned at the same location on the same machine. Personally, I get my scans done between 10 and 11 a.m., and I drink a few cups of black coffee in the morning and some water on the way to the scan. If I eat at all, it will be a few hours beforehand and will be only a little something, like a sausage patty or a couple of hard-boiled eggs. Wear comfortable clothes and be prepared to remove any jewelry or watches. For women, wear a sports bra instead of an underwire bra.

HOW ACCURATE ARE THE RESULTS?

Typical error rates are between 1 and 3 percent, making the DEXA scan one of the most accurate body composition scans available. They are much more accurate than at-home body composition scales or the body composition scanner at the gym. The only thing more accurate is an MRI. Be sure to follow the pre-scan procedures listed above to control for wild inaccuracies.

HOW TO READ THE RESULTS

DEXA is a three-component model that quantifies three primary metrics: bone, fat, and lean tissue. These components are then organized into additional metrics that are depicted throughout your report.

- **Total Mass:** Measured weight. It's the sum of your fat, lean, and BMC.
- **Fat Mass:** All fat mass including items like brain, bone marrow, etc.
- **Lean Mass:** Muscle mass, organs, blood, and stomach contents
- **BMC:** Bone mineral content; generally 3 to 5 percent of the total

Fat Free: The total of lean tissue and BMC

On the following pages are some examples of the reports I get when I do a DEXA scan. Keep in mind that the report you receive may look different.

I'm currently doing a DEXA scan every one to three months, and I find them to be an invaluable tool in my metabolic health journey.

BODY COMPOSITION HISTORY (REGION: TOTAL)

This is a standard body composition analysis page. It shows your current and previous scan data, including total body fat percentage, total mass, fat mass, lean mass, bone mineral content (BMC), and fat-free mass.

Measured Date	Total Body Fat %	Total Mass (lbs)	Fat Mass (lbs)	Lean Mass (lbs)	BMC (lbs)	Fat Free (lbs)
10/31/2024	31.3	149.5	46.8	97.1	5.6	102.7
10/03/2024	32.9	155.4	51.1	98.6	5.6	104.2
08/30/2024	32.7	159.0	52.0	101.3	5.6	107.0
...	...	...	...	...	...	...
09/16/2022	44.9	201.4	90.4	105.1	5.9	111.0

Measured Date	Total Mass (lbs)	Baseline (lbs)	Previous (lbs)	Fat Mass (lbs)	Baseline (lbs)	Previous (lbs)	Lean Mass (lbs)	Baseline (lbs)	Previous (lbs)
10/31/2024	**149.5**	−51.9	−5.9	**46.8**	−43.6	−4.3	**97.1**	−8.0	−1.5
10/03/2024	**155.4**	−46.0	−3.6	**51.1**	−39.3	−0.9	**98.6**	−6.5	−2.7
08/30/2024	**159.0**	−42.4	2.5	**52.0**	−38.4	0.0	**101.3**	−3.8	2.5
...	**...**	...		**...**	...		**...**	...	...
09/16/2022	**201.4**	baseline		**90.4**	baseline		**105.1**	baseline	

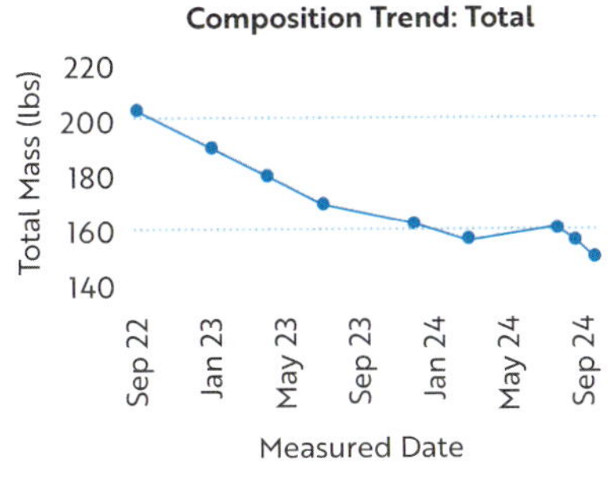

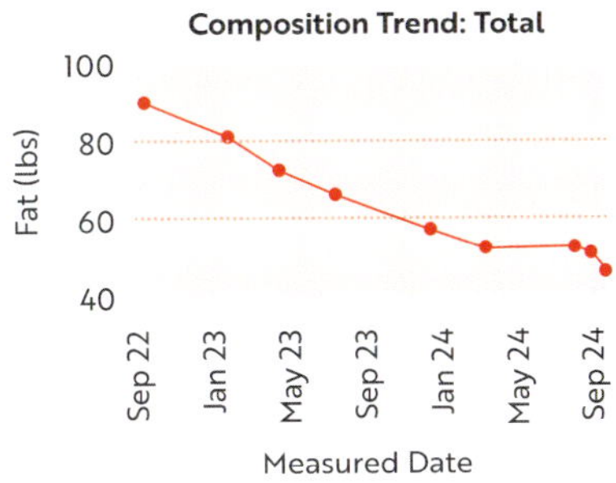

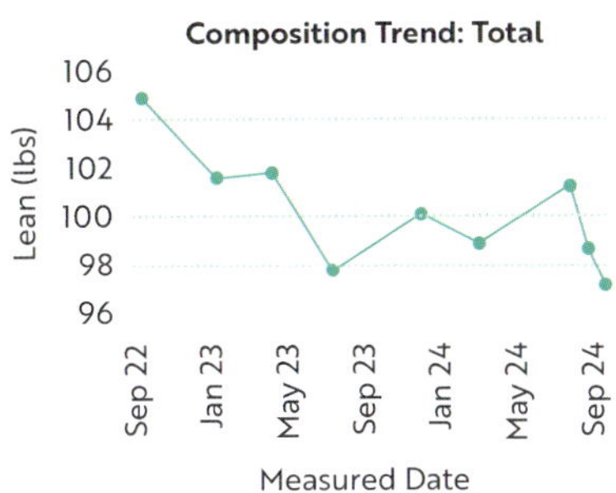

VISCERAL ADIPOSE TISSUE (VAT)

Visceral fat is the fat tucked around your organs in your belly. You want to keep it low—ideally under 1 pound. Your report may look different depending on the DEXA scan location, but it will still give you the information you need.

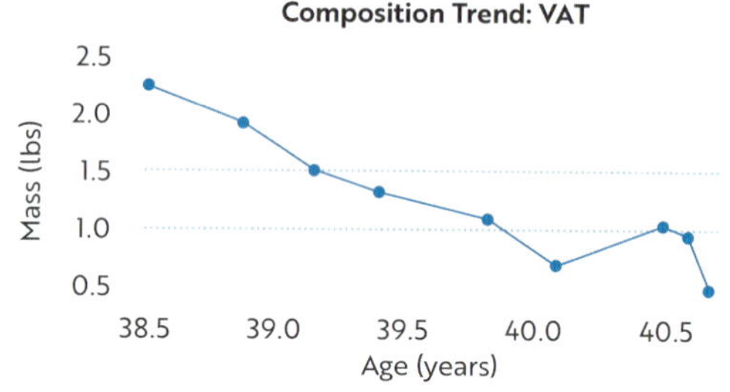

Date	Age	Fat Mass (lbs)	Volume (in³)
10/31/2024	40.6	0.51	15.00
10/03/2024	40.5	0.96	28.24
08/30/2024	40.4	1.03	30.17
04/02/2024	40.0	0.71	20.87
...	...	...	...
09/16/2022	38.5	2.24	65.78

HOW DOES YOUR VAT VOLUME COMPARE?

Adipose Tissue
1 Visceral
2 Subcutaneous

Ideal (Healthy)	Increased Risk (High)	At Risk (Very High)
0.00–52.00	52.15–112.10	112.10+
A VAT volume (in³) between the levels listed above is considered a healthy range. Continue to practice exercise and a balanced diet.	If your VAT volume (in³) is between the levels listed above, you are considered to be at an increased risk. Within this range, consider improving your diet and increasing exercise.	If your VAT volume (in³) is at or above the level listed above, your risk may be considered high. If you are within this range, consider consulting your physician.

TOTAL BODY BONE DENSITY REPORT

Total body bone density provides a snapshot of your overall skeletal health, helping you track bone strength, monitor changes over time, and support long-term wellness.

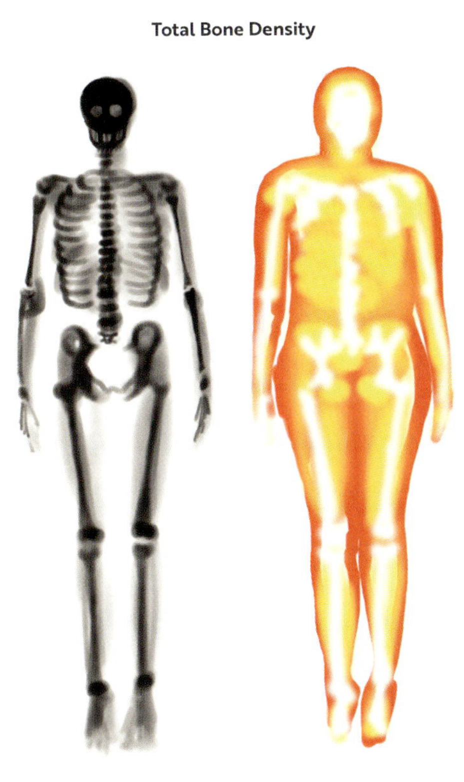

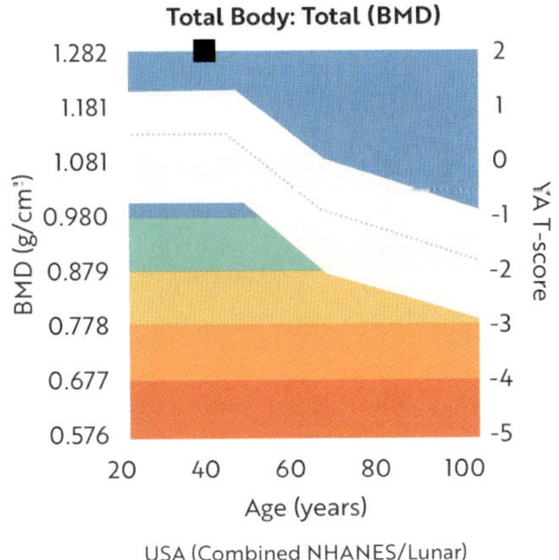

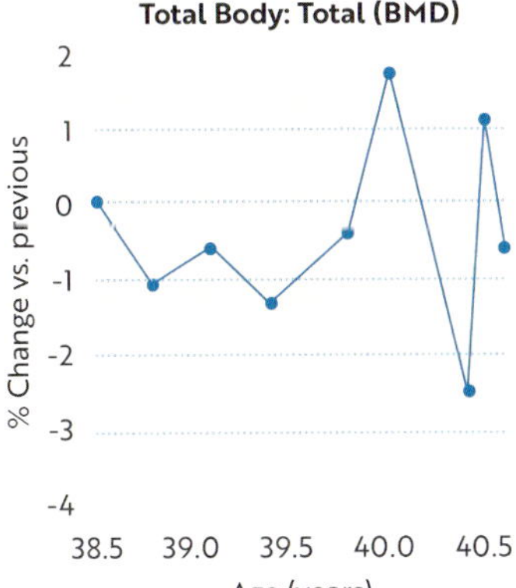

DENSITOMETRY: USA (COMBINED NHANES/LUNAR) (ENHANCED ANALYSIS)

Region	BMD (g/cm^2)	YA T-score	AM Z-score
Head	2.421	-	-
Arms	1.036	-	-
Legs	1.266	-	-
Trunk	1.007	-	-
Ribs	0.741	-	-
Spine	1.209	-	-
Pelvis	1.108	-	-
Total	1.271	1.9	1.6

Color Coding

Bone Lean

BODY COMPOSITION TRENDING REPORT

The body composition trending report shows changes in your fat, lean mass, and bone over time, helping you track progress and see long-term trends.

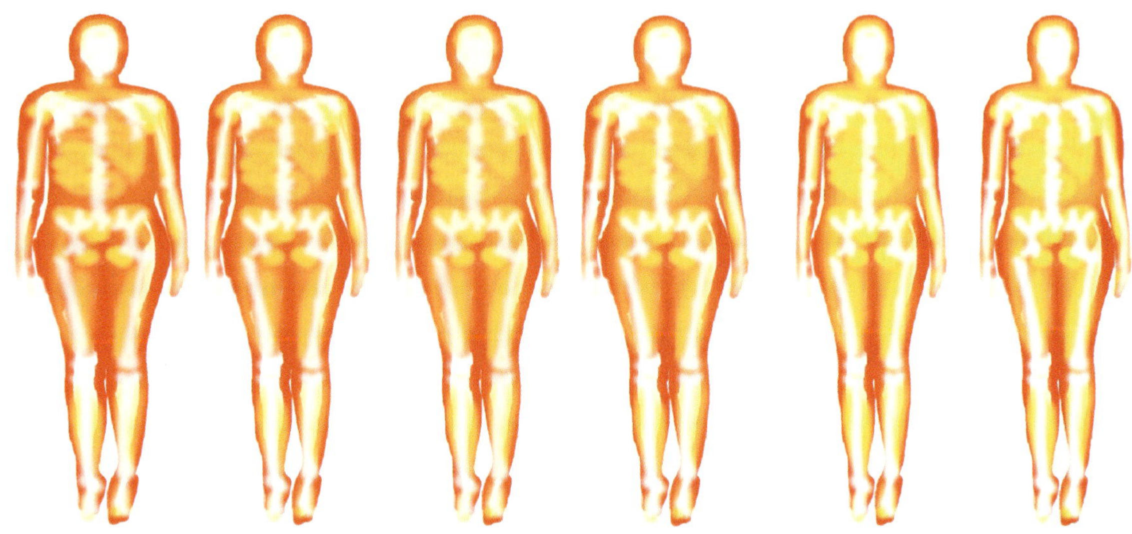

Measured Date	Total Mass (lbs)	Total Fat (%)	Total Fat (lbs)	Total Lean (lbs)	Trunk Fat (lbs)	Trunk Lean (lbs)	Arms Fat (lbs)	Arms Lean (lbs)	Legs Fat (lbs)	Legs Lean (lbs)
10/31/2024	149.5	31.3%	46.8	97.1	20.0	46.5	6.4	11.1	18.6	32.5
10/03/2024	155.4	32.9%	51.1	98.6	21.7	45.9	6.8	11.1	20.8	34.7
08/30/2024	159.0	32.7%	52.0	101.3	23.7	47.5	6.2	11.2	20.2	35.7
04/02/2024	156.5	33.3%	52.0	98.8	23.7	46.6	6.7	10.5	19.7	34.5
12/27/2023	162.7	35.0%	56.9	100.1	26.7	46.9	7.1	11.4	21.1	34.8
08/01/2023	169.4	39.0%	66.1	97.6	32.9	45.8	7.6	9.7	23.7	35.2
04/28/2023	180.2	40.3%	72.6	101.8	35.0	47.0	9.4	11.3	26.2	36.6
01/24/2023	188.4	43.0%	81.1	101.5	38.9	46.4	10.4	10.8	29.8	37.1
09/16/2022	201.4	44.9%	90.4	105.1	44.6	47.3	10.8	11.6	33.1	39.2

CONTINUOUS GLUCOSE MONITORING

As discussed in other parts of this book, high blood sugar is a tremendous problem in the general population. Unless you are diabetic, you probably have no insight into how food affects your glucose levels. But you don't need to be diabetic to take advantage of today's high-tech blood sugar management tools, like a continuous glucose monitor (CGM).

CGMs came onto the market in 1999 to continuously measure glucose levels and were a game changer for people with diabetes. The technology has improved rapidly since then. The newest prescription-grade CGMs are very accurate. And now, non-diabetics have discovered the value of CGMs and are using them to learn how different foods and lifestyle choices affect their glucose levels. I have been wearing a CGM since September 2022 and have tested all of the different brands and apps. I strongly recommend you wear one for at least a month. You can run experiments with food and lifestyle to see how your glucose responds.

HOW DO I GET A CONTINUOUS GLUCOSE MONITOR, AND HOW MUCH DOES IT COST?

It is easier than ever to get a CGM in the United States, even without a prescription. They are now available over the counter from the two largest CGM manufacturers in the US: Dexcom and Abbott. Dexcom's CGM is called Stelo, and Abbott's is called Lingo. You can order either one online without a prescription. The average cost is between $39 to $49 per sensor. I have tested both sensors and their apps; check out the comparison below:

Stelo (Dexcom)

- Works with Androids/iPhones
- 15 days, plus 12-hour grace period
- Very basic app
- Can only see current glucose level
- Moderately accurate readings
- No calibration
- Costs $89 per month

Lingo (Abbot)

- Works with iPhones
- 15 days, plus 12-hour grace period
- Excellent app
- Can look at historical data
- Moderately accurate readings
- No calibration
- Costs $89 per month

You can also get a prescription-grade CGM without a prescription through the multitude of non-diabetic CGM apps. Nutrisense, Levels, and Signos are the biggest names in non-diabetic continuous glucose monitoring and typically pair with the newest CGMs from Dexcom and Abbott.

HOW DO I USE A CGM?

CGM technology has come a long way, and the devices are very user-friendly. You receive instructions in the box and within whatever app you pair your device with. The instructions for applying a CGM are clear and easy to understand. Typically, you apply it to the back of your arm and keep it there for a specified period of time. Do not be scared! The application is virtually pain-free, and you will barely notice it's there. I always put a CGM patch over my CGM to help it stay in place for the full ten to fourteen days it is active.

Once you have applied the sensor, link it to the app you are using, following the instructions in the app. Most apps have some screens that explain how glucose measuring works and what to look for within the app. Do not worry; over the first few days of using the app, you will get the hang of it. These apps are not at all difficult to use once you've had a bit of practice.

WHAT ARE OPTIMAL GLUCOSE LEVELS?

Every glucose app has a slightly different angle when it comes to optimal levels, but here are the ranges to aim for when following a carnivore lifestyle:

- **Average glucose:** 75 to 95 mg/dL (4.17 to 5.28 mmol/L)
- **Time in range:** 100 percent
- **Variability:** 15 (0.83 mmol/L) or less
- **Max glucose:** Under 140 mg/dL (6.66 mmol/L)
- **Sleep average:** Under 90 mg/dL (5.0 mmol/L)
- **Morning average:** Under 90 mg/dL (5.0 mmol/L)

Remember that there will be some individual variation, and your numbers will change from day to day.

WHAT EXPERIMENTS CAN I RUN?

You can run experiments with different foods. You can try eating at different times of the day to see how it affects your glucose levels. You can try different forms of exercise to see how your glucose recovers after a workout. Saunas, hot tubs, and cold plunges are fun to experiment with. You could also have a cheat meal and see how much your glucose spikes. The world is your oyster, so figure out some fun experiments to run while wearing the sensor!

WHAT CAN AFFECT MY GLUCOSE LEVELS?

Your glucose levels can be influenced by so much more than food. Exercise, sleep, stress, travel, saunas, hydration levels, medications, supplements, fasting, exposure to pollutants, and more can have an impact. This is another reason I think it is important to wear a CGM for at least a month so you can learn how all of these things affect your glucose.

CGM MYTHS AND CAVEATS

There are some things to keep in mind when tracking your glucose with a CGM. First, CGMs measure interstitial fluid, not blood. This means that if you were to test your blood with a finger stick and then immediately look at your CGM, the numbers might differ a bit. If you take a finger stick, wait 15 minutes and then compare the reading to your CGM. If the CGM reading is within 5 to 10 points of the finger stick, I am happy with that. The value in wearing a CGM comes from being able to see your glucose all day instead of just a few times a day. With a CGM, you can identify patterns that you cannot see with a traditional finger stick.

Piggybacking off of that is manual calibration. If you are using a prescription-grade CGM like the Dexcom 7 or Libre 3, be sure to manually calibrate it to ensure accurate readings. Eight to twenty-four hours after applying your CGM, take a finger stick, wait 15 minutes, and then add that reading as a calibration in your CGM app. The app will update the data and adjust it to that calibration. It's only necessary to calibrate if your CGM readings are wildly off—more than ten to fifteen points different from your finger sticks. My husband has run into this issue. His CGM almost always reads twenty to twenty-five points higher than it should, so we always calibrate it. If you are getting CGM readings that seem off, test them against a finger stick and then calibrate accordingly. Unfortunately, Stelo and Lingo don't currently allow calibration, but if you pair them with the Nutrisense app, you can calibrate them through the app.

Next up is the effect of heat on the CGM. If you take a hot shower, go into a sauna or steam room, or soak in a hot tub, you may see a spike in your blood glucose. It may be a malfunction of the CGM, or it may be an actual glucose spike, but either way, it's nothing to worry about. Your glucose and the CGM readings will dip back to normal after you get out of the heat. Cold plunges can have a similar effect, though normally not as drastic.

Speaking of water, CGMs can be worn while swimming or bathing. Specifically, the Libre 2 and 3 can be immersed in up to three feet of water for thirty minutes, and the Dexcom 6 and 7 can be immersed in up to eight feet of water for twenty-four hours. Scuba divers have successfully used CGMs in up to eighty feet of water, but the monitor could fail. Try to time any diving excursions for when you will not be wearing a CGM so it doesn't go to waste if it fails.

A couple of people have said to me that it is unethical for a non-diabetic to wear a CGM because they would be taking a sensor from a diabetic. That is just silly, especially now that the Stelo and Lingo are available over the counter specifically for non-diabetics. There are more than enough CGMs available for anyone who wants one.

It's also important to remember your glucose levels are going to vary. The key is to keep glucose steady, without massive spikes and dips. One way to prevent a large spike is to consume protein at least ten minutes before eating any carbohydrates. Doing so will buffer your insulin response and cause a gentle rise in glucose as opposed to a massive spike. In general, you want to keep your glucose under 140 mg/dL (7.77 mmol/L) after eating. You will not typically see glucose this high when you are eating carnivore. But if you have a cheat meal and experience a spike above 140 mg/dL (7.77 mmol/L), that is okay! What's more important is that your glucose gets back under 140 mg/dL (7.77 mmol/L) within two hours of the spike. Remember that there is only about a teaspoon's worth of sugar in the form of glucose in your bloodstream at any time. If you eat a ton of sugar, you are going to see a spike.

Finally, while glucose tracking is valuable, it is just one of many measurement tools. Do not depend on it as your sole source of metabolic health data. Also, if you are becoming obsessed with your readings or experiencing anxiety over them, perhaps it is time to take a break from monitoring. The data is meant to be helpful, not all-consuming.

MEASURING KETONES AND THE BASICS OF KETOSIS

Ketosis is a metabolic state in which the body breaks down fat for energy instead of carbohydrates. The only way to know if you are in ketosis is to measure your ketone levels. Ketones (or ketone bodies) are acids your body makes when fat is its main energy source. The carnivore diet is a ketogenic diet, but to be in nutritional ketosis, you need to have detectable ketones in your bloodstream of at least 0.5 mmol/L. From here on out, when I say ketosis, I am referring to nutritional ketosis.

Why would you want to be in ketosis? When you have ketone levels over 0.5 mmol/L, you are burning fat. This could be the fat stores on your body, the fat you are eating, or a mix of the two. Ketones are a much more efficient fuel than glucose, and you will notice a difference in your energy levels and brain clarity when your ketones are elevated. Being in ketosis can help improve blood sugar levels and reduce your appetite, all while helping you lose weight.

People dealing with certain conditions, such as epilepsy, cancer, or mental health issues, will want to be in therapeutic ketosis. Typically, therapeutic ketosis is managed by a knowledgeable healthcare provider who can help the patient safely achieve the higher levels of ketones needed to manage these conditions.

Most people are not burning ketones as fuel because of the elevated amounts of carbohydrates they consume. On carnivore, you will eat very few carbs, if any. But you need to give your body time to become fat adapted, or fully adjusted to burning primarily fat instead of primarily glucose. This process takes time—typically up to three weeks—so if you aren't seeing any ketones when you test, or you are seeing very low ketone levels in the beginning, that's okay. Just give it time.

Here are the different ketone levels you can aim for:

Stage	Ketone Level (mmol/L)	Fat Burning
Not in ketosis **Not burning fat**	0–0.5	< 0.62g/h
Nutritional ketosis **Slight/moderate fat burning**	0.5–1.5	0.62–7.7g/h
Optimal zone **Efficient fat burning**	1.5–3.0	7.7–18.32g/h
Moderate high zone **Fast fat burning**	3.0–5.0	18.32–32.48g/h
High zone **Inefficient fat burning**	5.0–8.0	32.48–53.72g/h

Ketones are primarily measured through urine, breath, and blood. Let's weigh the pros and cons of each option for testing.

URINE

Urine testing is probably the easiest and most affordable way to measure ketone levels. A pack of 100 strips typically costs less than $10 and can be found online or at your local pharmacy. While convenient, I'm not a big fan—urine strips mainly detect acetoacetate, not the primary ketone, beta-hydroxybutyrate, so they aren't as accurate as blood testing. They also become less reliable after about a month on a low-carb diet. Still, their low cost makes them a practical choice for many people.

BREATH

Breath testing is more accurate than urine testing but can still fall prey to errors. Breath ketone meters measure acetone levels as an indirect indicator of ketone production. The key issues with breath measurements are variations in breathing techniques, food and drink consumption, alcohol use, mouthwash use, and device reliability, among other things. It is estimated that breath ketone meters have an error rate of up to 15 percent. Another downside is that you need to purchase the device itself, which can be pricey—typically anywhere from $40 to $300 depending on quality.

BLOOD

My favorite method for measuring ketones is to use a blood glucose meter. These meters measure beta-hydroxybutyrate levels and provide the most accurate results. Why bother with the other two options if you can go with the gold standard? You do have to purchase the meter along with the testing strips, which cost about $1 apiece. Blood ketone meters range in price from $20 to $215.

CONTINUOUS KETONE MONITORING

There is such a thing as a continuous ketone monitor, but these devices are not widely available as of this writing. I have evaluated some of the CKMs on the market and found them to be highly accurate. They will be game changers once they are readily available. I love that you do not have to stick your finger to find your ketone levels. For people trying to manage certain conditions with therapeutic ketosis, being able to see their current ketone levels on an app will make life so much easier. But at least for now, CKMs are not widely available.

WHEN AND HOW OFTEN SHOULD I MEASURE MY KETONES?

The most important thing is to be consistent. Some people like to test upon waking. Some test before and after meals. In the beginning, as you are learning about your personal ketone levels, it may be valuable to test several times a day. But as you continue on carnivore, you might only test as needed. It's really up to you.

WHAT IS THE DIFFERENCE BETWEEN KETOSIS AND KETOACIDOSIS?

Ketoacidosis is a life-threatening metabolic condition that occurs when the body produces too many ketones and the blood becomes acidic. It typically only affects people with type 1 diabetes, but it can affect those with type 2. Being in ketosis and experiencing ketoacidosis are not the same thing. Unfortunately, the fearmongering and confusion over this fact cause many diabetics to avoid ketogenic diets, even though they are the best diets they could be eating. You can go into remission from type 2 diabetes by eating an ultra-low-carb diet, and people with type 1 diabetes find it much easier to manage the condition using low-carb diets.

In general, you will not go into ketoacidosis if you are eating a ketogenic diet. Ketosis is a natural metabolic state. The levels of ketones in ketoacidosis are super high, and you will not approach those levels when you are doing a low-carb diet unless you are doing something incorrectly.

WILL I AUTOMATICALLY BE IN KETOSIS IF I AM NOT EATING ANY CARBS?

Not necessarily. Your body's ability to burn fat efficiently depends a lot on your metabolic health. I used to assume I was in ketosis if I wasn't eating any carbs until I found that to be untrue. After a high-carb cheat meal, it takes several days to a week for my ketone levels to return to at least 0.5 mmol/L. For my husband, who has some insulin resistance, it can take up to three weeks for his ketones to become detectable again. Don't just assume you are in ketosis. You need to measure to be sure.

WHAT LEVEL OF KETONES SHOULD I AIM FOR?

The ideal level of ketones will be different for each individual. As you measure ketones, you will begin to recognize a range where you feel your best. For example, I have the most energy and brain clarity when my ketones are between 1.5 and 4.0 mmol/L. Some people doing therapeutic ketosis aim for higher levels than that, but most report feeling great with anything over 1.0 mmol/L.

IODINE TESTING

Most people are deficient in iodine, which is essential for thyroid hormone production as well as proper cell and immune function. According to Dr. David Brownstein, without adequate iodine levels, life itself is not possible.[5]

It is a common misconception that you will get enough iodine from your diet alone or from seasoning your food with iodized salt. Iodine is part of the halide family, along with bromide, fluoride, and chloride. Only iodine is essential, while bromide, fluoride, and chloride are highly toxic to humans. Iodine and bromide are remarkably similar in chemical structure, so bromide molecules can fit into our iodine receptors. That is a problem, though, as the bromide does not do the same thing in our bodies as iodine. Bromide wreaks havoc on our systems and causes us to become iodine deficient. When we are iodine deficient, our metabolic health suffers.

There are several ways to evaluate for iodine deficiency, including skin, blood, and urine testing. The skin test is popular but not very accurate. In this test, you paint a small patch of iodine onto your skin and then check back

---

[5] David Brownstein, MD, *Iodine: Why You Need It, Why You Can't Live Without It* (Medical Alternative Press, 2008), 25.

twenty-four hours later. If the patch is gone, it's said that your body has absorbed the iodine, which tells you that you are deficient. If the patch remains, you have sufficient levels of iodine. The problem with this test is that most of the iodine evaporates. So, if nothing remains, it's not that your body has absorbed it; it has just evaporated. Also, even if this test were accurate, there is no way to know how deficient you are and how much you should supplement.

A much better way to test for iodine deficiency is a twenty-four-hour iodine loading test. You take an iodine tablet and then collect all your urine for twenty-four hours. Then you send a sample of that combined urine to a lab, where it is assessed to see how much of the iodine you excreted over that twenty-four-hour period. If you excreted 90 percent or more, you are likely sufficient in iodine and don't need to supplement much. If you excreted less than 90 percent, you are deficient.

You can order this test from the Hakala Labs website for $70. The company also offers bromide and fluoride testing. Here is a sample of the report you will receive:

URINE HALIDES

Iodine		Reference Range
24-hr excretion	42.77 mg	0–50mg/24 hours
% excretion/24 hr	85.5%	Iodine body sufficiency is achieved when the 24-hour urine collection contains 90 percent or more of the amount of iodine/iodide ingested.*

*However, if you excrete 90 percent or more and *are not* taking supplemental iodine, this may be caused by

- A symporter defect in which iodine is absorbed but not taken into the cells properly.
- An iodine organification problem where iodine gets into the cell but does not attach to the lipid complex for activation.
- Bromide, fluoride, and/or heavy metals interfering with the body's utilization of iodine.

If you have excreted more than 100 percent of the loading dose, there are two possible explanations:

- Iodine supplementation was not stopped at least forty-eight hours prior to the test.
- The reading of the total urine volume collected was incorrect.

I strongly recommend picking up a copy of Dr. Brownstein's book *Iodine: Why You Need It, Why You Can't Live Without It*. You will learn so much about the importance of iodine; I found the book hard to put down. This book and many others are in Appendix B.

GENETIC TESTING FOR MUTATIONS

About 40 percent of the population has a genetic mutation that impedes their ability to methylate B vitamins. This means that even if they consume a lot of B vitamin-rich foods, they are unable to break them down efficiently. Over time, this can lead to issues such as atrial fibrillation, elevated homocysteine levels (which increase the risk of chronic disease), heart disease, and much more.

The most commonly tested gene mutation is MTHFR, but you can also test for MTR, MTRR, AHCY, and COMT. These tests range from $60 to $600 and can be found online through a simple browser search.

Before pulling the trigger on an expensive genetic test, I recommend getting a homocysteine blood test done. If your homocysteine levels are in the double digits, begin supplementing with a high-quality methylated B vitamin complex and retest your homocysteine levels in a month (be sure to cease taking your B vitamins three days before the test so you don't skew the results). If your levels decline to the low single digits, you likely have one or several genetic mutations and will need to supplement with the methylated B complex for the rest of your life.

HEART TESTING

CAC SCAN

A coronary artery calcium (CAC) scan (also known as a calcium score) is a noninvasive CT scan that measures plaque buildup in the walls of the heart's arteries. These scans are typically inexpensive and can be scheduled without a doctor's referral. This information is valuable because it allows a doctor to assess your future cardiovascular risk with greater accuracy. I think everyone over the age of forty should get a baseline CAC scan and then retest every five to ten years depending on their score. These scans cost anywhere from $50 to $400 and are generally not covered by insurance (which is a shame, because they are an amazing diagnostic tool).

The goal is to have a score of zero, but in general, if your score is lower than eighty, you are in good shape. From test to test, you want it to stay the same or go up by only a few points. A drastic jump is an indicator that lifestyle changes are needed.

A question that I am asked often is, can your calcium score go down? The answer to that is unclear. Some cardiologists in the low-carb space have seen declining calcium scores in their patients, but the mechanism has not been studied enough to provide clear-cut answers as to how and why it is happening. I think it is possible using low-carbohydrate diets along with other lifestyle interventions, but I cannot prove that claim. Yet.

CCTA

Coronary computed tomography angiography (CCTA) is a noninvasive 3D imaging test that uses X-rays to create pictures of the heart and blood vessels. It shows the levels of calcified and noncalcified or soft plaques in your coronary arteries. Some people argue that this test is of more value than a CAC scan because it can detect the presence of both calcified and soft plaques. Regardless of the validity of that argument, CCTA scans are a bit more difficult to get because you typically need a referral from a cardiologist. In general, when looking at the results, the less plaque, the better.

There are many ways to measure your progress on carnivore, but I believe these are the most effective and accessible options available. You don't need to use all of these methods to lose weight and improve your metabolic health. However, choosing one or a few can help you track your progress more accurately and provide motivation during challenging times. For example, my husband was thrilled when his fasting insulin levels dropped into the single digits, and for me, seeing my visceral fat levels steadily decline over the past couple of years has reinforced the value of the carnivore diet.

Setting Up Your Own N-of-1 Experiments

If you want to run an experiment on yourself, pick a few of the measurement tools covered in this chapter and take some baseline measurements. Then do your experimental intervention for a set period and retest to see what happens! I have run many experiments on myself and my husband, including eating 100 cans of sardines in one month to see what would happen to my mercury levels and omegas, eating only Carnivore Bars for fourteen days to see what would happen to my blood work and weight, and using a continuous ketone monitor to test how different foods and lifestyle activities would affect my ketones. Be sure to pick one thing to test for a specific time period so you can confirm that the changes that occur are due to that one variable. The world is your oyster—try an N-of-1 experiment today!

PART 2

RECIPES

Icon Key

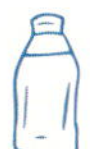

The recipe uses dairy other than butter, such as cheese or heavy cream.

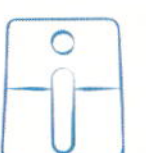

The recipe provides instructions for cooking in an air fryer.

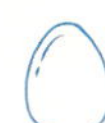

The recipe uses eggs.

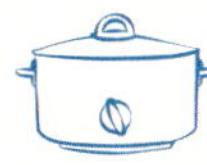

The recipe can be made in a slow cooker.

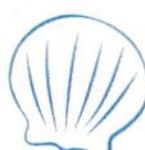

The recipe uses shellfish.

Note:

If an allergen icon is marked "optional," the recipe can be made without that ingredient.

Note:

If a cooking equipment icon is marked "optional," the recipe provides instructions for at least one other cooking method (such as the stovetop or oven).

The recipe can be made in 30 minutes or less.

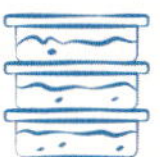

The recipe is good for meal prepping.

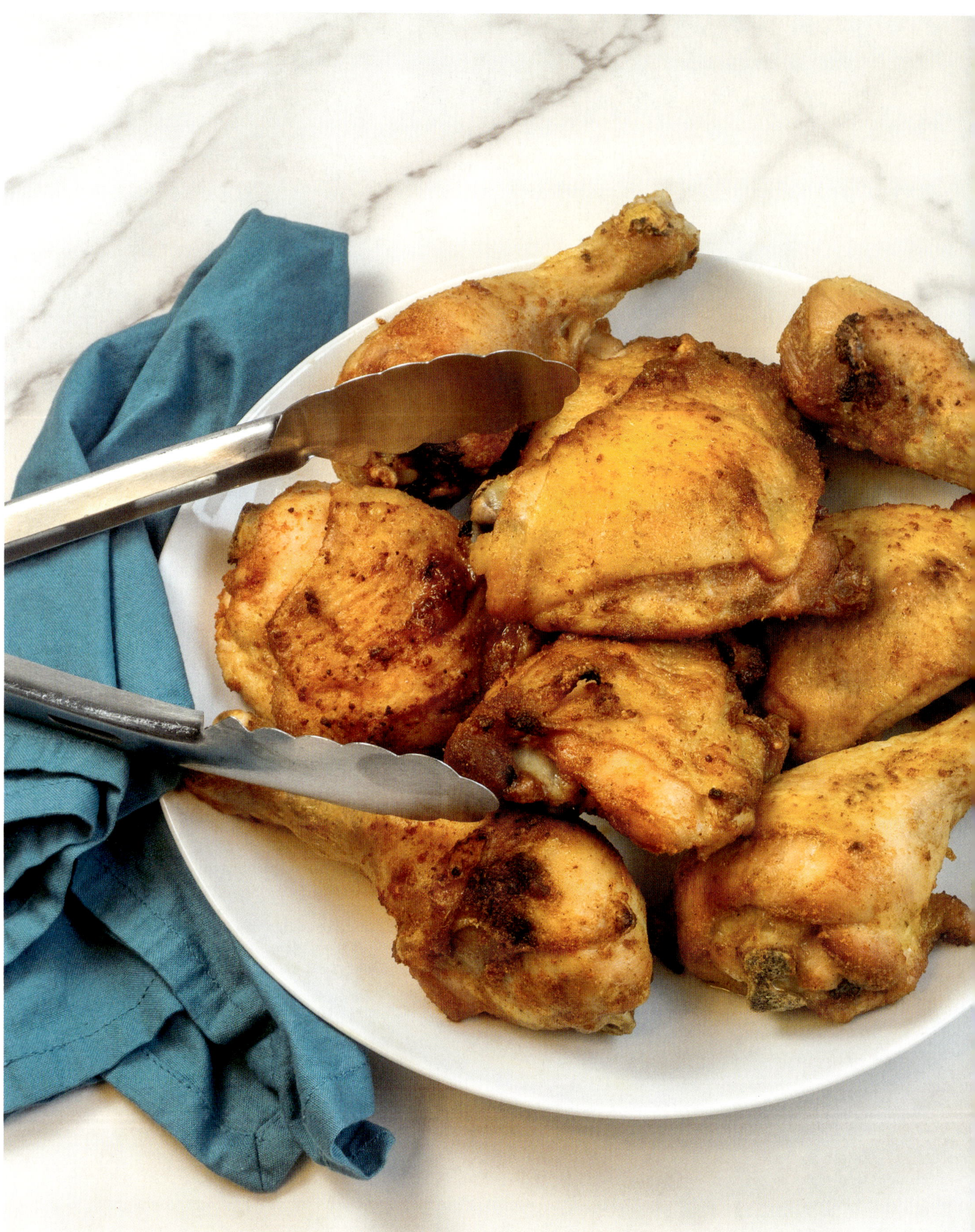

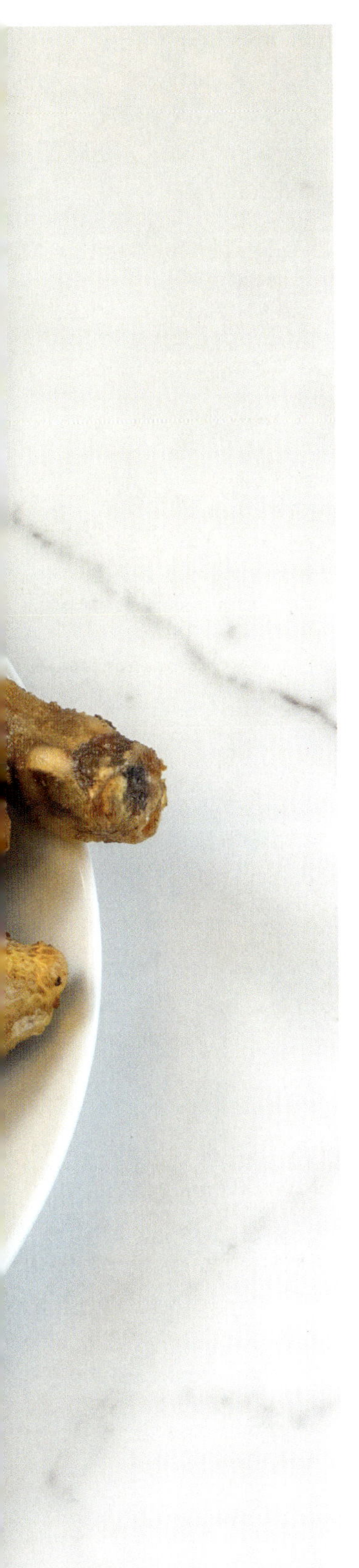

CHAPTER 9
CARNIVORE STAPLES

194 Rendered Tallow

197 Basted Ribeye

198 Prime Rib

201 Walleye

202 King Crab

205 Roasted Bone Marrow

206 Brisket

208 Burgers with Benefits

211 Crispy Baked Chicken Thighs & Drumsticks

212 Dehydrated Ground Meat

215 Egg Pudding

216 Cornish Hen

219 Slow Cooker Pot Roast

220 Wings

222 Pljeskavica (Serbian Burgers)

225 Ćevaps (Serbian Sausages)

YIELD: 2 cups (1 tablespoon per serving)

PREP TIME: 10 minutes

COOK TIME: 2 hours

RENDERED TALLOW

Rendering tallow is an essential skill on the carnivore diet. Tallow is simply rendered beef fat, and it's incredibly versatile in cooking. I save the excess fat I trim off steaks or get trimmings from my local butcher or grocery store. You can cook with it just like you would any other animal fat or incorporate it into recipes like my Whipped Tallow Bites (page 342). It's a great way to make use of every part of the animal and add rich flavor to your dishes.

2 pounds beef fat

1 Cut the fat into 1-inch cubes.

2 Place in a large cast-iron frying pan and cook over medium-low heat, ladling out the rendered liquid fat every 30 minutes.

3 Continue cooking down the fat until it is crispy and no longer releasing liquid fat, about 2 hours. You can eat these crispy fat bits or throw them in the air fryer to make them even crispier.

4 Strain the liquid fat through a fine-mesh strainer into a pint-sized glass storage container. Two pounds of fat will render down to 2 cups of tallow. Store in the fridge for up to 2 years.

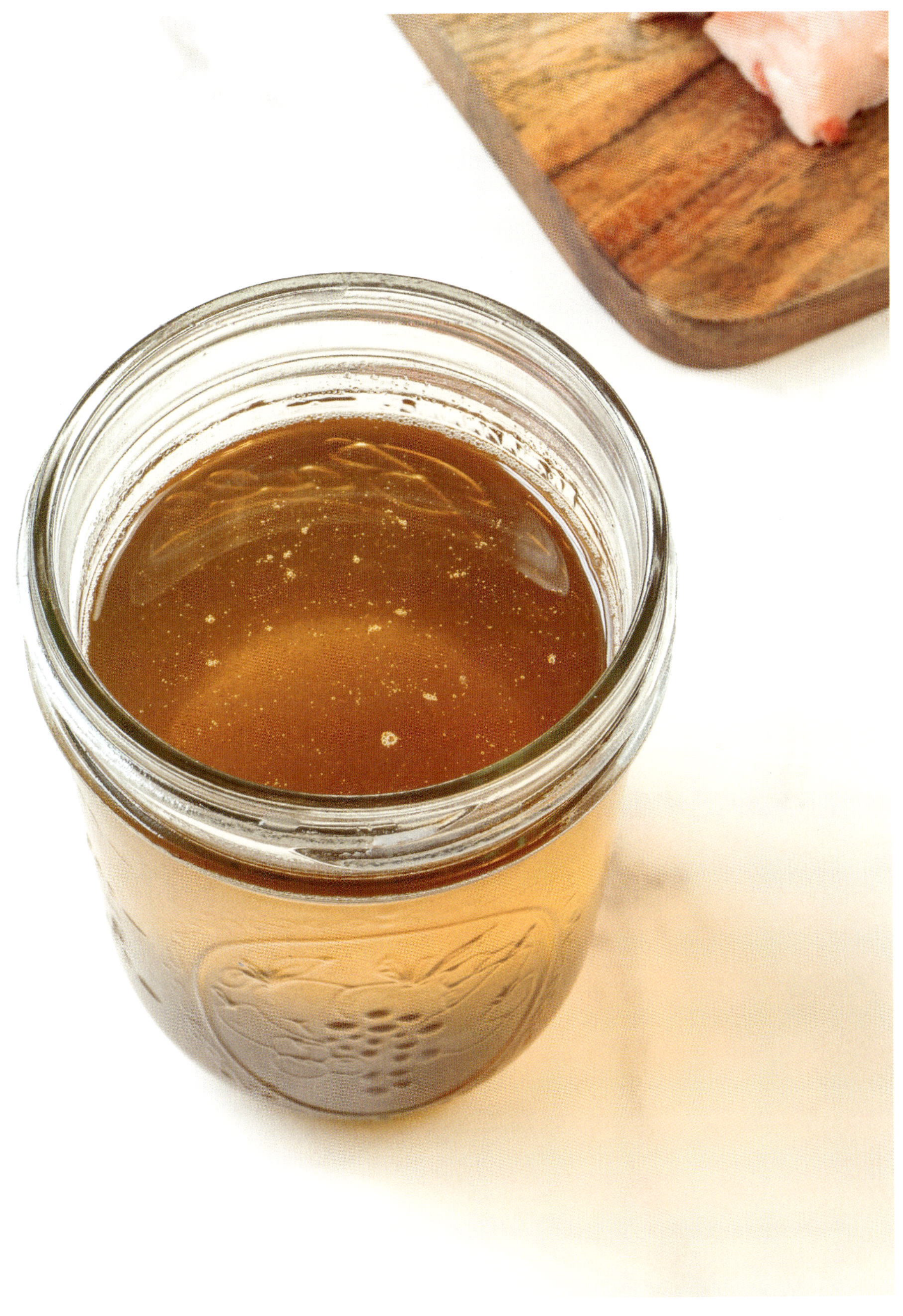

PER SERVING

calories: **115** | fat: **13g** | protein: **0g** | carbs: **0g** | macro split: **100/0/0**

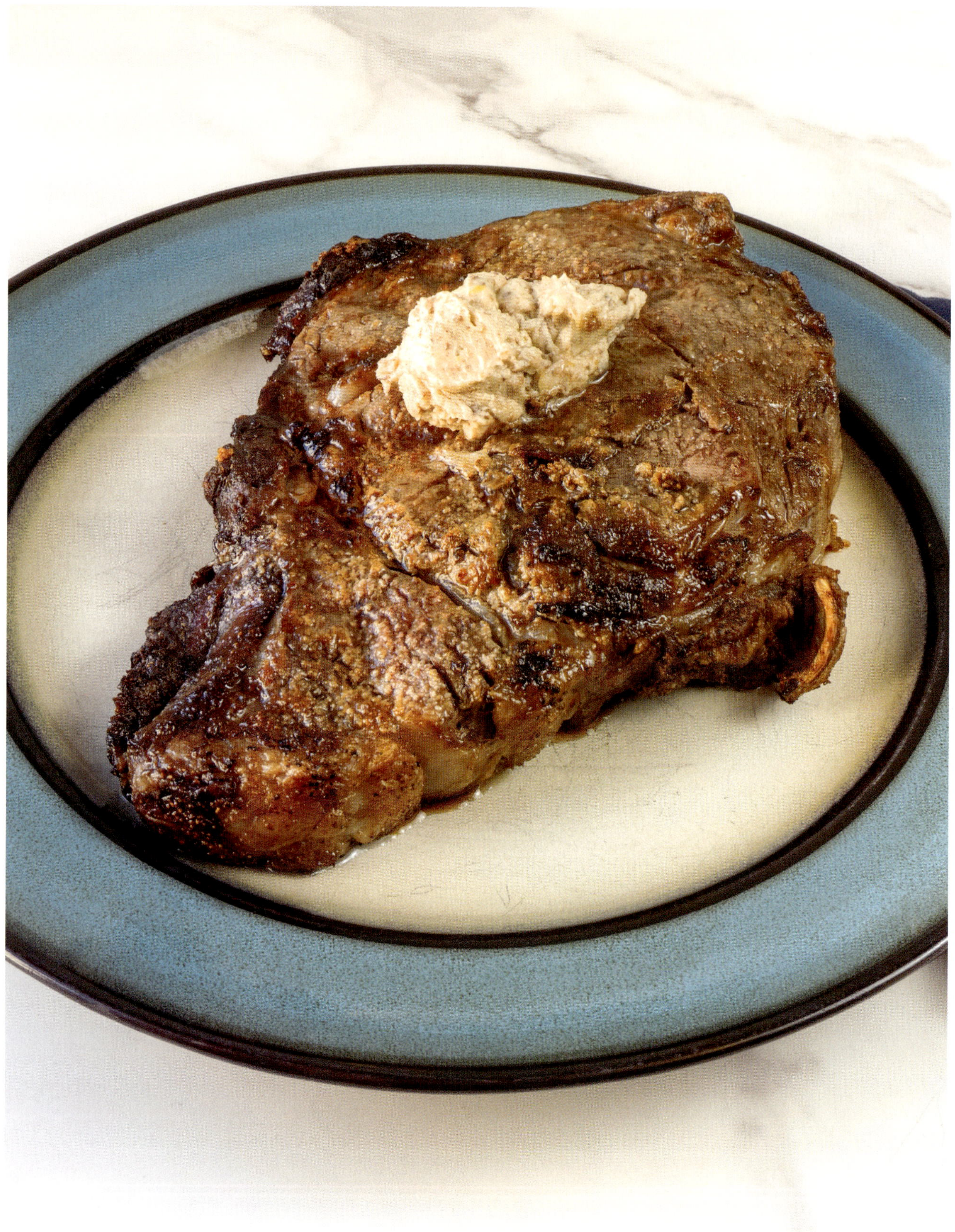

PER STEAK

calories: **1531** | fat: **128g** | protein: **95g** | carbs: **0g** | macro split: **75/25/0**

YIELD: 1 serving

PREP TIME: 5 minutes

COOK TIME: 15 minutes

BASTED RIBEYE

When I'm craving a special treat, I prepare ribeye this way. The combination of butter and bacon grease adds a rich, savory depth of flavor that makes every bite irresistible. This method doesn't take much longer than cooking a steak on the grill or in an air fryer, but the result tastes like you've spent hours perfecting it. It's a simple yet indulgent way to elevate your steak experience! I like to top mine with some Bone Marrow Butter (page 359).

1 (16-ounce) boneless ribeye steak, 1 to 1½ inches thick

1 teaspoon salt

1 teaspoon garlic powder (optional)

½ cup (1 stick) salted butter, divided

½ cup bacon grease

1. Preheat a large cast-iron or other heavy frying pan over medium-high heat.
2. While the pan is heating up, season the steak on both sides with the salt and garlic powder, if using. Insert a meat thermometer in the thickest part of the steak.
3. Put 1 tablespoon of the butter in the hot pan. Once the butter has melted and is smoking a bit, place the steak in the pan. Sear for 1 to 2 minutes on each side, until there is a nice golden brown crust on both sides.
4. Add the remaining butter and the bacon grease to the pan and lower the heat to medium. Using a spoon, baste the steak with the fat. Flip the steak at least once for even cooking and browning.
5. Cook to an internal temperature of 125°F for medium-rare or 130°F for medium, then remove the steak from the pan. Place on a cutting board or plate and allow to rest for 5 minutes before serving. The temperature will continue to rise a few degrees as it rests, so be sure to pull it from the pan once it reaches the desired temperature to avoid overcooking.

YIELD: 5 to 6 servings

PREP TIME: 15 minutes, plus 12 hours to marinate

COOK TIME: 2 hours 20 minutes to 3 hours 20 minutes

PRIME RIB

In our family, prime rib is a winter tradition, especially for New Year's Eve. Essentially, it's just a large ribeye, but roasting the beef low and slow with a rich coating of herb butter transforms this cut into a tender, melt-in-your-mouth delight.

½ cup (1 stick) salted butter

1½ tablespoons minced fresh rosemary

1 teaspoon salt

1 teaspoon ground white pepper

6 cloves garlic, peeled

1 (5- to 6-pound) bone-in prime rib

½ cup bacon grease

1 Put the butter in a small microwave-safe bowl and microwave for 30 seconds to soften. Then add the rosemary, salt, and pepper and mix with a spoon. Using a garlic press, squeeze the garlic into the bowl with the butter mixture and stir to incorporate.

2 Spread the herb butter all over the exterior of the prime rib. Place on a 13 by 9-inch sheet pan (aka quarter sheet pan) fitted with a wire rack and refrigerate uncovered for 12 to 16 hours. (Note: A smaller pan is ideal here because you are placing the pan in the fridge.)

3 Preheat the oven to 450°F. Remove the prime rib from the refrigerator and insert a meat thermometer. Place the prime rib in a large cast-iron or other oven-safe frying pan and bake for 20 minutes.

4 Turn the oven temperature down to 325°F and bake to an internal temperature of 125°F for medium-rare or 130°F for medium. This will take anywhere from 2 to 3 hours, depending on the exact size of the prime rib. Do not turn up the oven; low and slow heat is what you want.

5 Allow to rest for 10 to 15 minutes before carving. The temperature will continue to rise a few degrees, so be sure to remove it from the oven when it hits your desired temperature, or it will be overcooked.

6 Once it is done resting, carve with a sharp knife and serve.

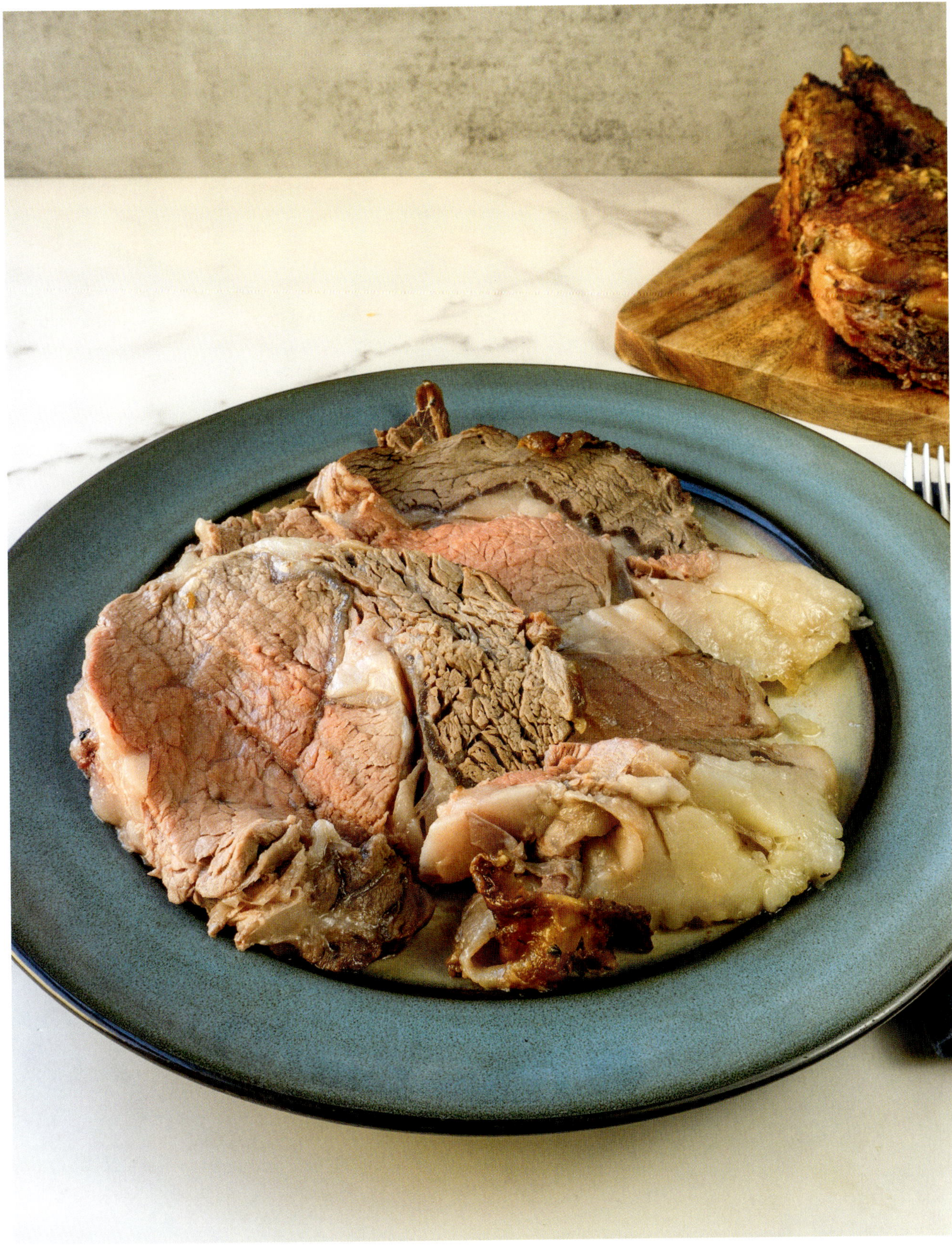

PER SERVING (1 pound)	calories: **1094**	fat: **78g**	protein: **88g**	carbs: **1g**	macro split: **66/33/0**

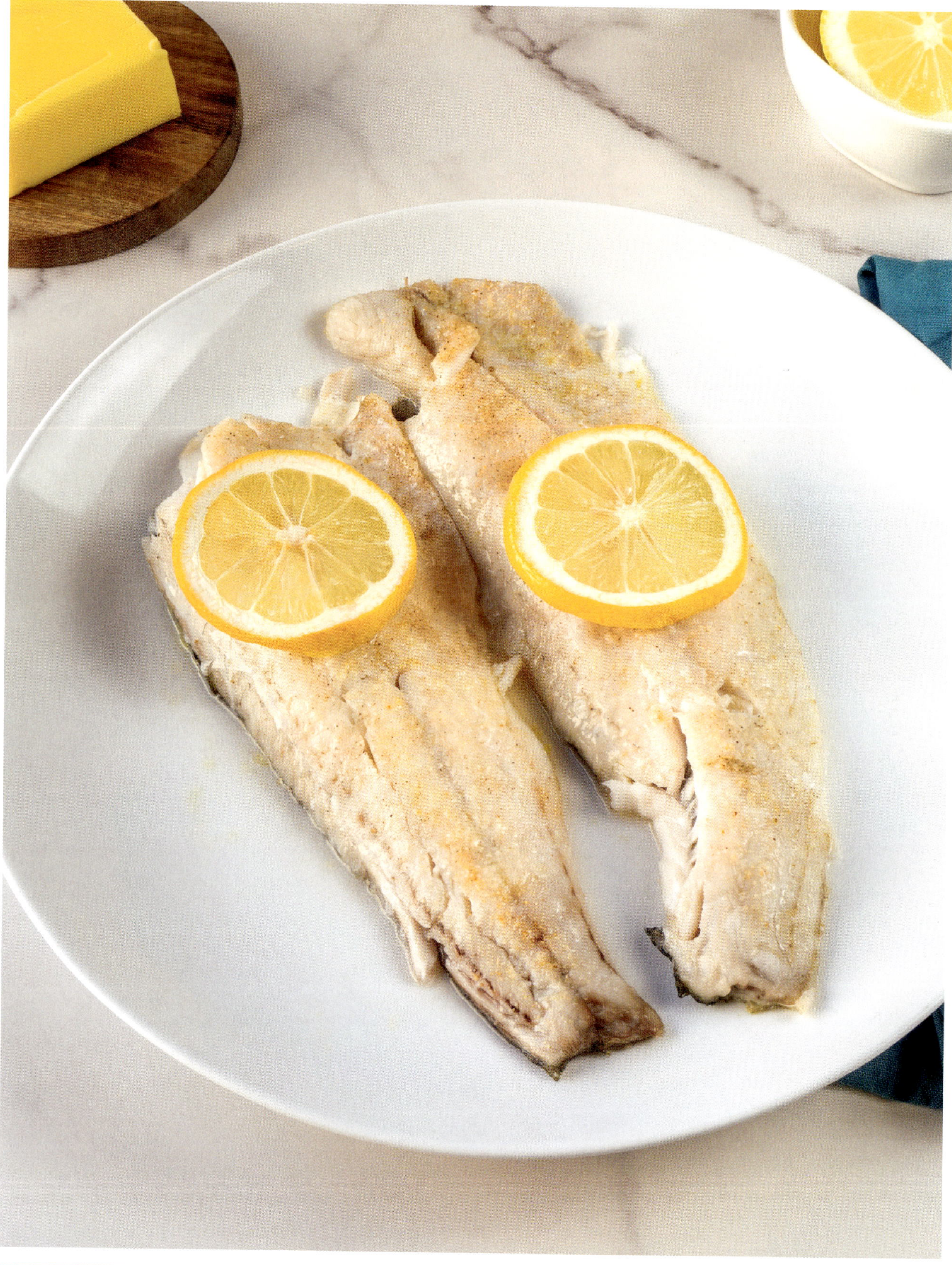

PER SERVING

calories: **311** | fat: **13g** | protein: **43g** | carbs: **0g** | macro split: **42/58/0**

YIELD: 2 servings

PREP TIME: 5 minutes

COOK TIME: 13 to 20 minutes, depending on method

WALLEYE

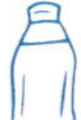

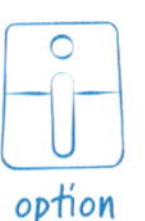

The first time I prepared walleye, I was pleasantly surprised by its bright, mild flavor. It's a delicate, flaky white fish that has a subtle sweetness to it, and when cooked with butter, it reminds me of fresh popcorn! Walleye is an excellent freshwater fish choice, offering a clean, non-fishy taste that even those who aren't big fish fans will enjoy. Plus, it's packed with omega-3s, making it a great addition to round out your carnivore diet. I always cook the fish in my air fryer because it is quick and easy, but you can use an oven as well; I have included instructions for both methods.

- 2 (8-ounce) fresh or frozen skin-on walleye fillets (thawed if frozen)
- 1 teaspoon salt
- 1 teaspoon ground white pepper
- 1 teaspoon garlic powder
- 2 tablespoons salted butter
- 2 to 4 lemon slices (optional)
- 1 tablespoon freshly squeezed lemon juice (optional)

1. If using the oven, preheat it to 400°F. Fit a sheet pan with a wire rack.
2. Lay the fish fillets skin side down on the wire rack or, if using an air fryer, in the air fryer basket (both fillets if you can fit them). Season the fillets with the salt, pepper, and garlic powder. Place 1 tablespoon of butter on each fillet, along with a lemon slice or two, if using.
3. Bake for 15 to 20 minutes or air-fry at 380°F for 12 to 13 minutes, until the fish is white and flaky.
4. Before serving, drizzle the lemon juice over the fillets, if desired.

YIELD: 2 servings

PREP TIME: 5 minutes

COOK TIME: 6 minutes

KING CRAB

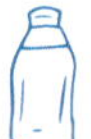

King crab is a special treat we look forward to every New Year's Eve. Though it's a bit pricey, we always splurge and pick up a few pounds to enjoy. This simple recipe is hearty enough to serve as a full meal on its own, or you can pair it with Prime Rib (page 198), like we do, for a truly indulgent feast. It's a festive way to kick off the new year with a delicious, memorable meal.

3 pounds fresh or frozen king crab legs, Alaskan or southern

6 tablespoons (¾ stick) salted butter, melted, for serving

1 lemon, halved, for serving

1. If the crab legs are frozen, allow them to thaw in the refrigerator for 4 to 6 hours.
2. Set a stockpot on the stove and place a wire rack inside it. You want to elevate the crab legs out of the water, so use whatever you have on hand (a metal steamer basket would also work). Pour in enough water to reach the top of the rack or whatever you use. Turn the heat to medium-high and bring the water to a boil.
3. Once the water is boiling, add the crab legs to the pot and cover. Steam for 5 to 6 minutes, until the meat is reddish pink and hot to the touch. Don't overcook it, or the meat will get rubbery.
4. Remove the crab legs from the pot and place on a large serving plate. Serve with the butter and lemon halves.

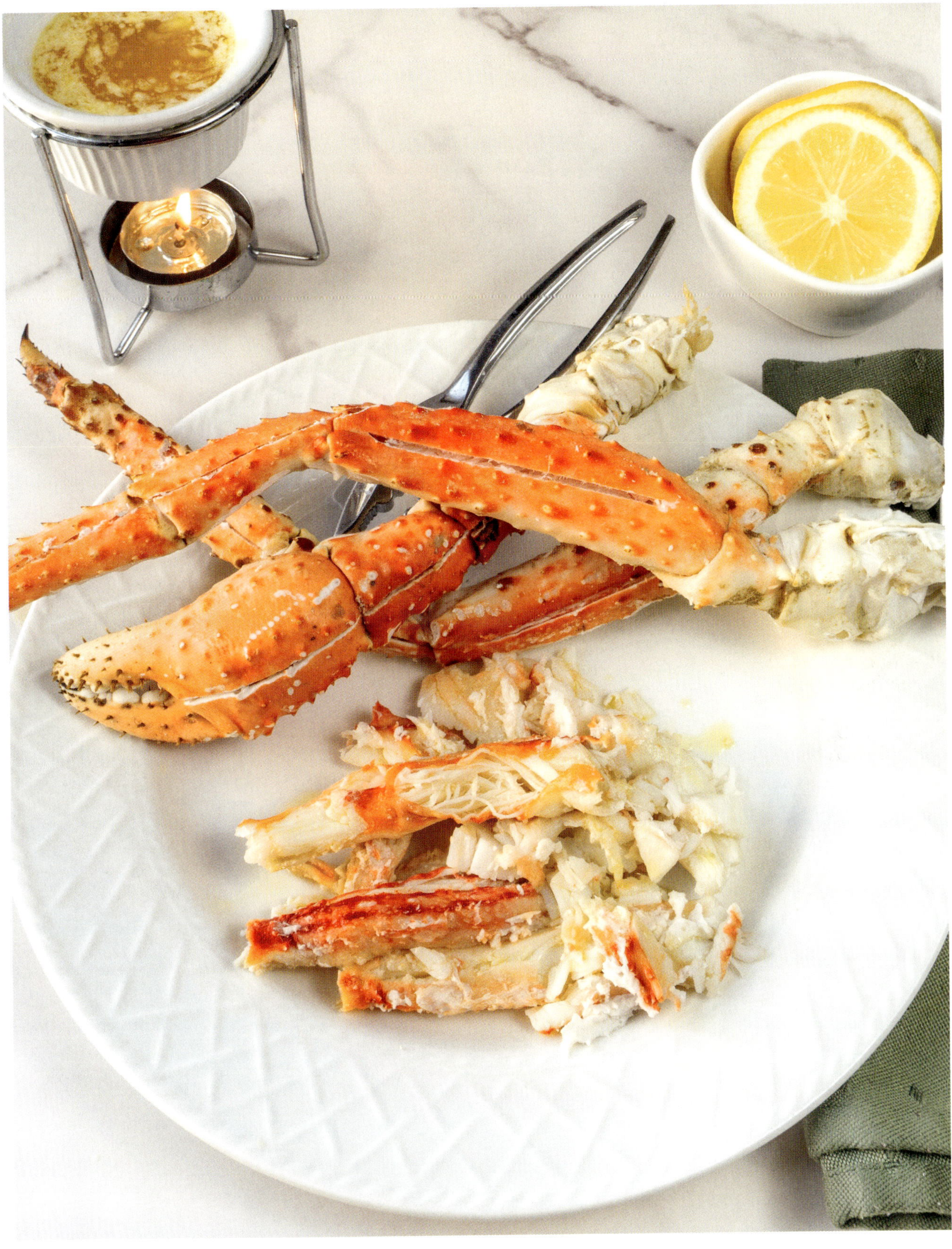

PER SERVING

calories: 690 | fat: 39g | protein: 77g | carbs: 0g | macro split: 53/47/0

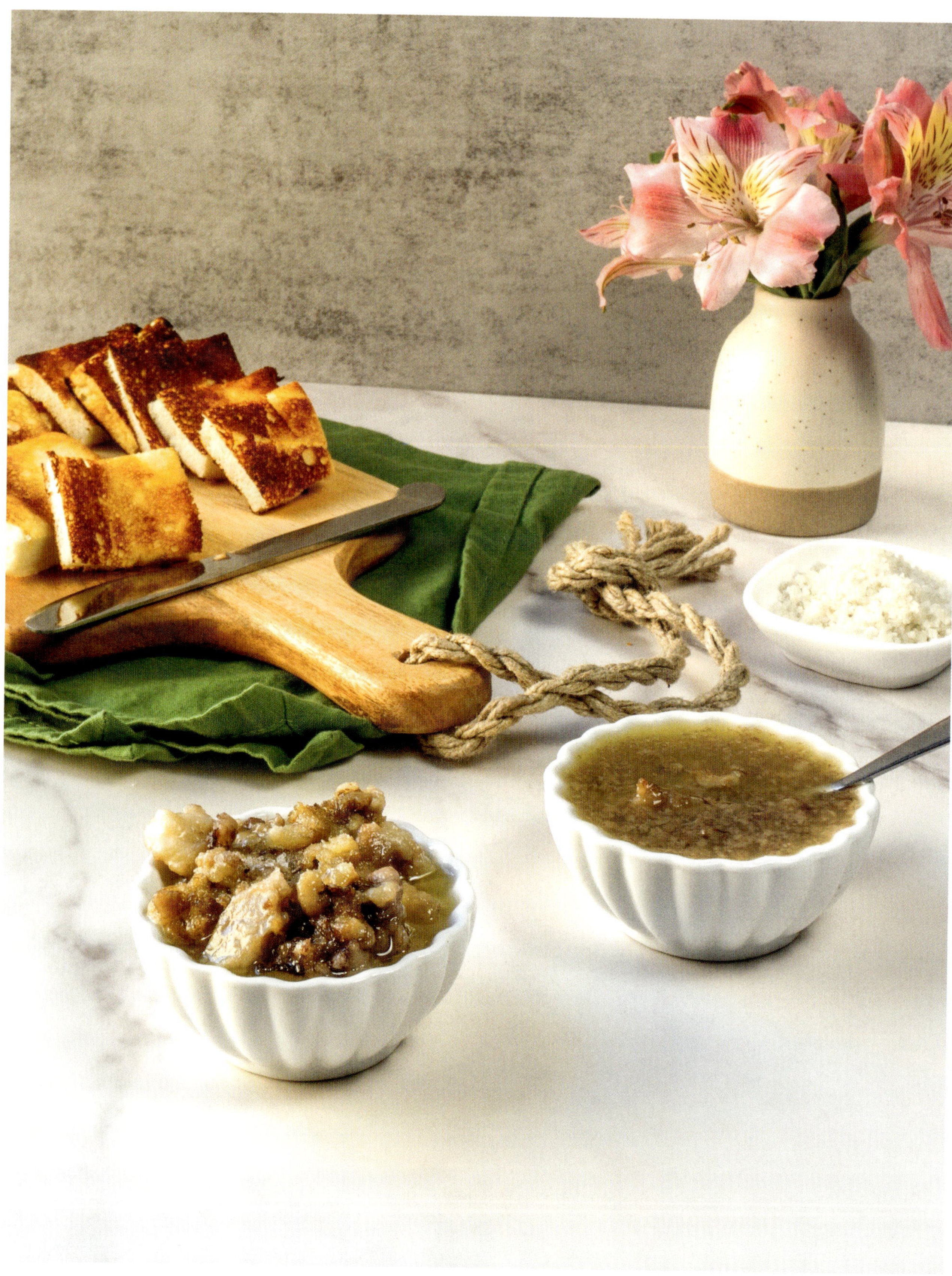

PER SERVING (1 tablespoon, marrow only)	calories: **104** | fat: **11g** | protein: **1g** | carbs: **0g** | macro split: **98/2/0**

YIELD: 4 servings

PREP TIME: 5 minutes

COOK TIME: 30 to 40 minutes, depending on cut of marrow bone used

ROASTED BONE MARROW

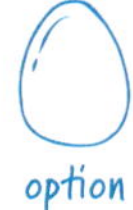

Whenever my husband and I spot bone marrow on a restaurant menu, we can't resist ordering it. As an ancestral food, bone marrow deserves a regular place in the human diet. Preparing it at home might seem a bit intimidating at first, but once you try it, you'll see it's surprisingly simple. You can enjoy the marrow as is with a spoon or—my preference—spread it on a slice of toasted cloud bread. The marrow can be scooped right out of the bone (bowl 1) or pureed (bowl 2). I like to sprinkle it with some sea salt (bowl 3).

8 beef marrow bones, cut crosswise or lengthwise into canoes

1 teaspoon salt

½ teaspoon garlic powder (optional)

Cloud Bread Loaf (page 372), sliced and toasted, for serving (optional)

1. Preheat the oven to 375°F. Fit a sheet pan with a wire rack. The rack will allow heat to circulate around the bones.
2. Place the marrow bones on the rack. If they are cut crosswise, place them standing up; if cut lengthwise, place them on the rack cut side up.
3. Bake for 30 to 40 minutes, depending on the thickness of the bones and the way they are cut. Canoe-cut bones will cook faster than cross-cut chunks. For canoe-cut bones, you can use the color of the marrow to determine doneness: When it turns a brownish gray color, the marrow is fully cooked. For cross-cut chunks, test for doneness by inserting a skewer through the length of the marrow. If it slides in easily, the marrow is done; if there is still some resistance, cook the bones a bit more.
4. To serve, spoon out all of the marrow into a bowl. With canoe-cut bones, you have the option of plating the bones so that the marrow can be spooned directly from the bones at the table.
5. Season with the salt and garlic powder, if using, and serve on toasted cloud bread, if desired.

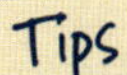

Reserve the liquid fat that collects in the sheet pan to make the bone marrow mayonnaise on page 355.

YIELD: 20 to 30 servings

PREP TIME: 10 minutes, plus 3 hours to marinate

COOK TIME: 6 to 12 hours

BRISKET

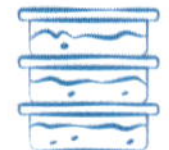

Brisket is my favorite barbecue meat, especially the fattier cuts, so I was eager to learn how to make it myself. For a carnivore, a smoker is an invaluable tool for outdoor cooking because it's so versatile, but brisket can also be made in the oven. I've included instructions for both methods to give you options. It is essential that you cook this cut of meat slowly, otherwise it will turn out dry and tough.

1 (10- to 15-pound) beef brisket

1 to 2 cups prepared yellow mustard (according to size of brisket)

10 to 15 tablespoons BBQ Spice Rub (page 347) (1 tablespoon per pound of brisket)

FOR THE SPRITZ:

1 cup apple cider vinegar

1 cup water

SPECIAL EQUIPMENT: Smoker, hardwood pellets or chips for smoke (optional)

1. Cut the brisket into two pieces if it will not fit into your smoker or oven. Remove any silverskin or excess fat (but not too much—the fat is the best part!).
2. Spread the mustard over one side of the brisket, then sprinkle the mustard-coated meat with half of the BBQ spice rub and pat down to create a "bark" or coating. Flip the brisket and repeat on the other side with the remaining mustard and spice rub.
3. Wrap in aluminum foil or butcher paper and refrigerate for 3 to 24 hours.
4. When ready to cook, preheat the smoker or oven to 225°F.
5. Unwrap the brisket(s) and insert a temperature probe(s) in the center. Place on a rack in the smoker or on a sheet pan in the oven. Make sure the point or thickest part of the brisket is closest to the heat source. Your goal is to cook this low and slow. It is going to take some time, typically a total of 6 to 12 hours. If using a smoker, add wood chips as needed to keep it nice and smoky.
6. After the first 3 to 4 hours in the smoker or oven, combine the vinegar and water in a clean, food-safe spray bottle and start spritzing the meat. Don't soak it; just spritz the edges a bit. Do this every 30 to 60 minutes to help the bark formation.
7. Once the internal temperature reaches 165°F to 175°F, pull the brisket and wrap it in unlined butcher paper, then place it back in the smoker or oven. If using a smoker, you no longer need to add wood chips.

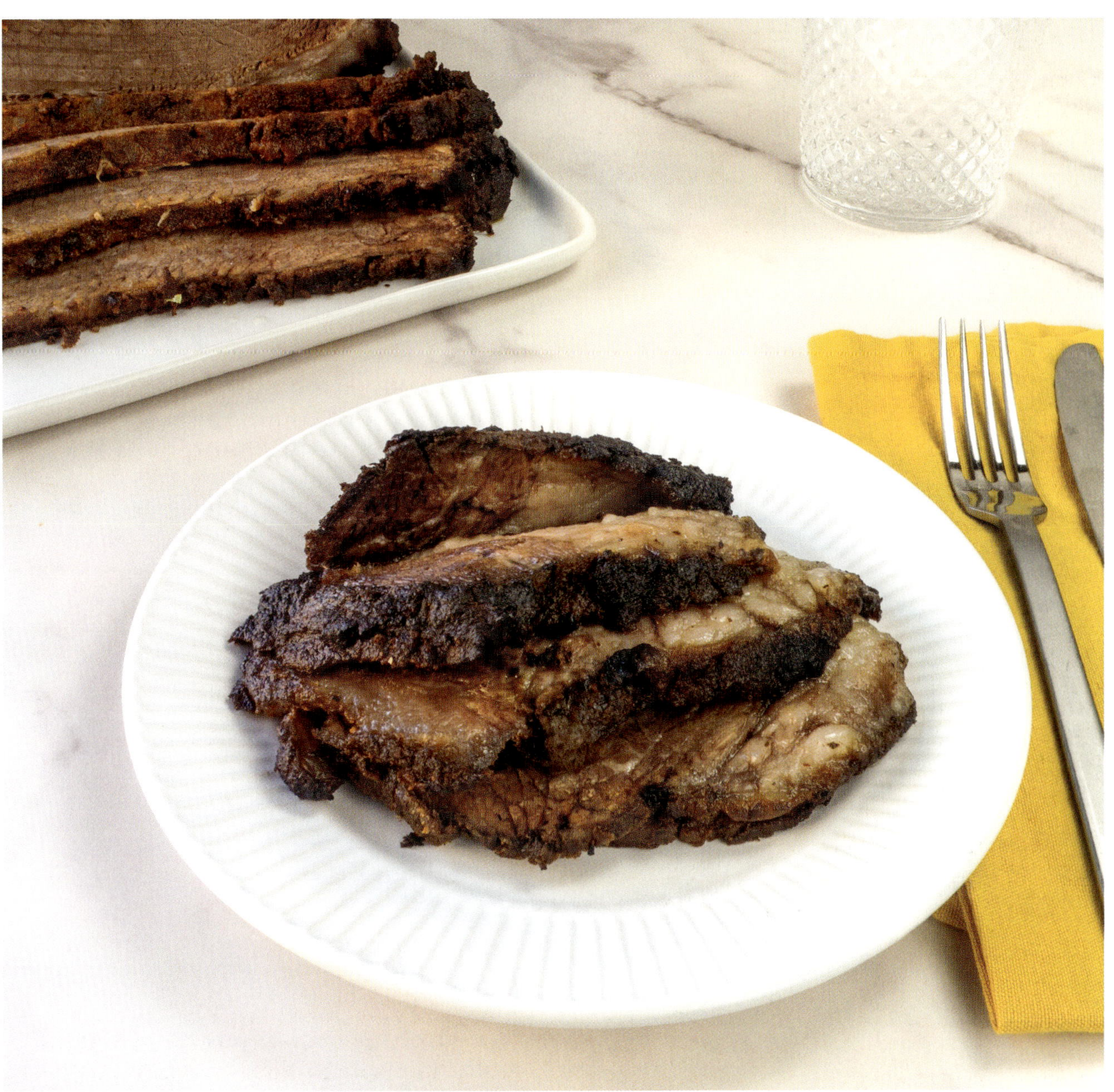

8 Continue to cook the brisket until it reaches 202°F to 205°F. Allow to rest, still wrapped, until the internal temperature has dropped to 180°F to 185°F. This could take up to an hour, depending on the exact size of your brisket. Then place it in the refrigerator to continue cooling; once the temperature reaches 140°F, it is ready to slice and serve. I like to cut the brisket into a few large chunks and then wrap each in aluminum foil or plastic wrap to store in the fridge for up to a week. Then I can pull a chunk out of the fridge and slice off whatever I am going to eat.

PER SERVING (8 ounces) calories: **595** | fat: **46g** | protein: **39g** | carbs: **0g** | macro split: **72/28/0**

YIELD: 8 burgers (1 per serving)

PREP TIME: 20 minutes

COOK TIME: 8 or 32 minutes, depending on method

BURGERS WITH BENEFITS

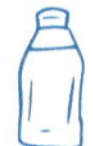

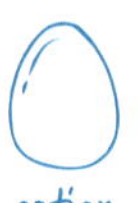

Everyone knows how to make a basic burger, but I love elevating this classic to something truly special. My favorite trick is rummaging through the fridge to find cheeses and meats to chop up and mix into the ground beef. The result? Flavor-packed patties with delicious surprises hidden inside. Today, I'm sharing three of my go-to variations: bacon cheddar, ham and cheese, and blue cheese bacon. Each one brings a unique twist to the beloved burger! You can eat these with a fork and knife or whip up some cloud buns for a handheld option. These are best cooked on the grill, but you could also use a frying pan on the stove.

2 pounds 80/20 ground beef

2 teaspoons salt

2 teaspoons garlic powder

8 Cloud Buns (page 372), split (optional)

FOR BACON CHEDDAR BURGERS:

1 cup chopped bacon (about 8 thick-cut strips)

1 cup diced cheddar cheese

8 slices cheddar cheese, for topping

FOR HAM AND CHEESE BURGERS:

1 cup diced ham

1 cup diced cheddar cheese

8 slices cheddar cheese, for topping

FOR BLUE CHEESE BACON BURGERS:

2 cups blue cheese crumbles, divided

1 cup chopped bacon (about 8 thick-cut strips)

1. Put the ground beef, salt, and garlic powder in a large bowl and mix thoroughly with your hands.
2. If you're making the bacon cheddar or ham and cheese burgers, add the first two ingredients listed for that variation (the chopped bacon and diced cheddar or the diced ham and cheese); if making the blue cheese bacon burgers, add 1 cup of the blue cheese crumbles and the chopped bacon. Thoroughly mix the add-ins into the beef.
3. Divide the meat mixture into eight evenly sized balls, then shape each ball into a 4-inch patty using your hands.
4. If grilling the burgers, preheat the grill to medium, then place the patties on the grill. Cook, uncovered, for 3 to 4 minutes, then flip and cook for another 3 to 4 minutes for medium-done burgers.

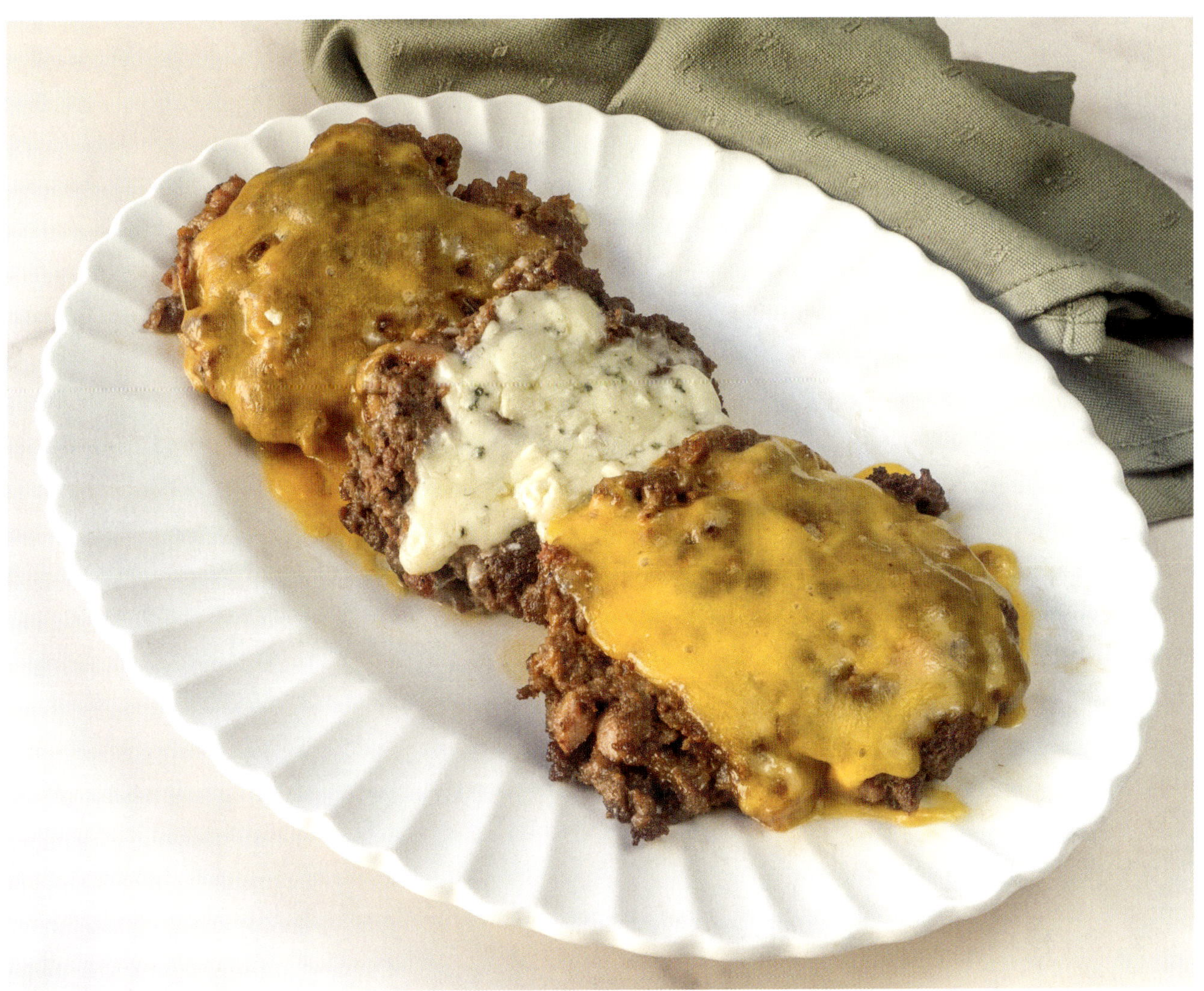

If cooking the burgers on the stovetop, preheat a large frying pan over medium heat. (The patties will release a lot of fat, so there is no need to add a cooking fat.) Cook two or three patties at a time for 3 to 4 minutes per side.

5 When the burgers are almost done, top each bacon cheddar or ham and cheese patty with a slice of cheddar cheese; if making the blue cheese bacon burgers, evenly top the patties with the remaining cup of blue cheese crumbles. Allow the cheese to melt, then remove the patties from the grill or frying pan. Serve as is or on cloud buns.

PER SERVING (bacon cheddar, no bun)	calories: **483** | fat: **39g** | protein: **30g** | carbs: **0g** | macro split: **74/26/0**
PER SERVING (ham and cheese, no bun)	calories: **442** | fat: **35g** | protein: **31g** | carbs: **0g** | macro split: **72/28/0**
PER SERVING (blue cheese bacon, no bun)	calories: **477** | fat: **37g** | protein: **20g** | carbs: **1g** | macro split: **73/26/0**

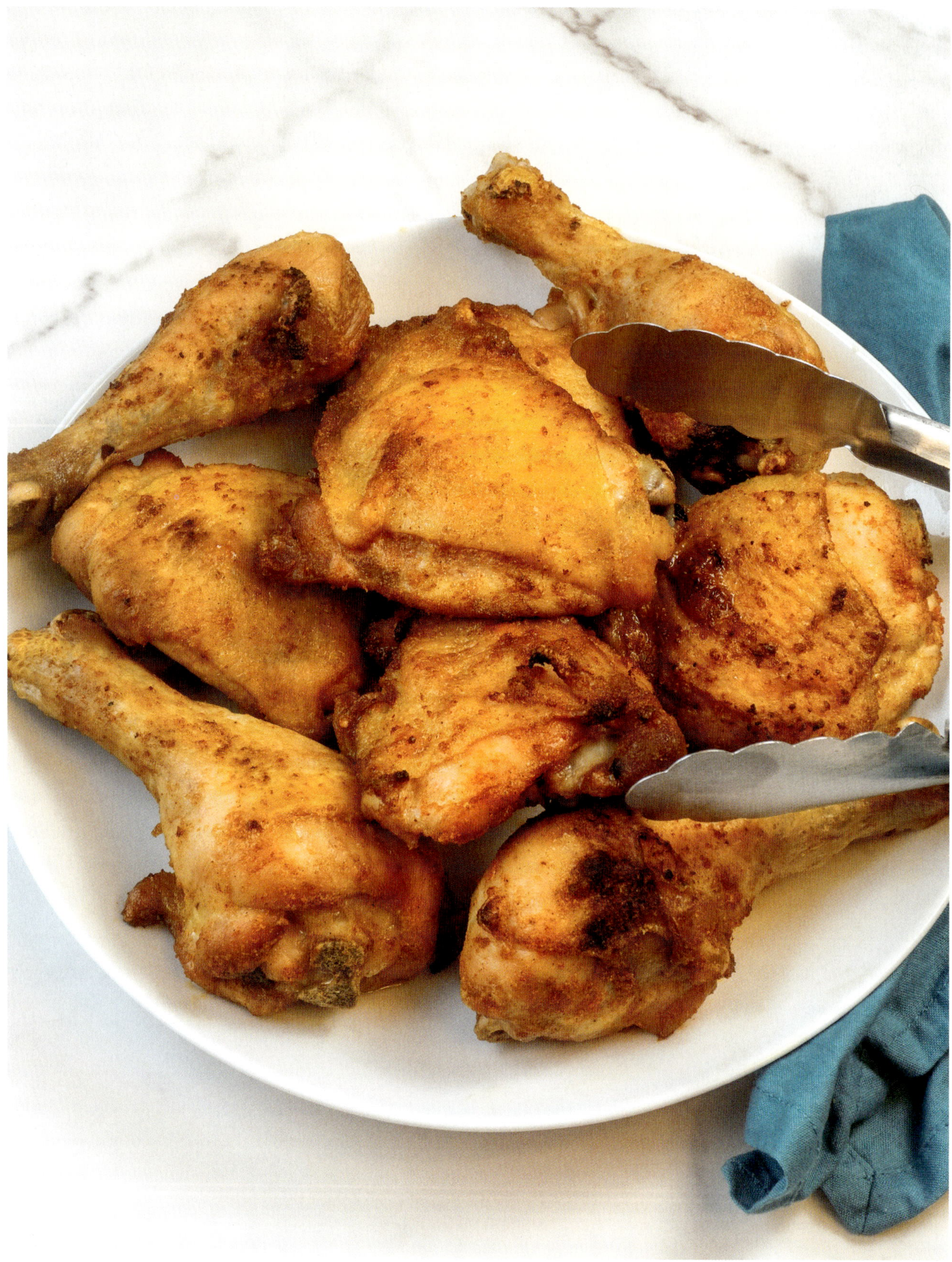

PER SERVING

calories: **352** | fat: **19g** | protein: **42g** | carbs: **0g** | macro split: **51/49/0**

YIELD: 6 servings

PREP TIME: 10 minutes

COOK TIME: 40 minutes

CRISPY BAKED CHICKEN THIGHS & DRUMSTICKS

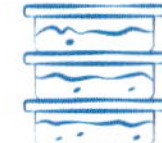

Enjoy perfectly baked bone-in chicken with irresistibly crispy skin. This recipe ensures tender, juicy meat with a golden, crunchy crust that's full of flavor—ideal for a quick weeknight meal or a crowd-pleasing main dish. I like to prepare a big batch of this chicken and keep it in the fridge for up to 5 days. I just reheat it in the microwave or air fryer, and sometimes I eat it cold!

6 bone-in, skin-on chicken thighs

6 chicken drumsticks

2 tablespoons avocado oil

2 to 4 tablespoons Chicken & Pork Seasoning (page 348)

1. Preheat the oven to 425°F. Fit a sheet pan with a wire rack and set aside.
2. Put the chicken thighs and drumsticks in a large bowl and cover with the avocado oil. Toss the chicken with your hands to ensure all sides are coated. Then add the Chicken & Pork Seasoning 1 tablespoon at a time, tossing after each addition to ensure the chicken is well coated. Use at least 2 tablespoons, or up to 4 tablespoons if you want your chicken extra flavorful.
3. Arrange the chicken on the wire rack and insert a meat thermometer into one of the thighs or drumsticks. Bake until the internal temperature reaches 160°F, 35 to 40 minutes, then turn the oven to broil and move the sheet pan to the top rack to crisp up the skin. Remove from the oven when the chicken reaches an internal temperature of 165°F.
4. Allow to cool for about 5 minutes, then serve.

YIELD: 2 cups (¼ cup per serving)

PREP TIME: 5 minutes

COOK TIME: 6 hours 10 minutes

DEHYDRATED GROUND MEAT

Learning to dehydrate ground meat is a valuable skill. I use dehydrated meat in a variety of recipes, including my Whipped Tallow Bites (page 342) and Butter Bites (page 333). It also makes a great coating for meats when ground into a powder. This excellent method for preserving meat allows it to keep for years stored in an airtight container in the refrigerator.

2 pounds 93/7 ground beef, lean pork, chicken, or turkey

1 teaspoon salt

1. Preheat the oven to 200°F. Put a layer of paper towels on a sheet pan and set aside.
2. Place the ground meat in a large frying pan and cook over medium-high heat, crumbling it with a spatula, until no pink remains, 7 to 10 minutes. Salt the meat halfway through cooking.
3. Drain the meat, then pour it onto the prepared sheet pan. Using more paper towels, press out as much of the remaining fat as possible.
4. Remove the paper towels and spread the cooked meat evenly on the pan. Break up any large pieces; you want the meat to be crumbled as finely as possible.
5. Bake for 2 hours.
6. At the 2-hour mark, remove the pan from the oven and move the meat around a bit. Return the pan to the oven and repeat two more times for a total cook time of 6 hours, stirring the meat at the 4-hour mark and then one final time after removing it from the oven. You will know the meat is fully dehydrated when no liquid remains and the meat is hard and crunchy.
7. Store in a glass container in the refrigerator indefinitely.

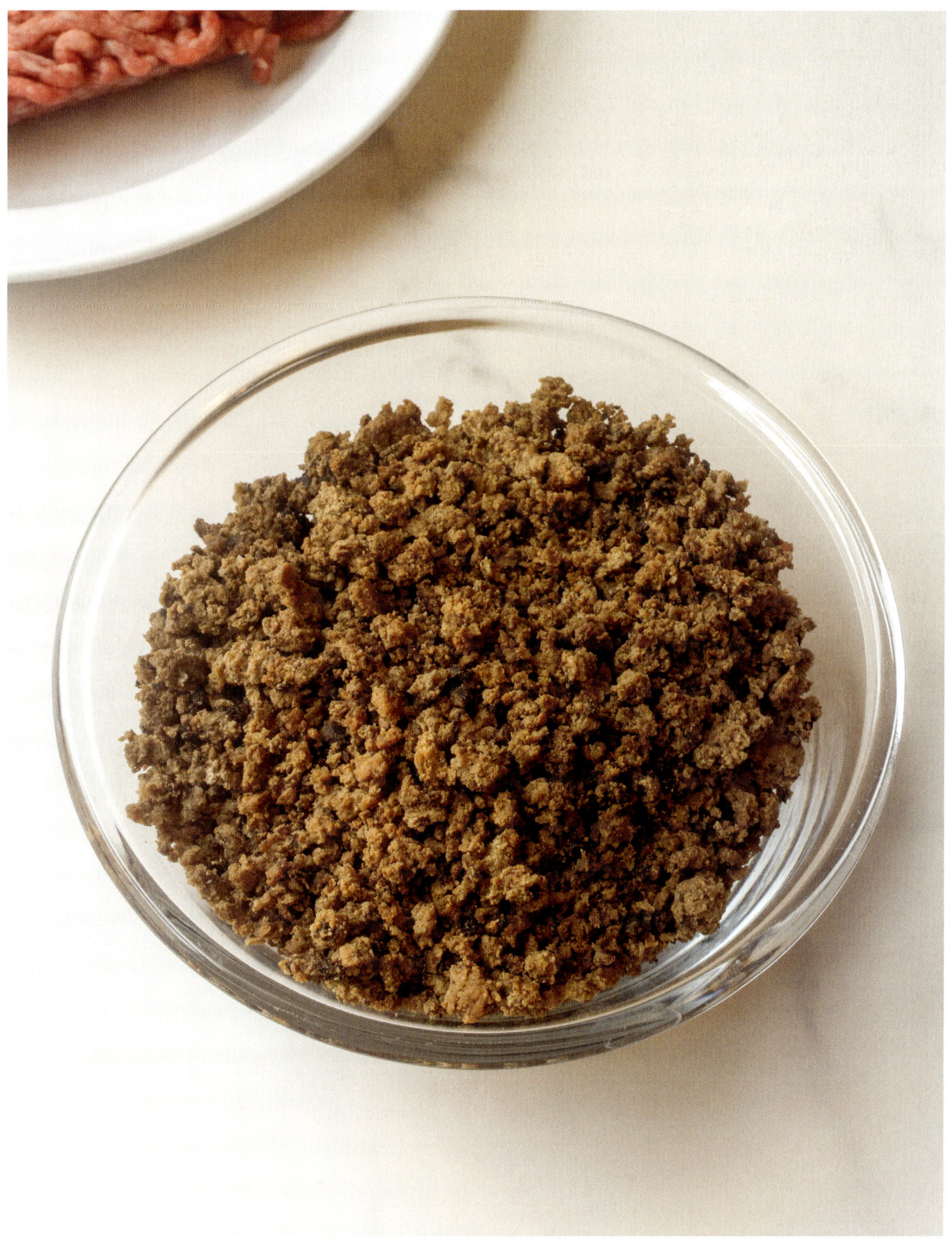

PER SERVING	calories: **172** | fat: **47g** | protein: **62g** | carbs: **0g** | macro split: **41/55/0**

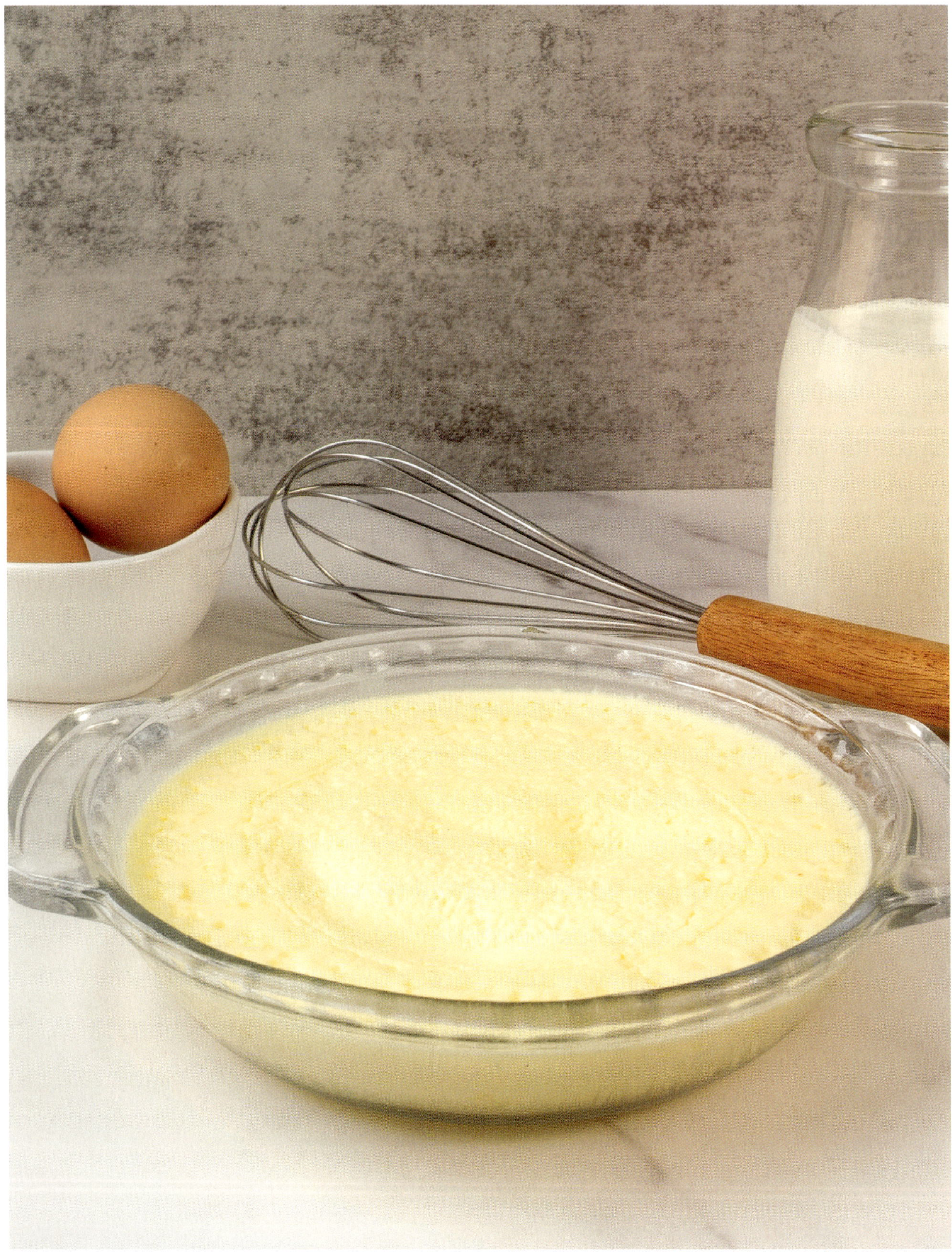

PER SERVING	calories: **551** | fat: **53g** | protein: **16g** | carbs: **4g** | macro split: **86/12/2**

YIELD: 1 serving

PREP TIME: 5 minutes

COOK TIME: 10 to 15 minutes

EGG PUDDING

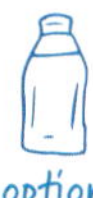

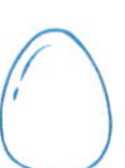

Egg pudding is an easy, versatile treat that can be made savory or sweet. I make mine with heavy cream, but if you're dairy free, bone broth or water will work just as well. For a simple topping, I love adding a dollop of plain mascarpone, but when I want something extra special with a touch of sweetness, I use my Whipped Cream & Mascarpone topping (page 341).

Salted butter, for the pie dish

2 large eggs

½ cup heavy cream, bone broth of choice, or water

SPECIAL EQUIPMENT: 6-inch wire rack, 6-inch glass pie pan

1. Grease a 6-inch glass pie dish with butter. Place a 6-inch wire rack in a 6- to 7-quart Dutch oven or soup pot. Fill the pot with water to just under the top of the rack. Set the pot on the stovetop over medium-high heat and bring the water to a boil.
2. Put the eggs and cream in a small bowl and whisk with a fork until combined.
3. Pour the egg mixture into the prepared pie dish. Set the dish on top of the wire rack in the pot and cover with a lid. Steam for 10 minutes.
4. After 10 minutes, remove the lid. Gently press the back of a spoon onto the surface of the pudding at the center. If the surface is still a bit liquid-y in the center, allow the pudding to cook for a few more minutes. It is done when the entire surface is no longer liquid-y.
5. Remove the pie dish from the pot and let the pudding cool for at least 10 minutes before eating.

YIELD: 2 servings

PREP TIME: 15 minutes, plus 3 hours to marinate

COOK TIME: 40 to 60 minutes, depending on method

CORNISH HEN

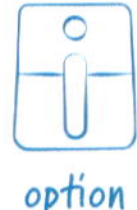

This recipe features perfectly crispy skin and tender, juicy meat seasoned with a dry rub and slathered with a rich rosemary garlic butter. Simple yet flavorful, it's an impressive dish that's perfect for a cozy dinner or a special occasion! You have the option of cooking the hens in the oven or in the air fryer.

2 Cornish game hens (about 4 pounds total)

FOR THE DRY RUB:

1 teaspoon salt

1 teaspoon ground white pepper

1 teaspoon garlic powder

1 teaspoon onion powder

1 teaspoon smoked paprika

FOR THE GARLIC BUTTER:

1 cup (2 sticks) salted butter, at room temperature

5 tablespoons chopped fresh rosemary

4 cloves garlic, crushed through a press

SPECIAL EQUIPMENT: Butcher's twine

1. Place a wire rack in a 13 by 9-inch sheet pan (aka quarter sheet pan). (Note: A smaller pan is ideal here because you will be placing the pan in the refrigerator.)
2. Pat the hens dry and set aside.
3. In a small bowl, mix together all of the ingredients for the dry rub. In a separate bowl, mix the butter with the rosemary and garlic until well blended.
4. Cover all sides of the hens as well as the inside of each cavity with the dry rub.
5. Slather the herbed garlic butter all over each hen, adding a bunch to each cavity. As best you can, try to get some under the skin as well.
6. Using butcher's twine, tie the legs together and tuck in the wings. Then place the hens on the wire rack and refrigerate uncovered for 3 to 12 hours.
7. If using the oven, place an oven rack in the bottom position and preheat the oven to 425°F. Insert a temperature probe into one of the hens and place the pan on the bottom rack of the oven. Pull from the oven when the internal temperature reaches 160°F to 163°F, 50 to 60 minutes.

   If using an air fryer, insert a temperature probe into one of the hens, set to air-fry mode at 330°F, and air-fry for 30 to 40 minutes, until they reach an internal temperature of 150°F. Then turn the heat up to 380°F and continue to cook for about 10 minutes, until the internal temperature reaches 160°F to 163°F.
8. Allow the birds to rest for 10 minutes before serving.

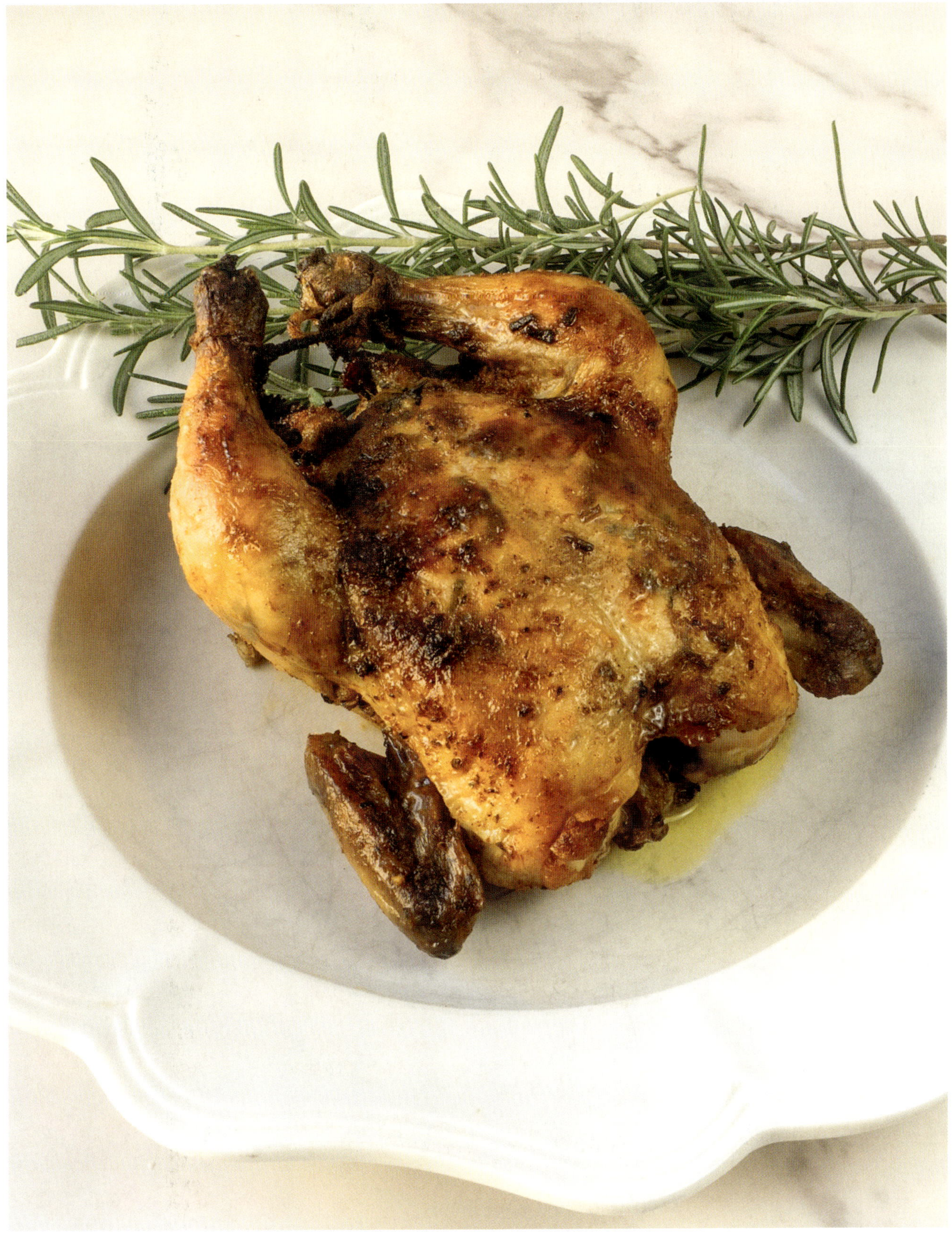

PER SERVING

calories: **670** | fat: **46g** | protein: **57g** | carbs: **0g** | macro split: **65/35/0**

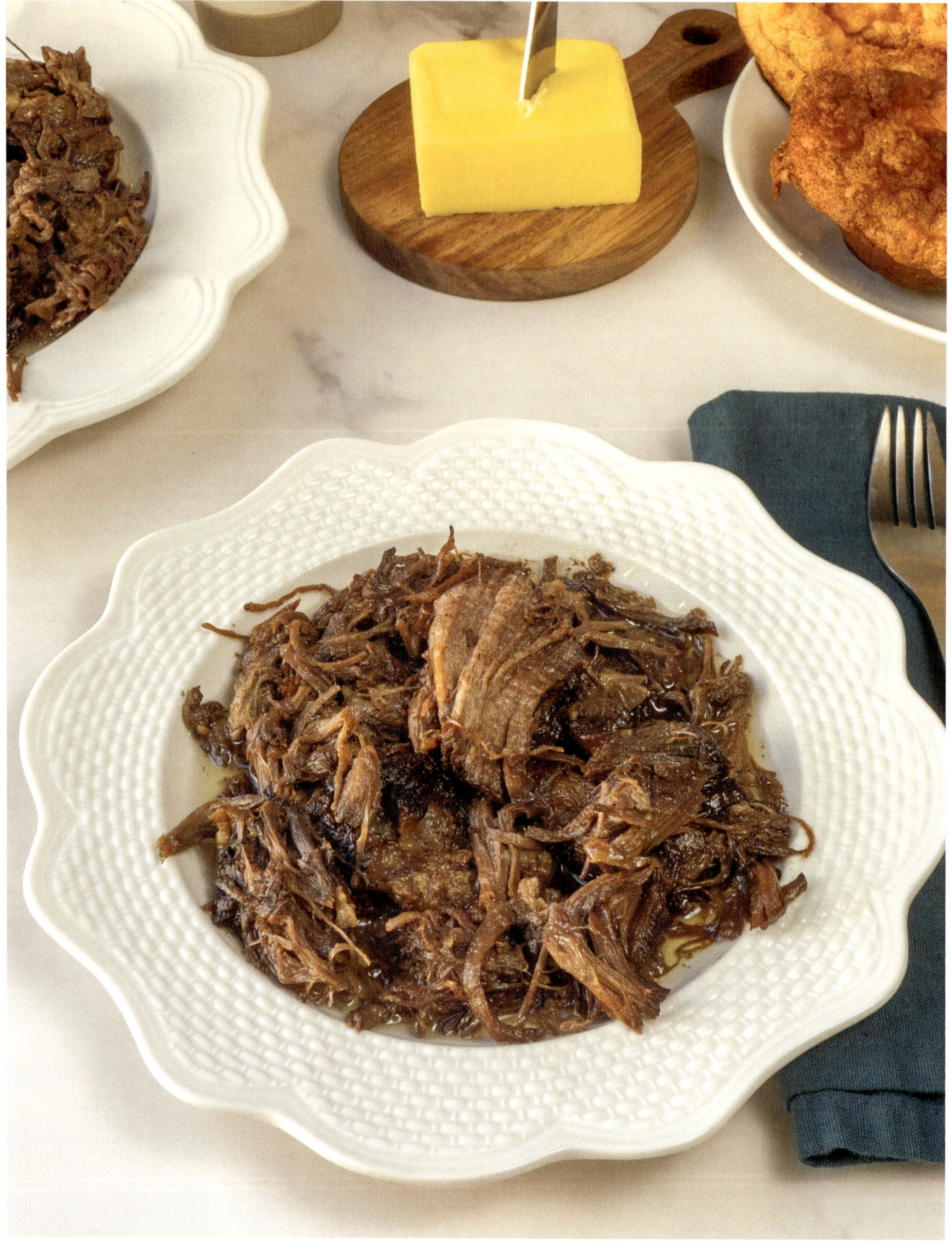

PER SERVING (8 ounces)	calories: **520** | fat: **40g** | protein: **38g** | carbs: **0g** | macro split: **70/30/0**

YIELD: 4 to 6 servings

PREP TIME: 15 minutes

COOK TIME: 6 to 8 hours

SLOW COOKER POT ROAST

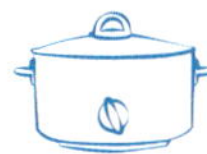
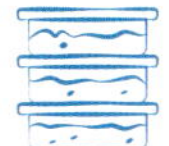

I grew up eating pot roast several times a month, and it was always a family favorite. The only difference between my mother's recipe and mine is that mine doesn't include any plants! I've kept all of the classic flavors, but I've adapted it to fit the carnivore diet. Searing the chuck roast before slow-cooking it really enhances its natural flavor and creates a delicious, caramelized crust. It makes a large batch, so you'll have plenty of leftovers to enjoy for several days, making it a perfect meal to prep in advance and savor throughout the week. I like to serve these with cloud buns (page 372) and butter. If you shred the meat, you can use the buns to make a sandwich (see page 270)!

1 (2- to 3-pound) chuck roast

2 teaspoons liquid smoke

2 teaspoons Worcestershire sauce

1 teaspoon salt

½ teaspoon ground white pepper

½ teaspoon garlic powder

½ teaspoon onion powder

1 tablespoon animal fat of choice (I like to use tallow)

1. Season the chuck roast on both sides with the liquid smoke, Worcestershire sauce, salt, pepper, garlic powder, and onion powder.
2. Preheat a large cast-iron pan or other heavy frying pan over medium-high heat. Add the animal fat to the pan. Once the fat is hot, place the chuck roast in the pan and sear on all sides, 5 to 7 minutes.
3. After searing, place the chuck roast in the slow cooker and cover with the lid. Turn the slow cooker to low and cook the chuck roast for 6 to 8 hours. It is done when it is very tender and falls apart with the slightest touch of a fork.
4. Serve immediately or store in a glass container in the refrigerator for up to 5 days. You can leave the meat in chunks or shred it. I like to pour some of the liquid from the slow cooker over the meat to keep it moist.

YIELD: 4 to 5 servings

PREP TIME: 5 minutes

COOK TIME: 20 to 40 minutes, depending on method

WINGS

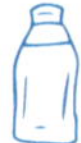

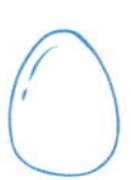

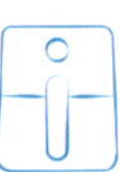

We used to order wings like these from a local restaurant, but once we realized how easy they are to make at home—and for a fraction of the cost—we never looked back. This recipe is perfect for the air fryer, which gives you beautifully crispy skin, but it works just as well in the oven. I've included instructions for both methods so you can choose your favorite way to enjoy them!

4 to 5 pounds whole chicken wings (see note)

1 tablespoon avocado oil or melted salted butter

1 teaspoon salt

1 teaspoon ground white pepper

1 teaspoon garlic powder

1 teaspoon onion powder

1 teaspoon smoked paprika

Buffalo sauce made with avocado oil, for dipping (optional)

Buttermilk Ranch Dressing (page 361) with blue cheese crumbles if desired, for dipping (optional)

1 If using the oven, preheat it to 425°F. Fit a sheet pan with a wire rack and set aside. Depending on the size of the wings and whether you're cooking 4 or 5 pounds, you may need two sheet pans. You need enough space to arrange the wings in a single layer without touching.

2 Put the wings in a large bowl and cover with the avocado oil. Toss the chicken with your hands to ensure every piece is coated.

3 Add the salt and spices to the bowl and toss the wings again until all sides are evenly coated.

4 If using the oven, arrange the wings on the wire rack and bake for 15 minutes, or until the skin is beginning to brown. Once you hit the 15-minute mark, turn the oven up to broil, move the pan to the top rack, and continue cooking for about 5 minutes to allow the skin to crisp up. The wings are done when the skin is golden brown and bubbly and the meat is no longer pink.

If using an air fryer, place as many wings as will fit comfortably (typically 6 to 8) in the air fryer basket, with the wing tips facing toward the center of the basket. Place the basket in the air fryer and set it to 420°F for 18 to 20 minutes. After 10 minutes, flip the wings. The wings are done when the meat is no longer pink and the skin is golden brown and bubbly. Repeat this process until you have cooked all of the wings.

5 Allow the wings to cool for 5 to 10 minutes before eating. I like to eat mine with Buffalo sauce, but you can also serve them with some of my Buttermilk Ranch Dressing, either as is or with some blue cheese crumbles mixed in to make a quick blue cheese dressing.

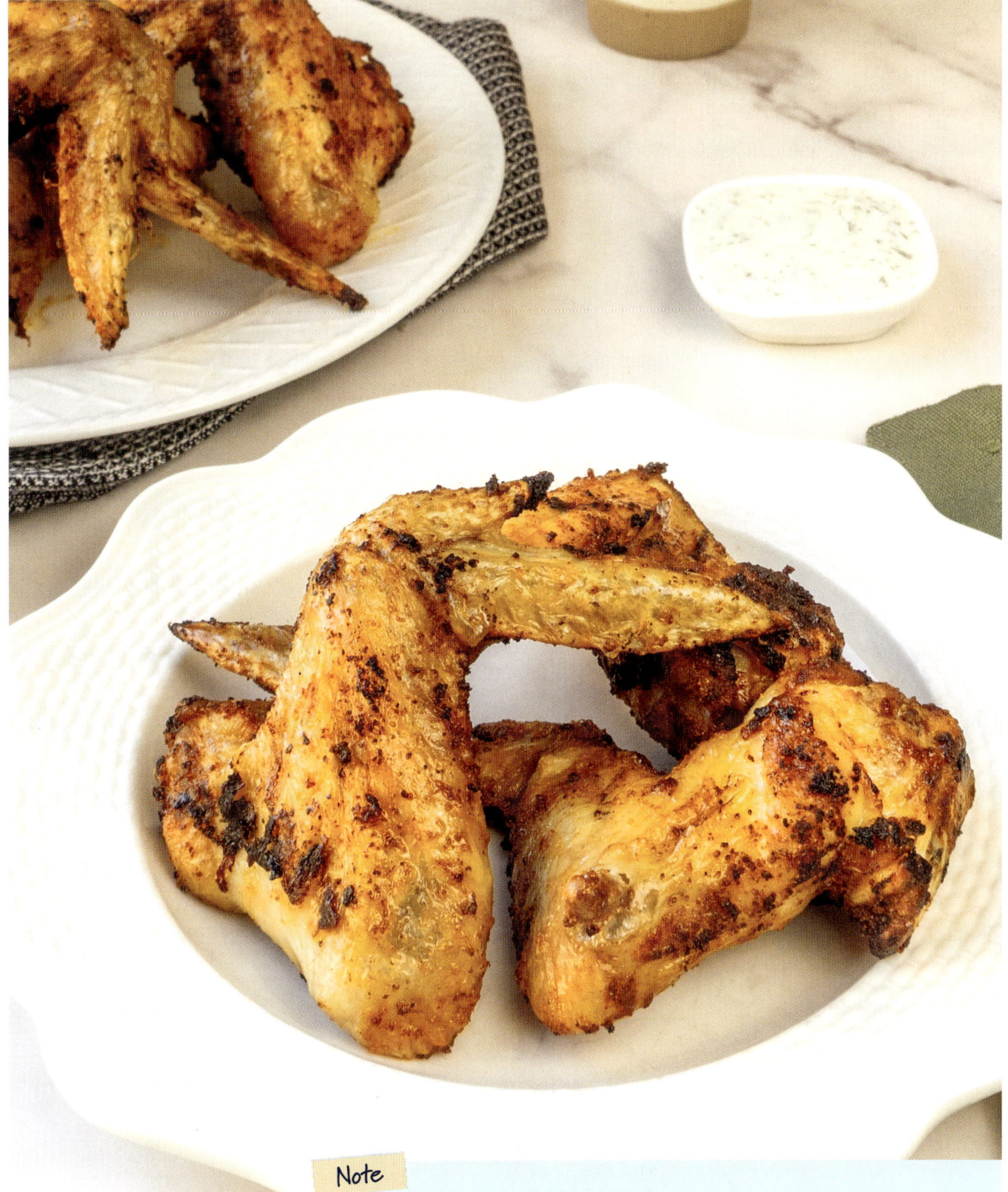

Note

I like to use the whole, or full, wing with the drumette (aka drummie), flat, and tip still attached.

PER SERVING (1 pound, weighed with bones in)	calories: **866** | fat: **58g** | protein: **79g** | carbs: **0g** | macro split: **62/38/0**

YIELD: 12 or 13 patties (1 per serving)

PREP TIME: 25 minutes, plus 3 hours to chill

COOK TIME: 10 or 40 minutes, depending on method

PLJESKAVICA (SERBIAN BURGERS)

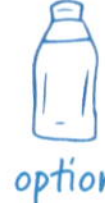

Pljeskavica are a flavorful Serbian take on the classic burger, traditionally grilled and served with round bread, kajmak (Serbian clotted cream), and chopped onions. On carnivore, we skip the bread and onions, letting the juicy spiced patty shine. Enjoy it with a dollop of creamy American Kajmak or on its own for a satisfying and unique twist on a classic. To more closely replicate the authentic Serbian experience, you could of course whip up a batch of cloud buns (page 372) and serve the patties in buns. If you don't want to fire up the grill, you have the option of cooking these in a frying pan on the stove.

- 2½ pounds 70/30 or 80/20 ground beef (see note)
- 2½ pounds ground pork, lamb, or veal
- 1 tablespoon minced garlic
- 2 tablespoons salt
- 1 teaspoon ground black pepper
- ¾ cup avocado oil or extra-virgin olive oil
- ¾ cup warm water
- 2 large mild or hot chili peppers, such as banana peppers or jalapeños (optional)
- 1 medium white or yellow onion (optional)
- 1 tablespoon animal fat of choice (for stovetop method)
- Sliced cheese of choice, for topping (optional)
- American Kajmak (page 357), for serving (optional)

1. Put the ground meats, garlic, salt, and black pepper in a stand mixer. Turn the speed to medium-low and slowly add the oil and warm water. Continue mixing until the mixture is smooth like a dough. (Note: If you don't own a stand mixer, you can also do this with a large bowl and an electric hand mixer.)
2. If using the chili peppers, remove the seeds and membranes. Finely chop the peppers and/or onion, if using, and add to the meat mixture. Mix on medium-low speed until fully incorporated.
3. Leaving the meat mixture in the mixing bowl, put the meat in the fridge for at least 3 hours but ideally overnight.
4. Once ready to form into patties, pull the meat mixture from the fridge and remix it in the stand mixer (or with a handheld mixer) for about 30 seconds.
5. Fill a small bowl with fresh water and set to the side. Wet your hands, take 6 ounces of the meat mixture, and shape into a thin, 6-inch-diameter patty. Wetting your hands allows you to shape the meat more easily. You should be able to make twelve or thirteen pljeskavica.
6. If grilling the patties, preheat a grill to medium heat. Grill until both sides are well browned and the patties have shrunk a bit, 7 to 10 minutes total.

   If cooking the patties on the stovetop, preheat a large frying pan over medium heat. When hot, drop in the animal fat

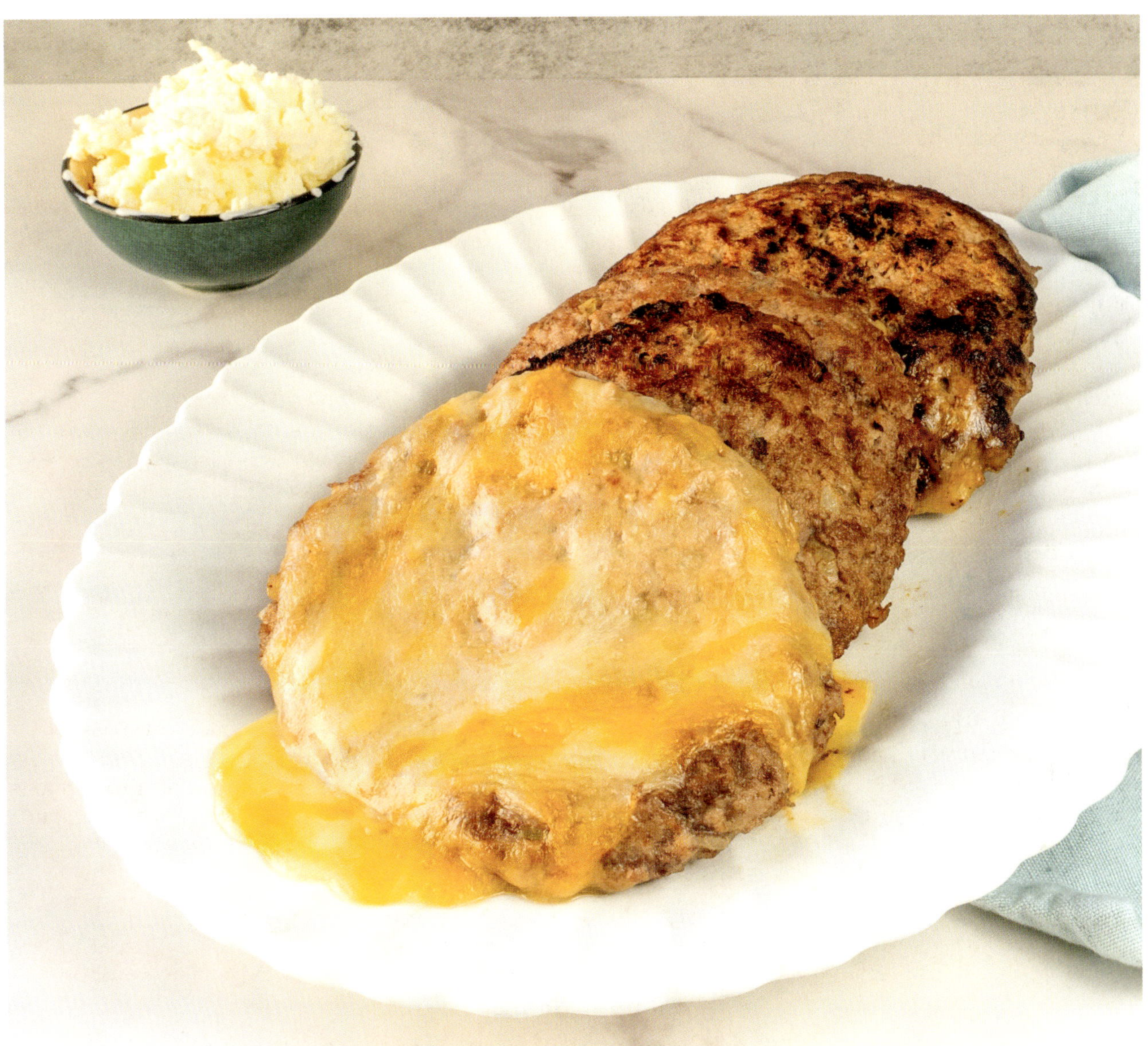

and add the patties in batches to avoid crowding. Cook until the patties have shrunk a bit and both sides are well browned, 7 to 10 minutes total.

7 If topping with cheese, add the cheese slice(s) 1 to 2 minutes before the patties are done. Serve with American Kajmak or plain.

Note

For this recipe, 70/30 ground beef is ideal. If you can't find it, 80/20 will do.

PER SERVING (using 70/30 ground beef, grilled)

calories: **720** | fat: **68g** | protein: **27g** | carbs: **1g** | macro split: **85/15/0**

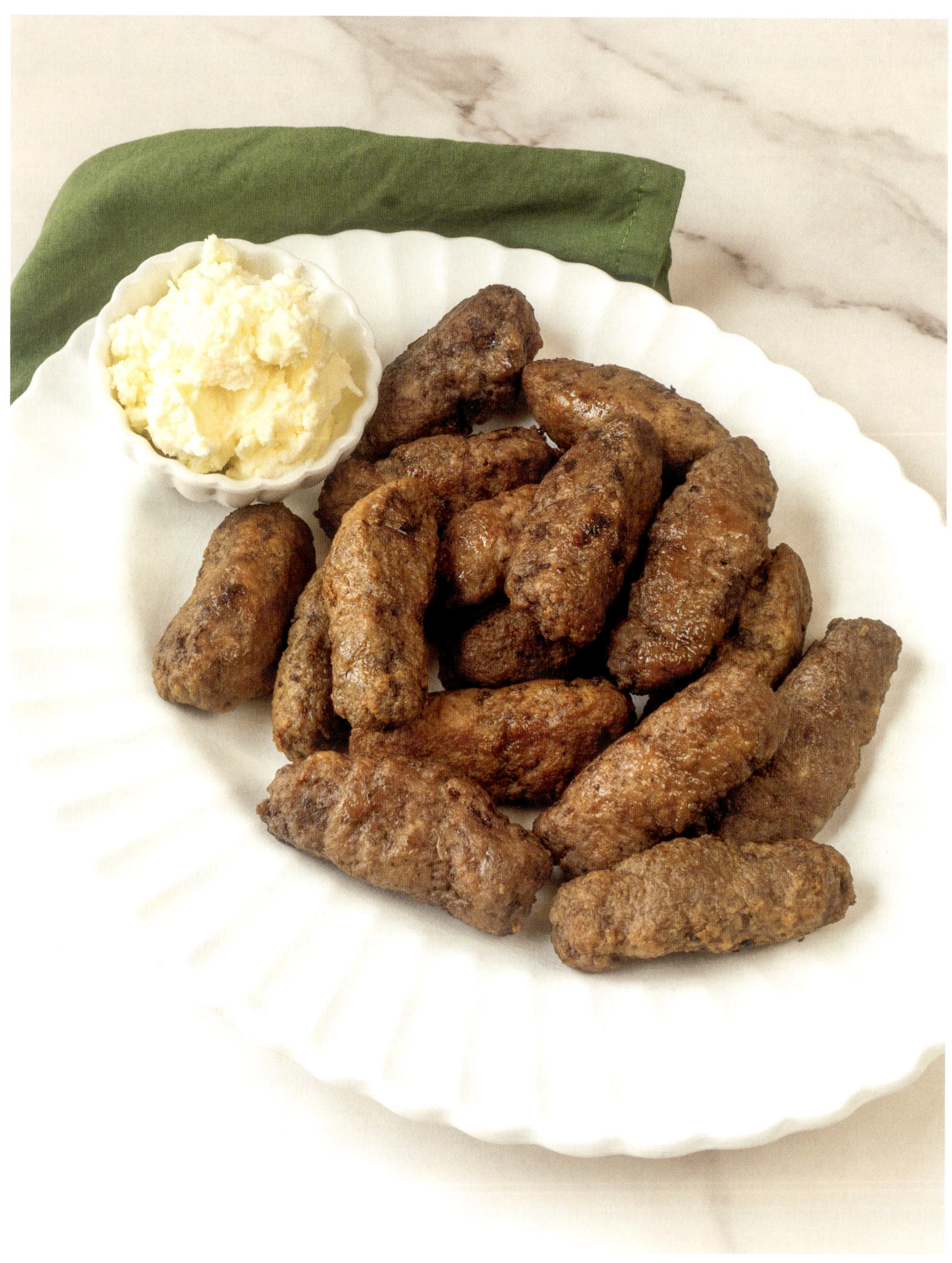

PER SERVING (using 70/30 ground beef)	calories: **1729** | fat: **163g** | protein: **64g** | carbs: **2g** | macro split: **85/15/0**

YIELD: about 40 ćevaps (8 per serving)

PREP TIME: 25 minutes, plus 3 hours to chill

COOK TIME: 10 or 20 minutes, depending on method

ĆEVAPS (SERBIAN SAUSAGES)

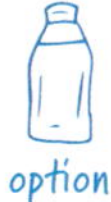

Ćevaps are small, flavorful Serbian sausages made without casing, traditionally served alongside bread, kajmak (Serbian clotted cream), and chopped onions. A full serving typically includes eight ćevaps, while a half serving consists of five. These bite-sized sausages are a delicious and satisfying staple of Serbian cuisine!

- 2½ pounds 70/30 or 80/20 ground beef (see note, page 223)
- 2½ pounds ground pork, lamb, or veal
- 1 tablespoon minced garlic
- 2 tablespoons salt
- 1 teaspoon ground black pepper
- ¾ cup avocado oil or extra-virgin olive oil
- ¾ cup warm water
- 1 tablespoon animal fat of choice, plus extra as needed (for stovetop method)
- American Kajmak (page 357), for dipping (optional)

1. Put the ground meats, garlic, salt, and pepper in a stand mixer. Turn the speed to medium-low and slowly add the oil and warm water. Continue mixing until the mixture is smooth like a dough. (Note: If you don't own a stand mixer, you can also do this with a large bowl and an electric hand mixer.)
2. Leaving the meat mixture in the mixing bowl, put the meat in the fridge for at least 3 hours but ideally overnight.
3. Once ready to form into sausages, pull the meat mixture from the fridge and remix it in the stand mixer (or with a hand mixer) for about 30 seconds.
4. Fill a small bowl with fresh water and set to the side. Wet your hands, take 2 ounces of the meat mixture, and roll in your hands into a sausage shape. You're aiming for sausages about 3 inches long and ½ inch thick. Wetting your hands allows you to roll the meat more easily. You should be able to make eight ćevaps per pound of meat.
5. If grilling the sausages, preheat a grill to medium heat. Grill the sausages until they shrink a bit and are well browned on all sides, 7 to 10 minutes total.

   If cooking the sausages on the stovetop, preheat a large frying pan over medium heat. When hot, drop in the fat and add the sausages in batches to avoid crowding. Cook until they shrink a bit and are well browned on all sides, 7 to 10 minutes total. When cooking the second batch of ćevaps, you may need to add more fat to the pan.
6. Serve with American Kajmak or plain.

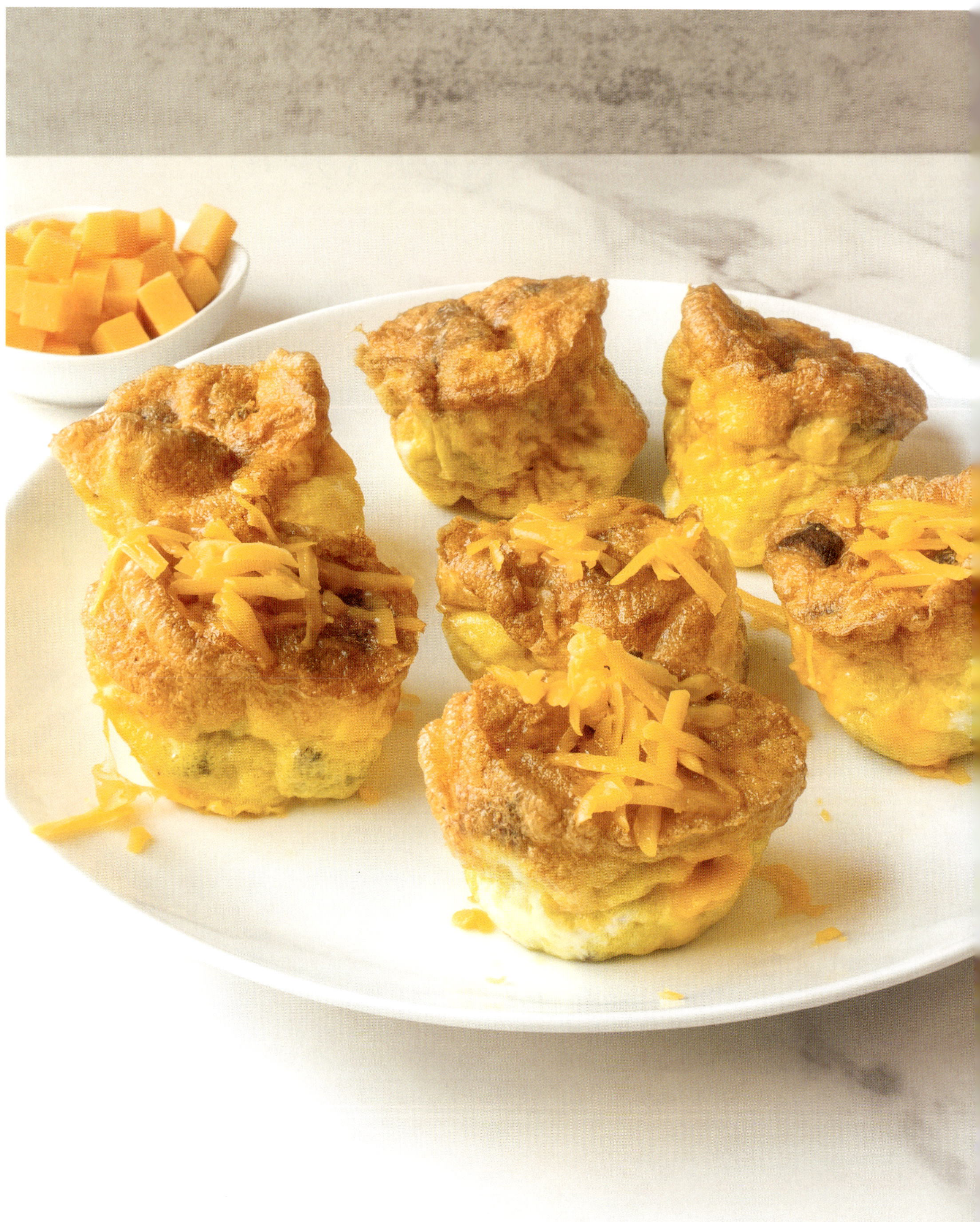

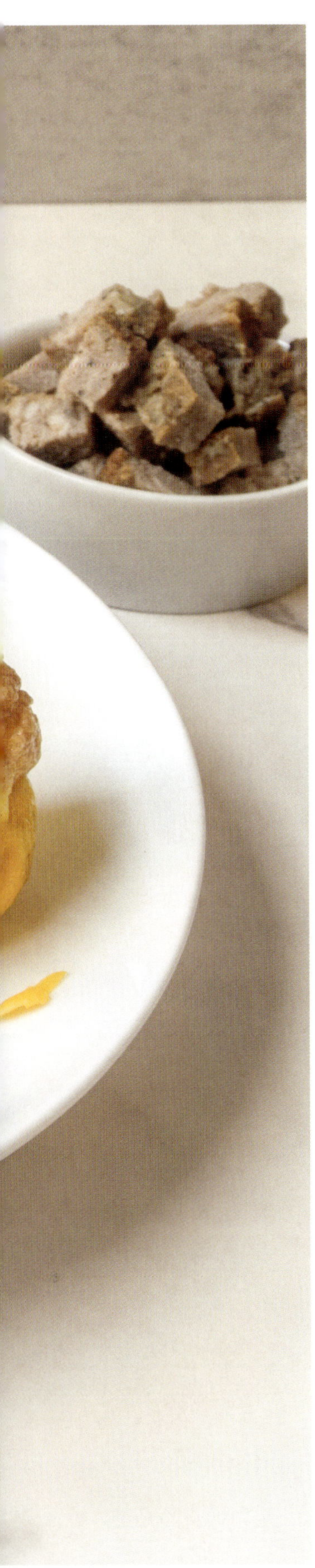

CHAPTER 10
BREAKFAST

228 Breakfast Casserole

231 Soufflé Omelet

232 Air Fryer Egg Bites

235 Ground Beef & Eggs

236 Soft-Boiled Eggs

239 Sweet Cream Cheese–Filled Crepes

240 Carnivore Cinnamon Rolls

243 Bacon, Egg & Cheese Sandwich

YIELD: 6 servings

PREP TIME: 10 minutes (not including time to cook ground beef)

COOK TIME: 30 minutes

BREAKFAST CASSEROLE

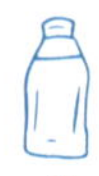

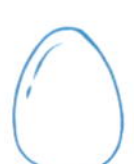
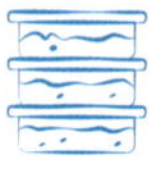

This quick and easy recipe is excellent for meal prep. It reheats well and allows you to use up leftover meats. You simply cook up a pound of ground beef and add eggs and whatever leftover meat(s) you have lying around in the fridge. Anything is fine here: bacon, breakfast sausage, steak, chicken, pork chops, kielbasa . . .

- Bacon grease or salted butter, for the dish
- 1 to 2 cups coarsely chopped leftover cooked meat(s) of choice
- 1 pound 80/20 ground beef, cooked and drained
- 1 dozen large eggs
- 1 teaspoon salt
- 1 teaspoon garlic powder (optional)
- ¼ cup heavy cream (optional)
- 1 cup shredded cheddar cheese, divided (optional)

1. Preheat the oven to 350°F. Grease a 13 by 9-inch baking dish with bacon grease or butter.
2. Put the chopped leftover meat and cooked ground beef in the prepared dish, spreading them into an even layer.
3. Crack the eggs into a medium mixing bowl, then add the salt and garlic powder, if using, and mix well with a fork, whisk, or immersion blender. If you are using dairy, add the cream and mix until blended.
4. Pour the egg mixture over the meat. If adding cheese, sprinkle ½ cup onto the top of the egg/meat mixture.
5. Bake for 25 to 30 minutes, until a toothpick comes out clean when inserted in the center of the casserole.
6. If using cheese, sprinkle the remaining ½ cup of cheese over the casserole and put the pan back into the oven until the cheese is fully melted.
7. Let the casserole rest for 10 minutes, then enjoy!

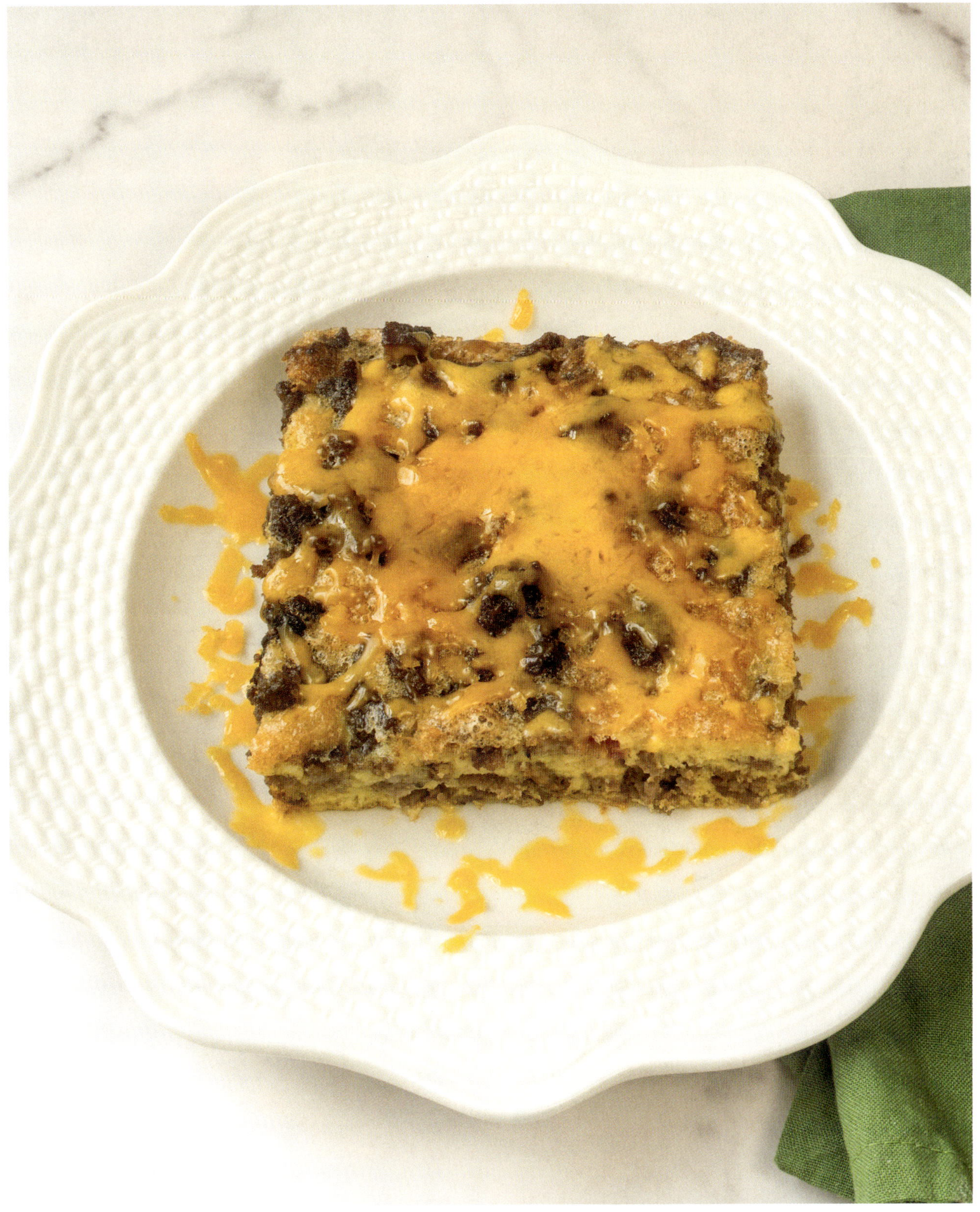

PER SERVING (without dairy)	calories: **458** | fat: **35g** | protein: **34g** | carbs: **0g** | macro split: **70/30/0**
PER SERVING (with dairy)	calories: **565** | fat: **44g** | protein: **39g** | carbs: **2g** | macro split: **71/28/1**

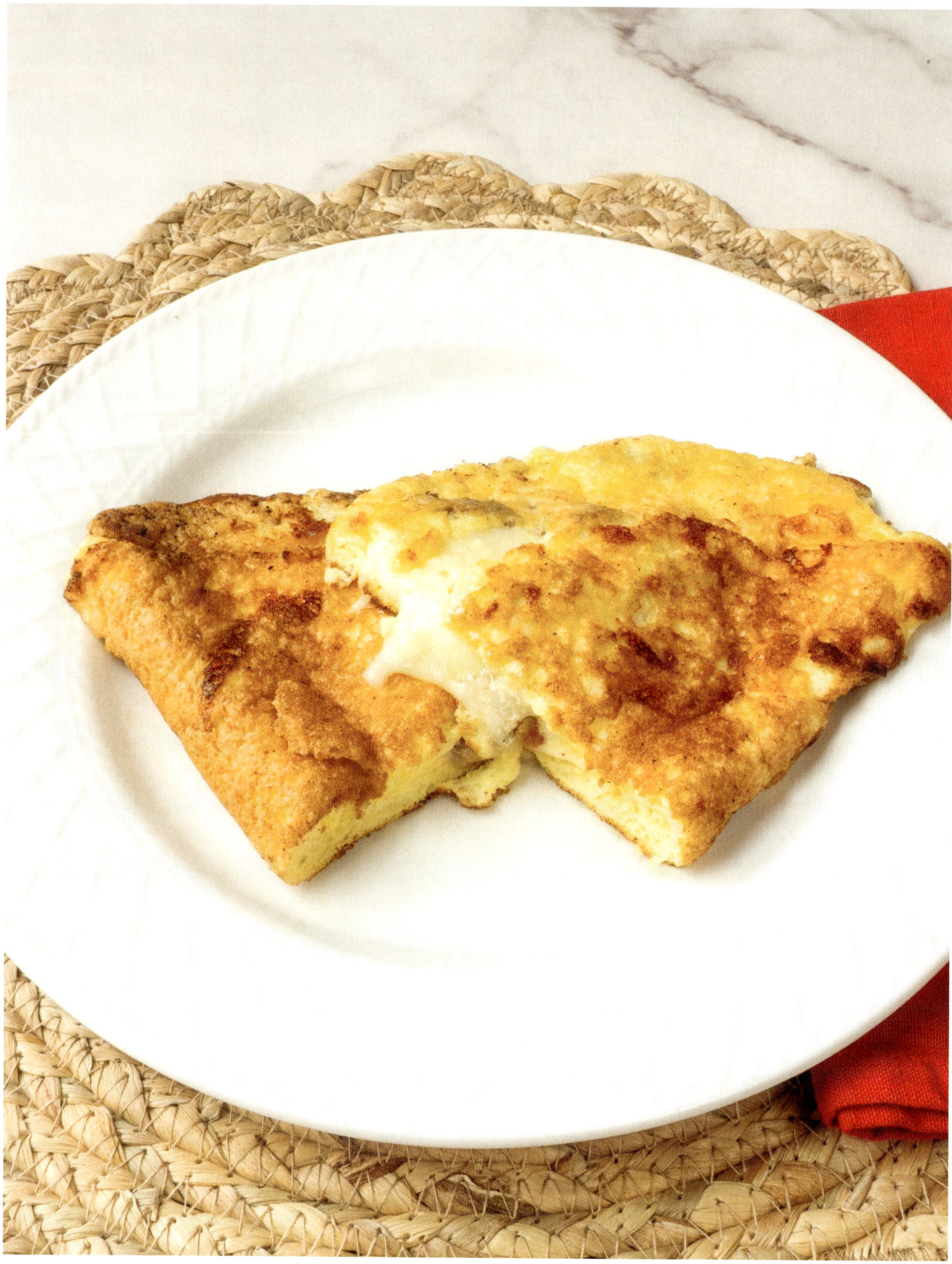

PER SERVING	calories: **610** | fat: **48g** | protein: **39g** | carbs: **3g** | macro split: **72/26/2**

YIELD: 1 serving

PREP TIME: 10 minutes (not including time to cook meat)

COOK TIME: 8 minutes

SOUFFLÉ OMELET

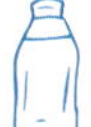
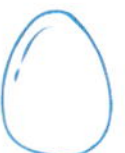

This delightful soufflé-style omelet is light as air and irresistibly tender. Made with a few simple ingredients and a quick, easy method, it's perfect for breakfast, brunch, or any time you're craving a cozy, comforting dish. The only trick is to be sure to whip the egg whites to the stiff peak stage. With an electric mixer, this is the work of just 3 or 4 minutes. The result? An omelet with a soft, fluffy texture that simply melts in your mouth.

2 large eggs, yolks and whites separated

Pinch of salt

Pinch of ground white pepper

½ cup shredded mozzarella cheese, divided

1 tablespoon salted butter

¼ cup crumbled cooked bacon or coarsely chopped cooked breakfast sausage

1. Put the egg whites, salt, and white pepper in a large metal or glass bowl or the bowl of a stand mixer fitted with the whisk attachment. Using a hand mixer or the stand mixer, whip the whites at high speed until stiff peaks form. (You'll know the egg whites are sufficiently stiff when they hold a peak on their own when you dip in a spoon and lift it straight up.)
2. Whisk the egg yolks in a small bowl and then fold them into the egg white mixture along with ¼ cup of the mozzarella cheese.
3. Melt the butter in a 9-inch frying pan over medium heat. When the butter starts bubbling, scoop the egg white mixture into the pan, spread it out with a silicone spatula, and cook for 3 to 4 minutes, until the bottom is browning and holds its shape. Then sprinkle on the meat and remaining mozzarella cheese and fold the egg white mixture over onto itself, making an omelet.
4. Flip the omelet and cook for few more minutes, until both sides are golden brown.
5. Serve immediately.

YIELD: 8 egg bites (4 per serving)

PREP TIME: 10 minutes

COOK TIME: 15 minutes

AIR FRYER EGG BITES

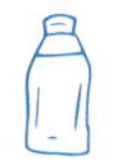

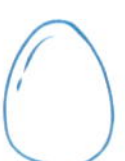
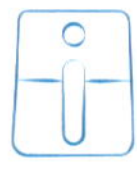

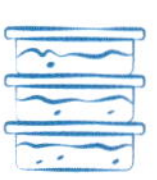

I love recipes that help me use up leftovers! One of my favorites is chopping up any extra breakfast meats I have and adding them to egg bites. This quick and easy breakfast can be prepped ahead of time, so all you need to do is reheat a few in the microwave for a convenient grab-and-go meal.

1 teaspoon salted butter, melted, or cooking spray

8 large eggs

2 tablespoons half-and-half (optional)

⅛ teaspoon salt

⅛ teaspoon ground white pepper

⅛ teaspoon garlic powder

⅛ teaspoon smoked paprika

½ cup finely chopped leftover cooked meat(s), such as bacon, sausage, ground beef, and/or ham

½ cup chopped or shredded cheddar cheese (optional)

TOPPINGS (OPTIONAL):

¼ cup shredded cheddar cheese

¼ cup full-fat sour cream

SPECIAL EQUIPMENT:
8 silicone muffin cups

1. Paint the insides of the silicone muffin cups with the melted butter, or grease with cooking spray.
2. Crack the eggs into a 2-cup or larger liquid measuring cup and add the half-and-half, if using. Mix well with a fork, whisk, or immersion blender, then add the salt and spices and continue to mix until frothy.
3. Distribute the chopped meat and the cheese, if using, evenly among the muffin cups. Then pour the egg mixture into the cups, filling each about three-quarters of the way full.
4. Carefully place the muffin cups in the air fryer basket and set it to 350°F for 13 to 15 minutes. After 5 minutes, open up the air fryer and use a fork to stir each egg bite. The top will have formed a crust, but the inside will still be liquid, so you want to stir that around. Repeat the stirring at the 10-minute mark. The egg bites are done when the centers are cooked through and the tops are a nice golden color.
5. Top with the additional shredded cheddar and/or sour cream, if desired, and serve.

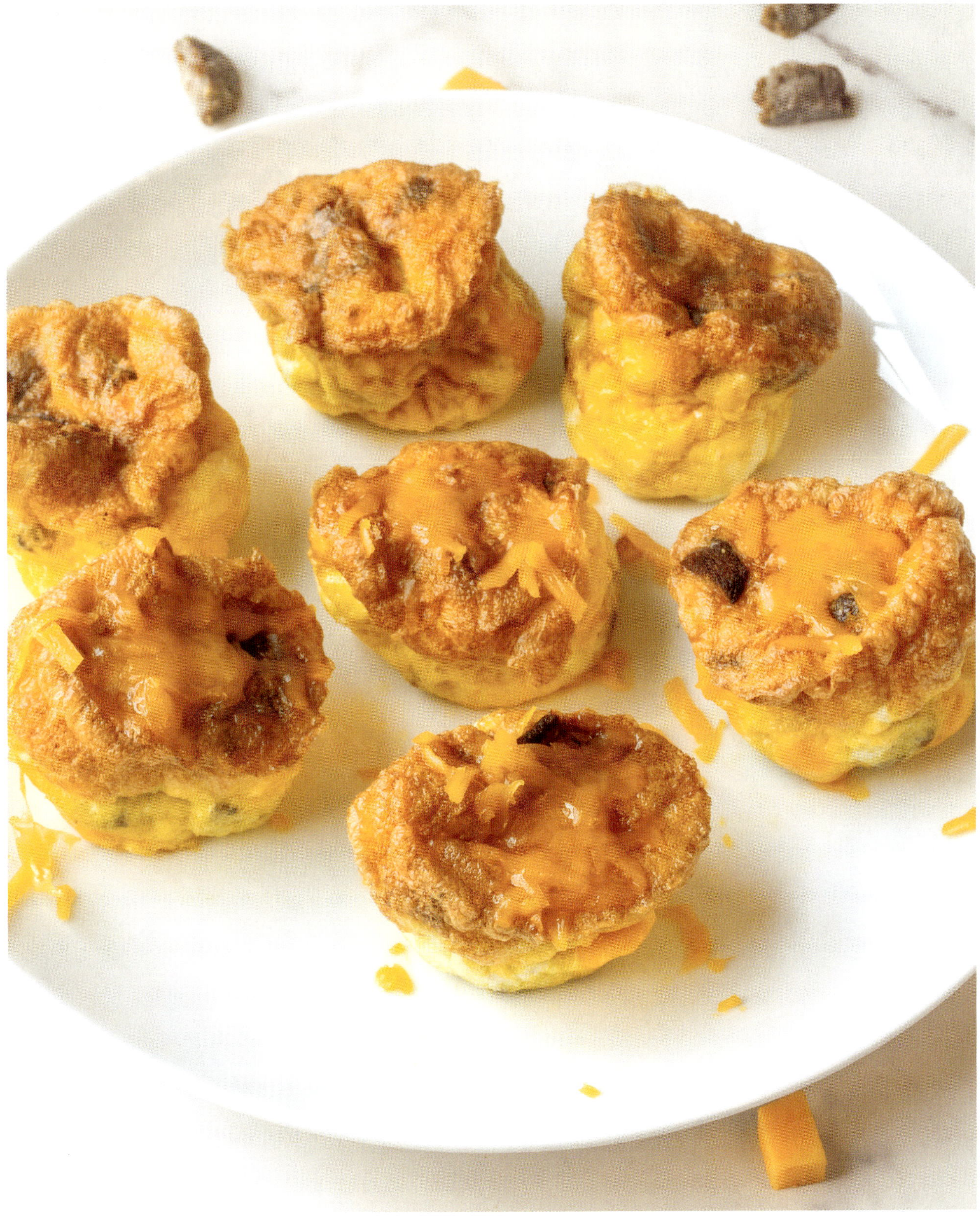

PER SERVING (with dairy)	calories: **528** | fat: **33g** | protein: **43g** | carbs: **2.5g** | macro split: **62/36/2**
PER SERVING (without dairy)	calories: **451** | fat: **26g** | protein: **39g** | carbs: **1g** | macro split: **59/39/1**

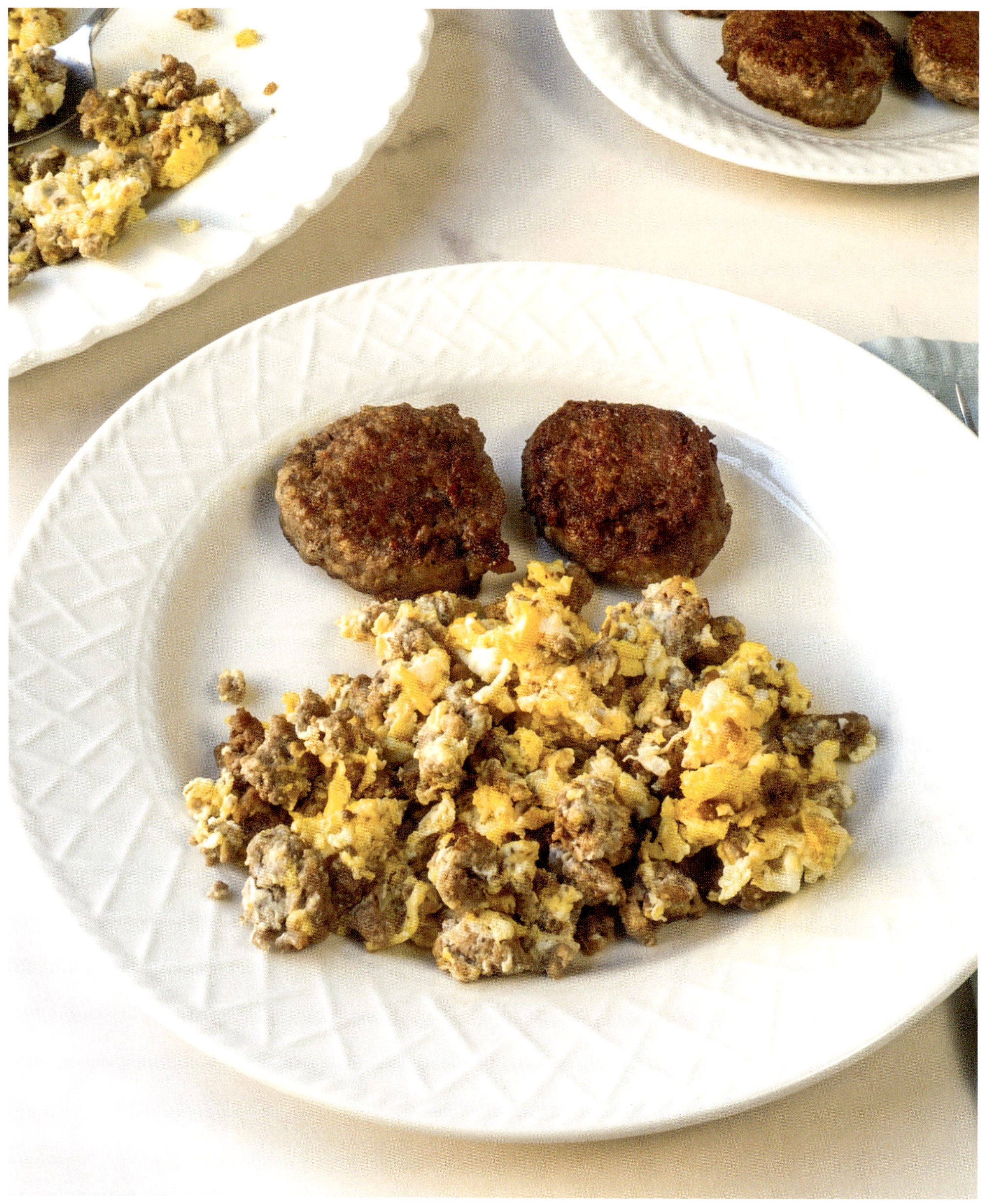

PER SERVING (without dairy)	calories: **430** | fat: **32g** | protein: **32g** | carbs: **1g** | macro split: **69/30/1**
PER SERVING (with dairy)	calories: **450** | fat: **33g** | protein: **32g** | carbs: **1g** | macro split: **69/30/1**

YIELD: 2 servings

PREP TIME: 5 minutes

COOK TIME: 15 minutes

GROUND BEEF & EGGS

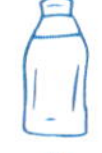

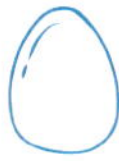

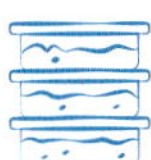

This simple carnivore breakfast classic is easy to cook and makes great leftovers. I like to serve this dish with a side of breakfast sausage or bacon. Whether you're feeding a crowd or meal-prepping for the week, it's a versatile option that never disappoints. Plus, it reheats beautifully, so you can enjoy it just as much the next day!

1 pound 80/20 ground beef

1 teaspoon salt

1 teaspoon garlic powder

8 large eggs

1 tablespoon half-and-half (optional)

1. Brown the ground beef in a large frying pan over medium heat, crumbling it as it cooks, 7 to 10 minutes. About halfway through cooking, add the salt and garlic powder and mix to distribute the seasoning throughout. The beef is done when there is no pink remaining. Turn off the heat and drain about half of the fat from the pan; set the pan aside.
2. Crack the eggs into a medium bowl and beat with a fork, whisk, or immersion blender until the whites and yolks are fully mixed together. Add the half-and-half, if using, and mix to combine.
3. Add the beaten eggs to the pan with the ground beef and set over medium heat. Move the eggs around with a silicone spatula and cook until the eggs are light and fluffy.
4. Season with salt to taste and enjoy!

YIELD: 12 eggs

PREP TIME: 2 minutes

COOK TIME: 7 to 8 minutes

SOFT-BOILED EGGS

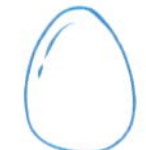

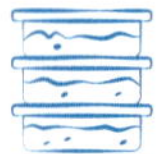

I always keep a container of soft-boiled eggs in my refrigerator. I eat them for breakfast or as a quick snack. Transferring the cooked eggs to an ice bath is essential for making the eggs super easy to peel. I prefer soft-boiled eggs with slightly runny yolks; if you prefer just set and very moist yolks (aka "jammy"), just cook them a bit longer (times for both options are included below). You can use this same method to make hard-boiled eggs; see the variation below the recipe. Note that the cooking times are based on using refrigerated eggs.

1 dozen large eggs

1. Fill a large saucepan two-thirds of the way full with water and bring to a rolling boil.
2. While the water is coming to a boil, make an ice bath in a large mixing bowl by filling it halfway with ice and water. Set aside.
3. Once the water is at a rolling boil, take a mesh skimmer (aka spider skimmer) and gently lower the eggs into the boiling water.
4. Set a timer for 6 minutes 45 seconds to 7 minutes for runny soft-boiled eggs, or 7 minutes 30 seconds to 8 minutes for jammy soft-boiled eggs.
5. When the timer goes off, use the mesh strainer to lift the eggs from the boiling water. Take a spoon and crack one side of each egg and then place them in the ice bath for at least 5 minutes. This will stop the cooking.
6. Cracking each egg before placing it in the ice bath will make peeling the shells much easier. Peel each egg and enjoy!

VARIATION:

Hard-Boiled Eggs. Use this same method, but set the timer for 9 to 10 minutes.

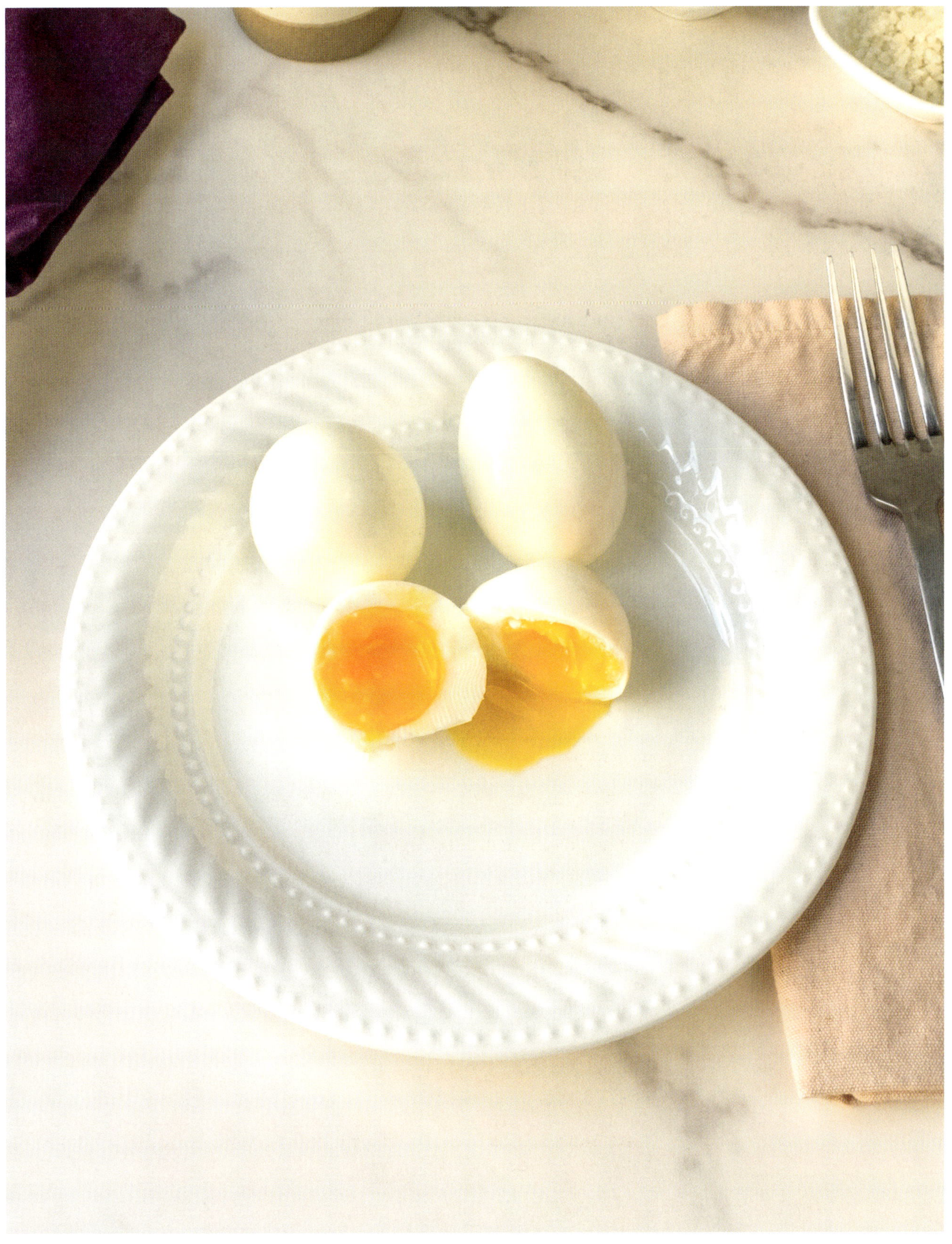

PER EGG

calories: **78** | fat: **5g** | protein: **6g** | carbs: **1g** | macro split: **63/34/3**

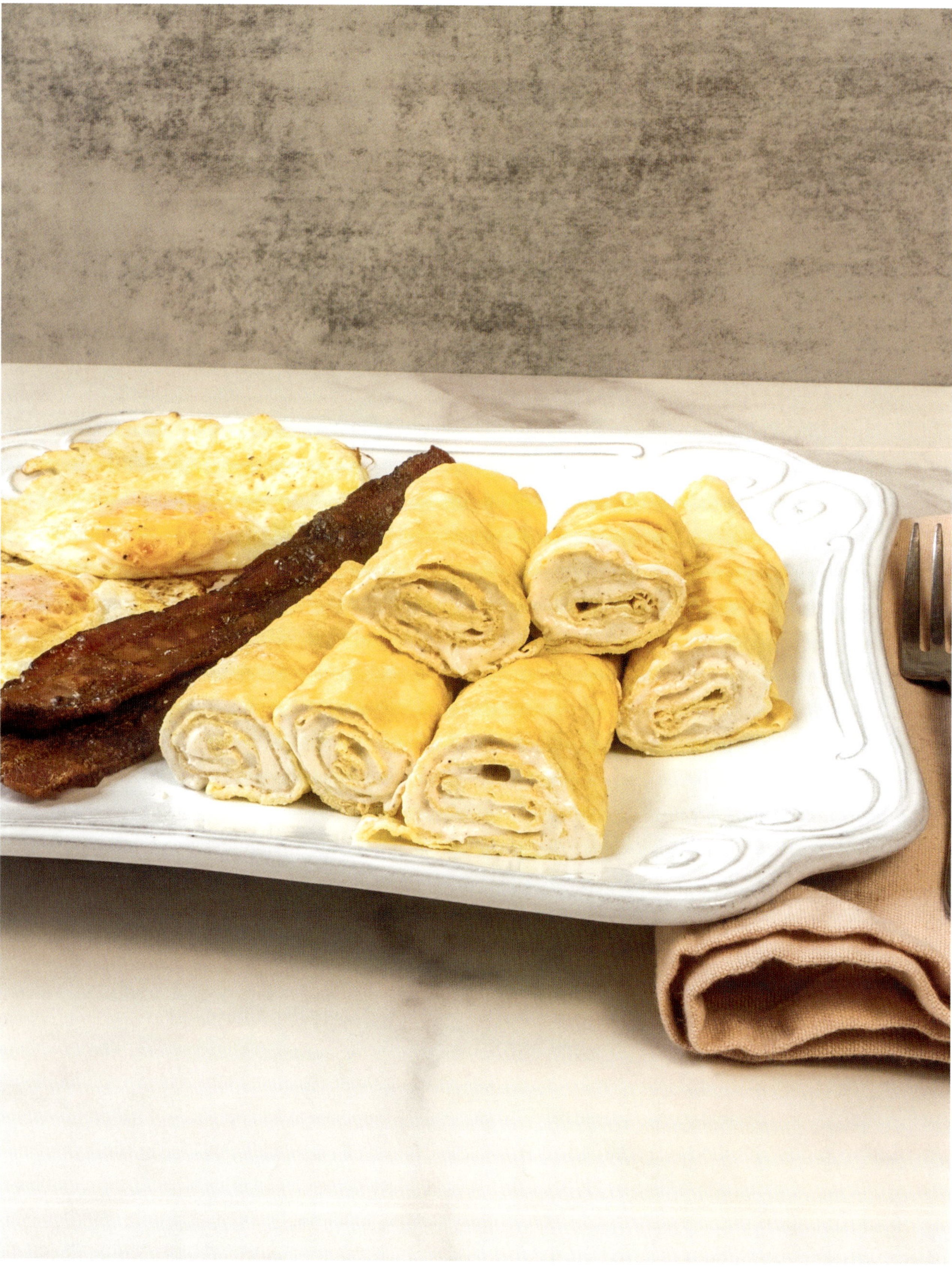

PER SERVING	calories: **1004** | fat: **85g** | protein: **48g** | carbs: **12g** | macro split: **76/19/5**

YIELD: 2 servings

PREP TIME: 10 minutes (not including time to make crepes)

SWEET CREAM CHEESE–FILLED CREPES

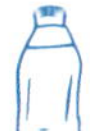
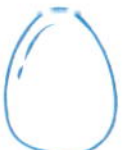

These indulgent sweet crepes are so delicious, you might forget they're carnivore! The allulose is optional, but I love to add it—it gives the crepes that classic sweetness, making them taste just like the traditional version. You can serve these on their own or with a side of bacon, eggs, or other breakfast items. Once you've made the crepes, this recipe comes together very quickly. All you need to remember is to set the cream cheese on the counter ahead of time to soften.

1½ (8-ounce packages) full-fat cream cheese, at room temperature

¼ cup powdered allulose or other sugar substitute, such as stevia or monkfruit (optional)

½ teaspoon ground cinnamon

2 batches Carnivore Crepes (page 364)

1 tablespoon salted butter, melted

1. Put the cream cheese, allulose (if using), and cinnamon in a medium bowl and stir until the allulose and cinnamon are distributed throughout the cream cheese.
2. Place a crepe on a plate. Take about 2 tablespoons of the cream cheese filling and spread it over the entire crepe using the back of a spoon. Then roll the crepe up and place on another plate. Repeat with the remaining crepes and filling to make a total of six filled crepes, dividing the crepes evenly between two plates.
3. Pour the melted butter over the crepes, dividing it evenly between both servings. I like to cut the crepes in half before serving, but that is up to you.

YIELD: 9 rolls (1 per serving)

PREP TIME: 10 minutes (not including time to make crepes)

COOK TIME: 20 minutes

CARNIVORE CINNAMON ROLLS

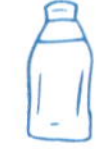
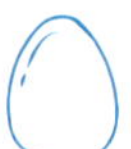

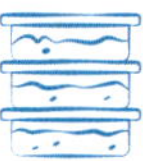

Occasionally, I crave a special treat that feels truly indulgent. That's when I turn to these cinnamon rolls—a decadent delight that satisfies my sweet tooth without breaking my commitment to the carnivore lifestyle. Made with simple, animal-based ingredients, they're fully carnivore and absolutely delicious. Best of all, I can enjoy them guilt-free, knowing they align perfectly with my dietary goals while still delivering that warm, cinnamon-spiced comfort I love.

FOR THE ROLLS:

1 (8-ounce) package plus 2 tablespoons full-fat cream cheese, at room temperature

6 tablespoons powdered allulose or other sweetener of choice

2 teaspoons ground cinnamon, plus extra for sprinkling

3 batches Carnivore Crepes (page 364) (see note)

2 tablespoons salted butter, melted

FOR THE ICING (OPTIONAL):

¼ cup plus 1 tablespoon Swerve confectioners' sugar

2 tablespoons heavy cream

⅛ teaspoon vanilla extract

1. Preheat the oven to 350°F. Have on hand a 9-inch pie pan.
2. In a medium bowl, mix the cream cheese, allulose, and cinnamon with a spoon or silicone spatula until smooth. Then place one crepe on a plate, take 2 tablespoons of the cream cheese mixture, and spread on the entire crepe with the back of a spoon. Roll the crepe into a traditional cylinder shape, then roll the cylinder like a pinwheel and place in the pie pan with the open end of the roll placed against the edge of the pan to prevent it from unrolling. Repeat this process with the other eight crepes and remaining cream cheese mixture.
3. Pour the melted butter over the tops of the cinnamon rolls.
4. If using icing, mix the ingredients together in a small bowl until well blended, then spread the icing on top of the rolls.
5. Sprinkle each roll with a bit of cinnamon.
6. Bake uncovered for 15 to 20 minutes, until bubbly and heated through. Allow to cool for 5 minutes and then enjoy! These will keep for up to a week in the refrigerator. I reheat them in the microwave (30 seconds for one roll) or toaster oven (10 minutes).

Note:

You will need to make nine crepes, or a triple batch, for these cinnamon rolls. Once you've made the crepes, this recipe comes together fairly quickly. You can cook the crepes up to a few days ahead of time. To make them more pliable, pop them in the microwave for 15 to 30 seconds.

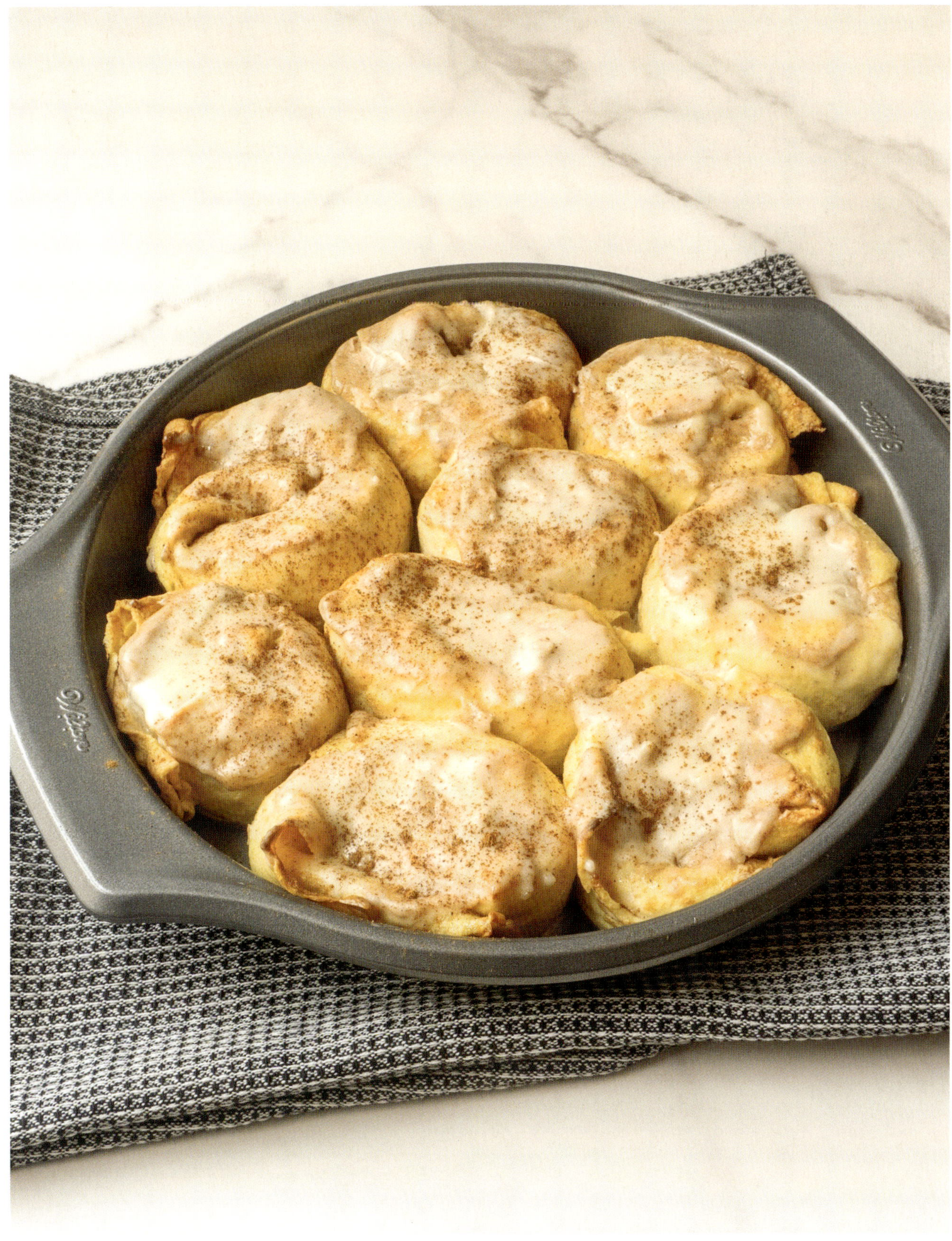

PER SERVING (with icing) | calories: **331** | fat: **28g** | protein: **16g** | carbs: **3g** | macro split: **77/20/3**

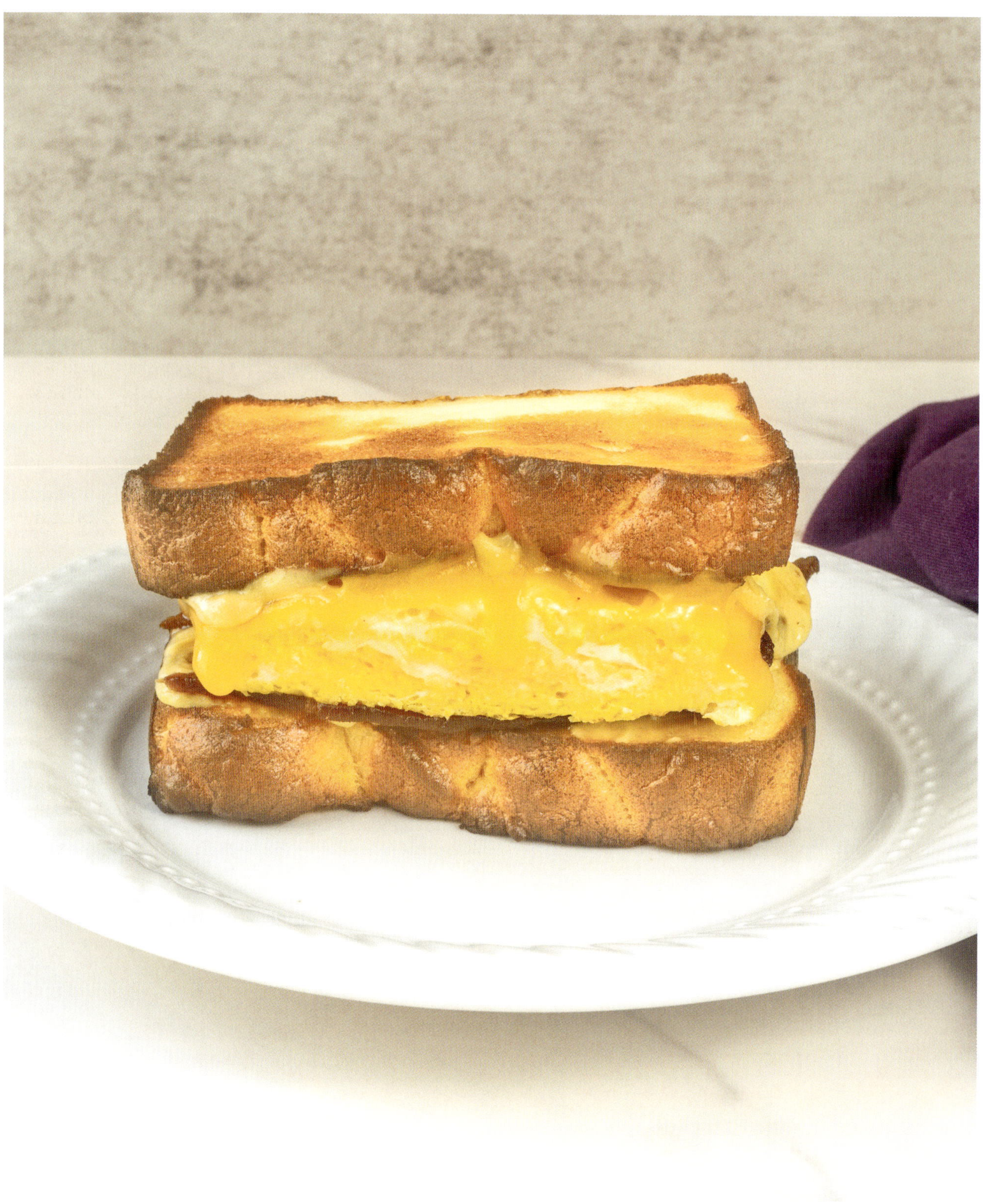

PER SANDWICH (with cloud bread)	calories: **723** | fat: **57g** | protein: **44g** | carbs: **4g** | macro split: **73/25/2**
PER SANDWICH (with chaffles)	calories: **883** | fat: **73g** | protein: **49g** | carbs: **4g** | macro split: **75/23/2**

YIELD: 1 sandwich

PREP TIME: 5 minutes (not including time to make bread or cook bacon)

COOK TIME: 5 minutes

BACON, EGG & CHEESE SANDWICH

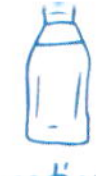

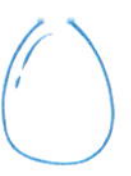

The classic bacon, egg, and cheese sandwich was one of my favorites, but it's not something I could enjoy anymore on the carnivore diet—until I discovered a bread substitute. Now, with cloud bread or chaffles, I can indulge in this delicious sandwich once again, with all of the flavors I love, without compromising my dietary lifestyle.

2 tablespoons store-bought avocado oil mayonnaise or Bacon Mayonnaise (page 352)

2 slices Cloud Bread Loaf (page 372), toasted, or 2 Chaffles (page 368)

2 large eggs

Pinch of salt

Pinch of ground white pepper

1 tablespoon salted butter

2 slices cheddar cheese

2 strips bacon, cooked

1. Spread 1 tablespoon of mayo on each piece of cloud bread or each chaffle. Set aside on a plate.
2. Crack the eggs into a small bowl, add the salt and pepper, and mix well with a fork.
3. In a small frying pan, melt the butter over medium heat. Pour in the eggs and scramble until done to your liking. Then top the eggs with the cheese slices and shape into the size of the bread slices or chaffles.
4. Layer the bacon strips on one slice of bread or chaffle. Using a spatula, place the eggs and cheese on the bacon, then top with the other slice of bread or chaffle, mayo side down.

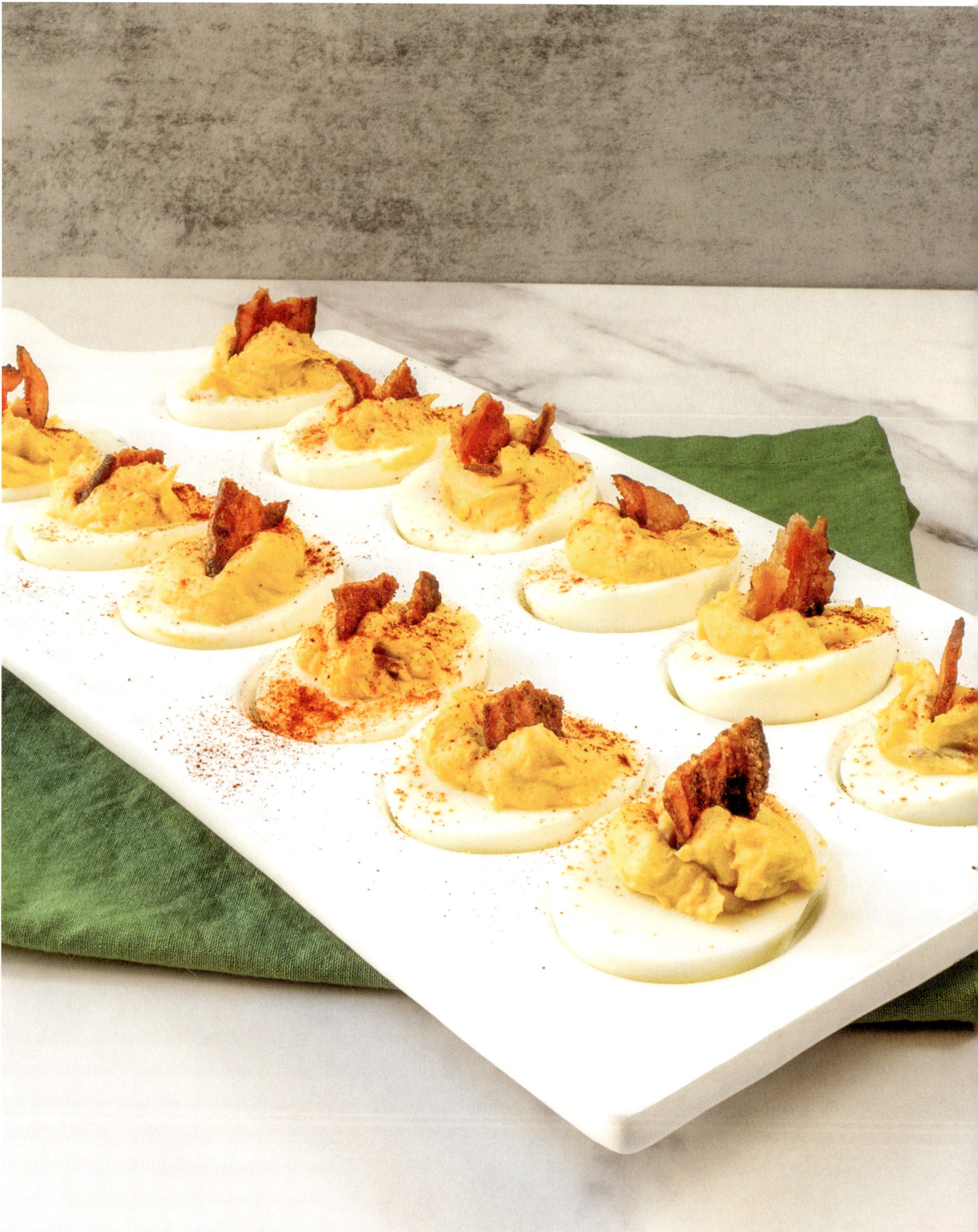

CHAPTER 11
APPETIZERS

246 Cheesy Pepperoni Chips

249 Air Fryer Sausage Rosemary Cream Cheese Bites

250 Chicken Sliders with Spicy Mayo

253 Deviled Eggs

254 Meat Lover's Pizza Roll-Ups

257 Cvarci (Serbian Pork Cracklings)

258 Pihtije (Meat Jelly)

YIELD: 24 chips (12 per serving)

PREP TIME: 10 minutes

COOK TIME: 5 minutes

CHEESY PEPPERONI CHIPS

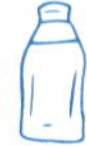
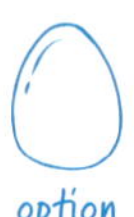

These little chips are addictive, simple, and delightfully crispy! I like to pair them with my Buttermilk Ranch Dressing for dipping, but you could use low-carb marinara for a keto substitute.

24 pepperoni slices

4 ounces (½ cup) shredded sharp cheddar cheese

Buttermilk Ranch Dressing (page 361), for dipping (optional)

SPECIAL EQUIPMENT:

24-well mini muffin pan

1. Preheat the oven to 400°F.
2. Place a pepperoni slice in each mini muffin cup, then fill the wells halfway with the cheese.
3. Bake for 4 to 5 minutes, until the cheese is melted. Allow to cool for 5 to 10 minutes before removing from the pan. The grease from the pepperoni allows these to release easily.
4. Enjoy on their own or dipped in ranch dressing.

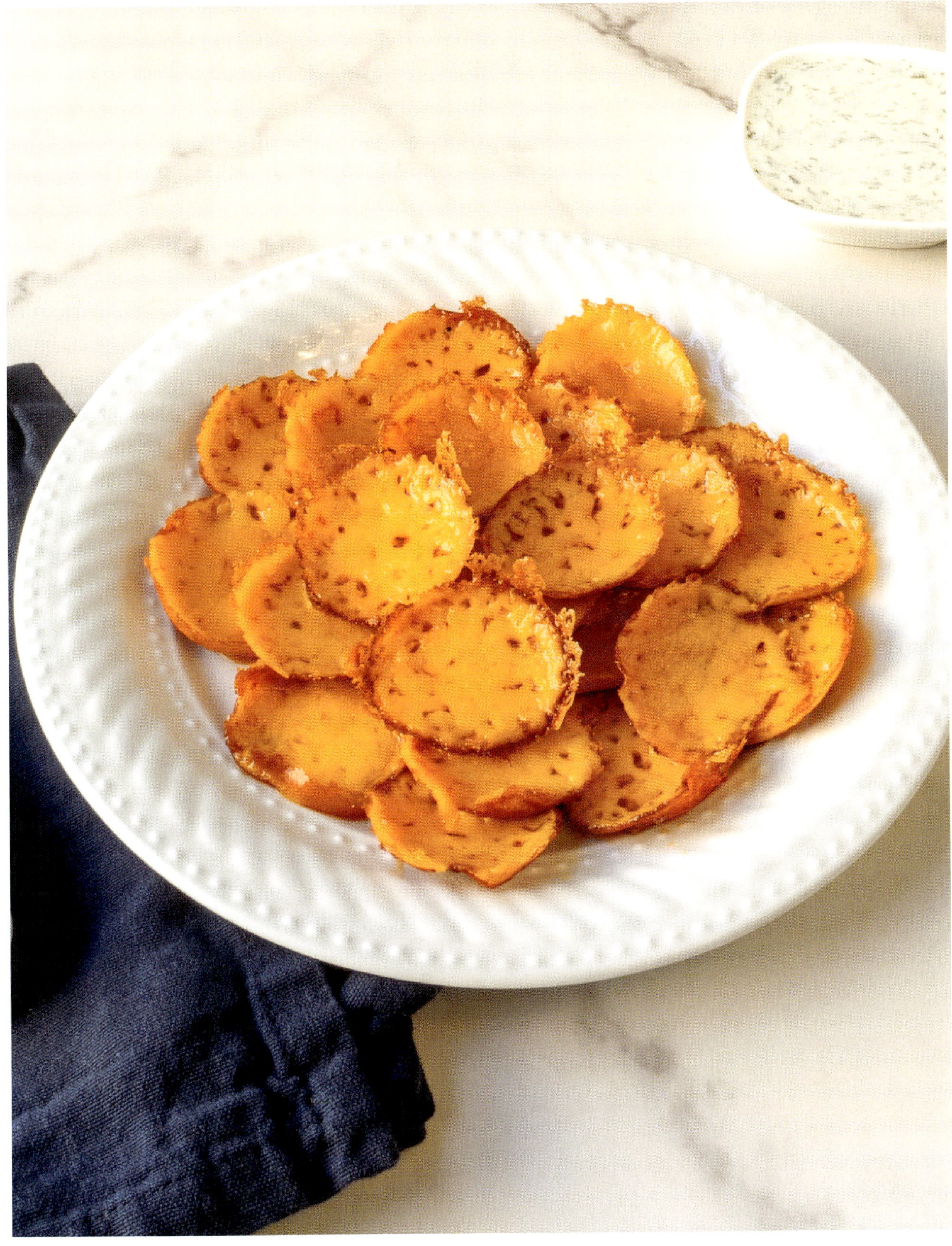

PER SERVING

calories: **344** | fat: **30g** | protein: **19g** | carbs: **2g** | macro split: **76/22/2**

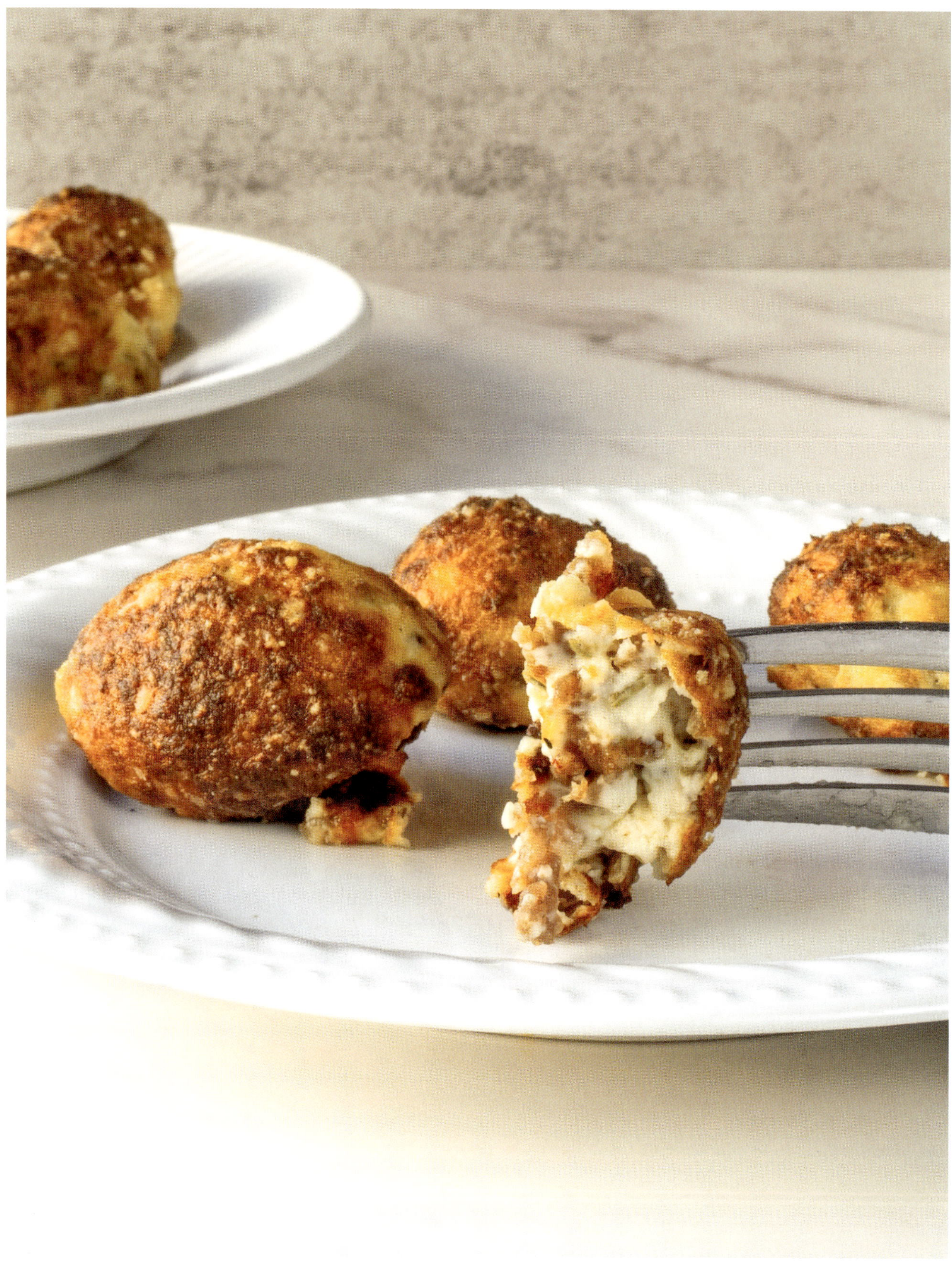

PER SERVING

calories: **340** | fat: **29g** | protein: **19g** | carbs: **2g** | macro split: **75/22/3**

YIELD: 10 to 14 bites (3 per serving)

PREP TIME: 15 minutes (not including time to cook sausage)

COOK TIME: 10 minutes

AIR FRYER SAUSAGE ROSEMARY CREAM CHEESE BITES

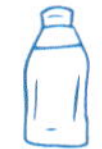
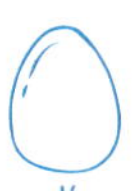

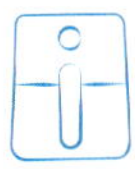

These cheese bites are a savory carnivore-friendly treat, blending rich sausage with creamy cheese and aromatic rosemary for a burst of flavor in every bite. With minimal ingredients, they're simple to make and perfect as a high-protein snack or appetizer.

1 (8-ounce) package full-fat cream cheese, at room temperature

1 cup cooked bulk Italian sausage (mild)

¼ teaspoon garlic powder

⅛ teaspoon onion powder

⅛ teaspoon ground white pepper

⅛ teaspoon dried rosemary needles

⅛ teaspoon salt

2 ounces (2 tablespoons) grated Pecorino Romano cheese, for coating

Buttermilk Ranch Dressing (page 361) or low-carb marinara for keto version, for serving (optional)

1. Put the cream cheese, cooked sausage, spices, rosemary, and salt in a large mixing bowl and mix with your hands until thoroughly combined.
2. Scoop up 1 to 2 tablespoons of the cream cheese and sausage mixture and roll it between your palms to form a smooth 1-inch ball. Repeat with the remaining mixture, making a total of ten to fourteen balls.
3. Take each ball and roll it in the Pecorino Romano cheese until it is fully covered. The coating doesn't have to be thick, but make sure the cheese covers all sides of the cream cheese ball.
4. Place the balls in an air fryer, making sure they have a bit of space between them. You will likely have to cook them in two or three batches.
5. Air-fry at 400°F for 8 to 10 minutes, until the balls are crispy and brown on the outside. Allow to cool for a couple of minutes before eating.
6. Serve as is or, if you wish, with a side of ranch or marinara.

YIELD: 6 sliders (3 per serving)

PREP TIME: 10 minutes (not including time to make flatbread or mayo or cook bacon)

COOK TIME: 20 minutes

CHICKEN SLIDERS WITH SPICY MAYO

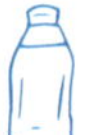
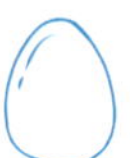

This cheap and easy appetizer, using rotisserie chicken, is super simple to whip up. I recommend making the flatbreads into small rounds so they're perfectly shaped for sliders, but you can also cut the baked rectangular flatbreads into square pieces if you prefer. These can be stored in the refrigerator for up to 5 days, but I recommend eating them immediately for the best taste and texture.

1 cup chopped rotisserie chicken (dark or white meat or a mix)

¾ cup shredded cheddar cheese

1 large egg

½ cup chopped cooked bacon

Pinch of salt

Pinch of ground black pepper

3 tablespoons Spicy Mayonnaise (page 356)

12 Individual Cottage Cheese Flatbread Rounds, or 2 Cottage Cheese Flatbreads cut into 12 equal squares (page 371), for buns

1. Preheat the oven to 350°F. Line a sheet pan with parchment paper or a silicone baking mat.
2. Put the chicken, cheese, egg, bacon, salt, and pepper in a medium bowl and mix well.
3. Scoop up one-sixth (3 to 4 tablespoons) of the chicken mixture, roll it into a ball between your palms, and then flatten the ball out into a patty about 3 inches in diameter. Place on the prepared pan. Repeat with the rest of the chicken mixture to make a total of six patties.
4. Bake the patties for 20 minutes, or until golden brown and crispy. Allow to cool for 5 minutes.
5. Assemble the sliders: Slather the spicy mayo on all of the buns. Then place one of the chicken patties on each bun and top with the other bun. Enjoy immediately.

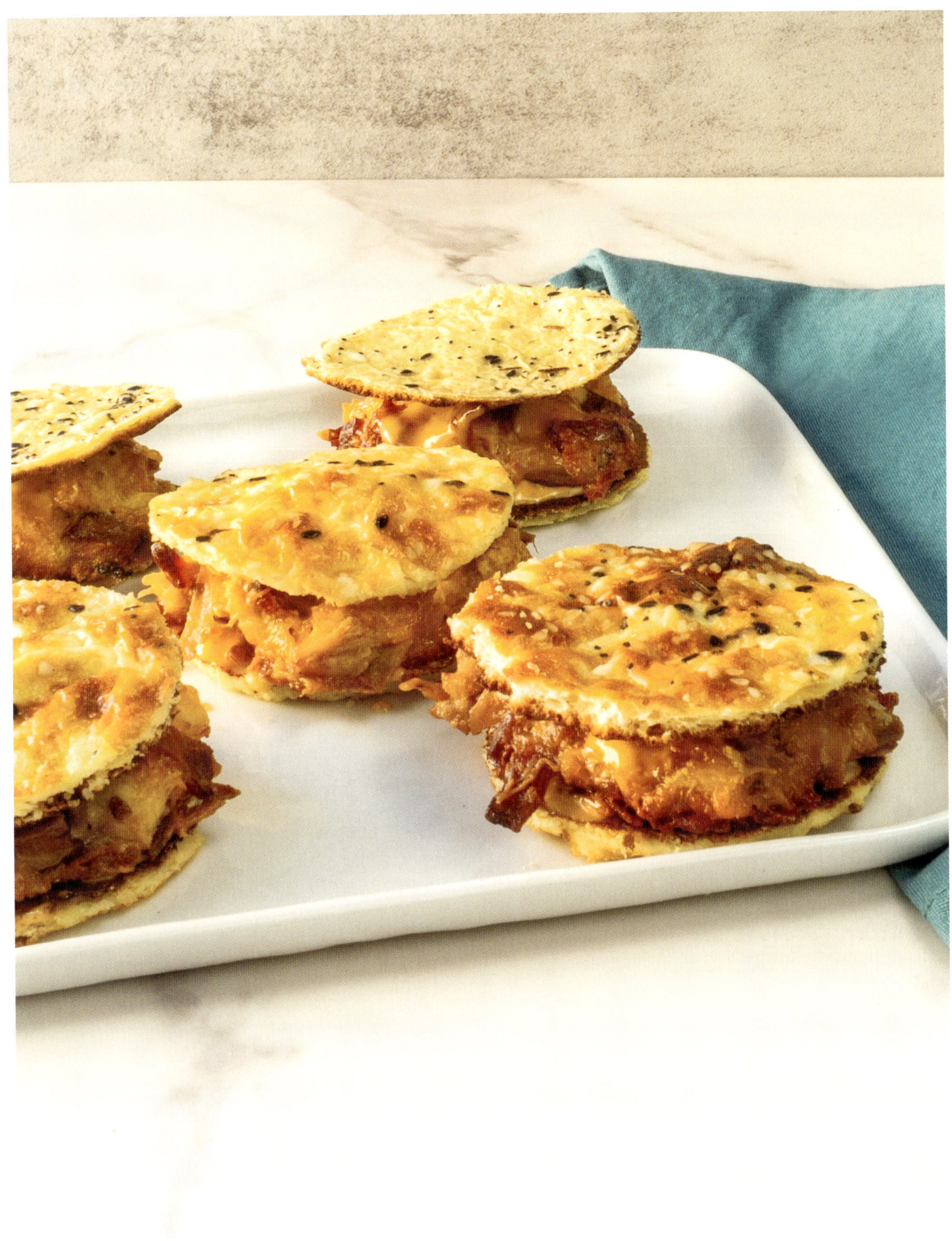

PER SERVING calories: **993** | fat: **72g** | protein: **75g** | carbs: **14g** | macro split: **64/30/6**

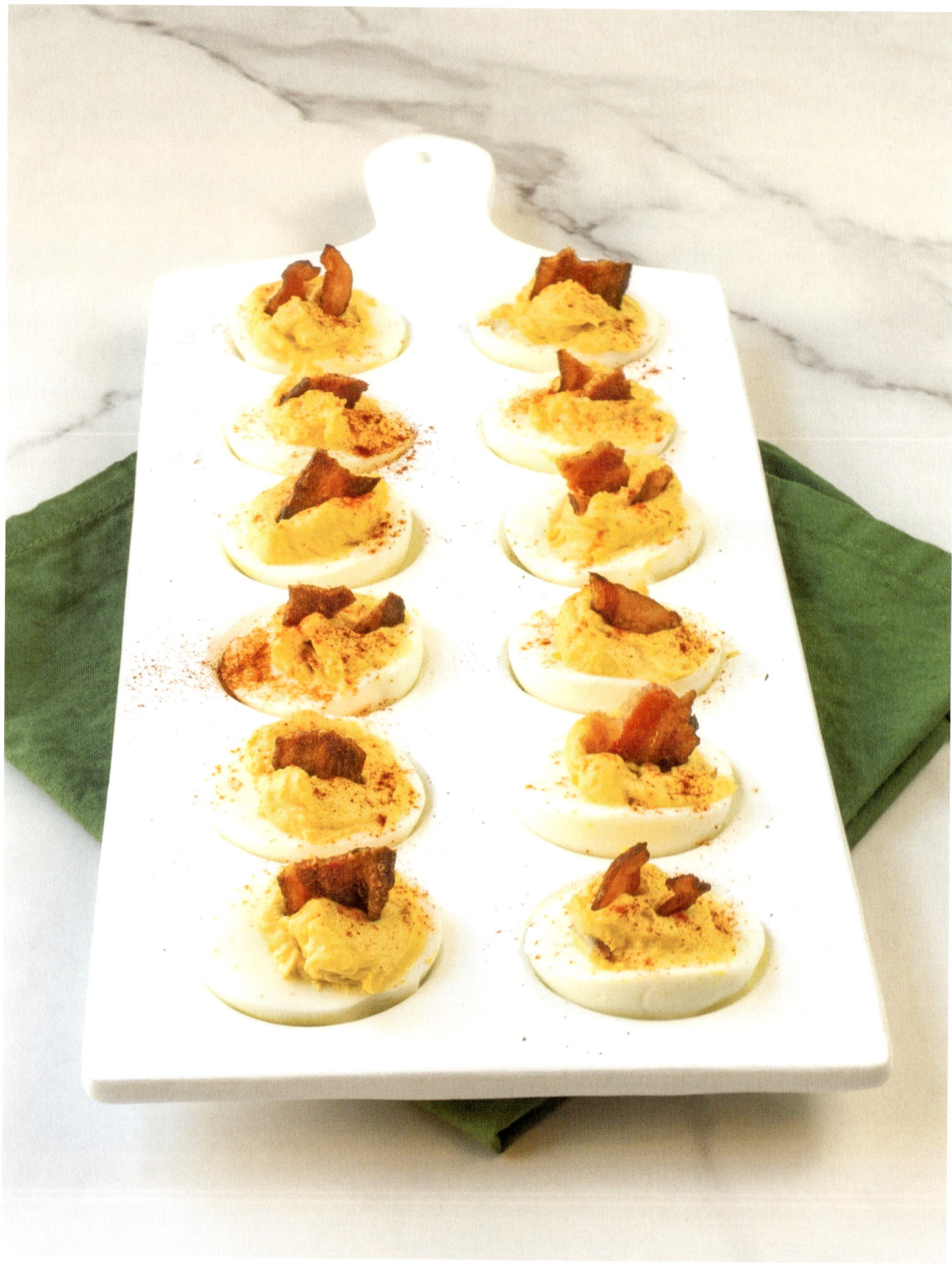

PER SERVING

calories: **242** | fat: **20g** | protein: **12g** | carbs: **1g** | macro split: **78/21/1**

YIELD: 12 deviled egg halves (3 per serving)

PREP TIME: 10 minutes (not including time to make mayonnaise or cook eggs and bacon)

DEVILED EGGS

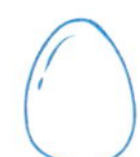

I make these deviled eggs with my bacon mayo, but they'd taste fantastic with store-bought avocado oil mayo, too. I could easily finish a whole plate myself—and I wouldn't feel the least bit guilty about it! If that describes you, I suggest you invest in a deviled egg platter for serving. I'm not normally a fan of one-off kitchen tools, but an egg platter is highly practical! Not only do these platters make for a pretty display, but the egg-shaped indentations keep the deviled eggs from sliding off and onto the floor.

6 large hard-boiled eggs (see page 236)

Salt

¼ cup Bacon Mayonnaise (page 352)

1 teaspoon Dijon mustard

3 teaspoons apple cider vinegar

⅛ teaspoon smoked paprika, plus extra for garnish

1 to 2 strips bacon, cooked until crispy and cut into ½-inch pieces

SPECIAL EQUIPMENT: Deviled egg platter (optional)

1. Cut the hard-boiled eggs in half lengthwise and carefully spoon the yolks into a small mixing bowl. Set the whites on a serving platter, ideally one designed for deviled eggs, and sprinkle with a pinch of salt. (If you don't have a deviled egg platter, cut a small amount off the bottom of each egg white half to create a flat surface; this will help keep them from sliding off the platter.)
2. Mix the egg yolks with the bacon mayo, mustard, vinegar, smoked paprika, and ⅛ teaspoon of salt until smooth.
3. Evenly spoon the egg yolk mixture into the cavities in the egg white halves.
4. Top each deviled egg with some of the crispy bacon pieces, garnish with a sprinkle of smoked paprika, and enjoy!

YIELD: 6 roll-ups (3 per serving)

PREP TIME: 10 minutes (not including time to cook sausage and bacon)

COOK TIME: 8 minutes

MEAT LOVER'S PIZZA ROLL-UPS

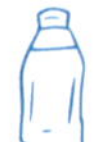

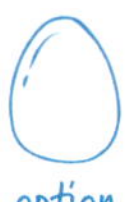

Who doesn't love pizza? These roll-ups are quick to assemble and cook in under 10 minutes. They might be gone in less than a minute, but that's all good—they're fully carnivore with only 6 grams of carbs per serving! I like to serve them with a side of ranch, but you can use marinara if you're going for a keto-friendly option.

6 large pepperoni slices (2 to 3 inches in diameter)

2 cups shredded whole-milk mozzarella (see note)

¼ cup cooked Italian sausage (removed from casings)

¼ cup crumbled cooked bacon

Italian seasoning (optional)

Buttermilk Ranch Dressing (page 361) or low-carb marinara sauce, for dipping (optional)

1. Preheat the oven to 375°F. Line a sheet pan with parchment paper or a silicone baking mat.
2. Place the pepperoni slices on the prepared pan, leaving some space between them. Evenly top each pepperoni slice with one-sixth each of the cheese, sausage, and bacon, in that order. (For the cheese, you'll use about ⅓ cup for each stack, and for the Italian sausage and bacon, about 2 teaspoons of each.) Sprinkle each stack with some Italian seasoning, if using.
3. Bake the stacks for 8 minutes, or until the cheese is bubbly and melted.
4. Allow to cool for 2 minutes. Then roll each stack into a crepe shape and serve immediately with ranch dressing or marinara sauce, if desired. For visual interest, you can roll some pepperoni side out and some cheese side out.

Note:

Be sure to use whole-milk mozzarella for this recipe; part-skim mozzarella won't melt correctly.

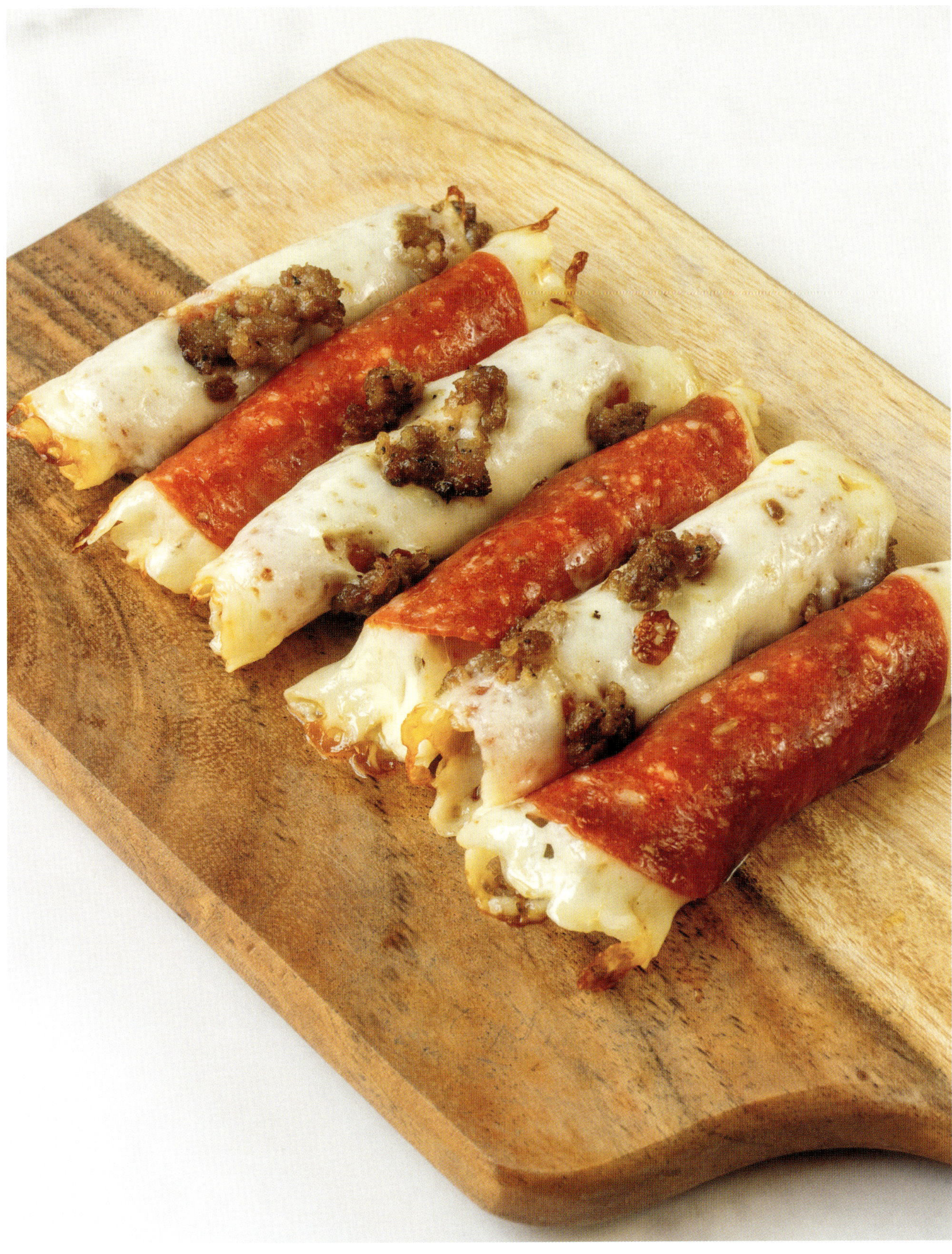

PER SERVING	calories: **690** | fat: **54g** | protein: **41g** | carbs: **6g** | macro split: **72/25/3**

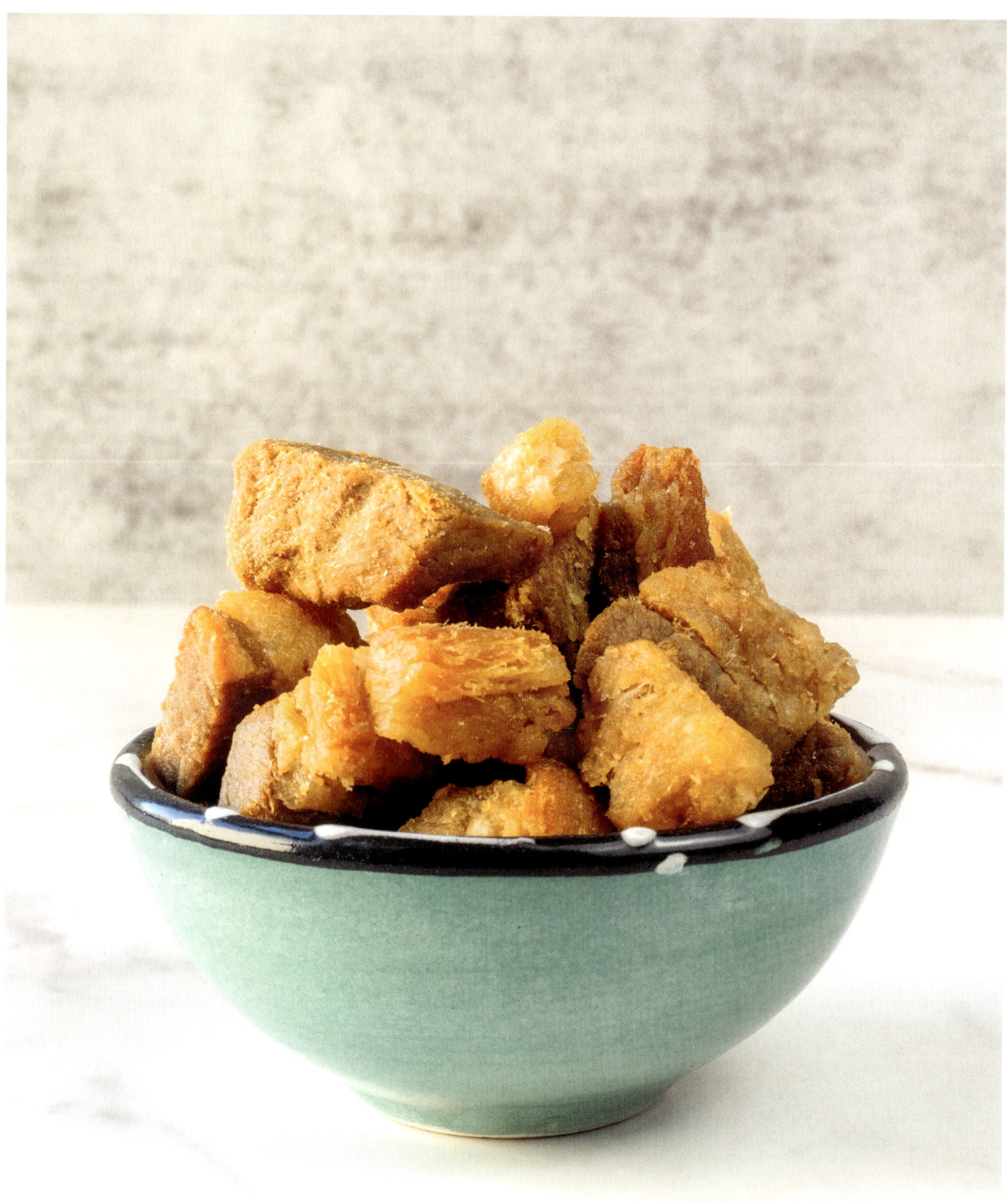

PER SERVING

calories: **587** | fat: **60g** | protein: **11g** | carbs: **0g** | macro split: **93/7/0**

YIELD: 3 to 4 cups (¼ cup per serving)

PREP TIME: 10 minutes

COOK TIME: 3 hours

CVARCI (SERBIAN PORK CRACKLINGS)

This traditional Serbian dish is prepared in the fall after the pork harvest. While most of the fat is rendered into lard, the tender bits of meat and fat left behind are turned into a crispy, delicious snack or appetizer. Think of it as pork belly popcorn. It requires time and patience to cook, but when done right, these morsels are melt-in-your-mouth perfection. Because these can't be made quickly, it doesn't make sense to make a small batch; instead, I suggest you make this when you are having friends or family over and want to introduce them to a classic Eastern European dish that doubles as the perfect carnivore snack.

3 to 4 pounds pork belly (the fattiest you can find)

4 cups lard

Salt

1. Rinse the pork belly and cut into 1-inch cubes. Put the cubes in a stockpot or large soup pot and place on the stovetop.
2. Melt the lard until soft and add to the pot with the pork belly. Turn the heat under the pot to high and cook until the lard starts to boil. Once at a boil, turn the heat to low and gently simmer, stirring occasionally, until the pieces of pork belly have shrunk to about a quarter of their original size. This will take 2 to 2½ hours. The chunks of pork belly will be swimming in the lard as they cook.
3. When the pork belly pieces are reduced, turn the heat up to medium-high to crisp them up, stirring every few minutes. This will take anywhere from 5 to 15 minutes. They will be done when they are no longer soft on the outside and have a golden crust, and they will float to the top.
4. Using a mesh skimmer (aka spider skimmer), remove the pork belly from the lard and spread out in a single layer on some paper towels. Season with salt to taste while they are still hot.
5. These are best served fresh and hot, but they will keep in an airtight container in the refrigerator for a few days.

YIELD: twenty-eight 1-inch meat jellies (4 per serving)

PREP TIME: 15 minutes, plus overnight to chill

COOK TIME: 5 to 6 hours

PIHTIJE (MEAT JELLY)

Pihtije, or meat jelly, is a traditional Serbian winter dish enjoyed when people crave hearty animal fats. Often served as an appetizer at Slava (a patron saint celebration) or as a side, it's made from various bone-in meats saved and frozen throughout the year, along with smoked meats from the fall harvest. The essential ingredients are pork or beef bones with meat, as they provide the necessary cartilage for the jelly to set. Adding a piece of fresh veal on the bone enhances the dish but isn't required. Some people eat this with jalapeños, hot sauce, or Sriracha.

4 pounds smoked ham hocks

2½ pounds fresh beef or pork feet

2 to 3 pounds bone-in veal, any cut (optional)

2 gallons plus up to 2 quarts water, divided

2 tablespoons minced garlic

Salt, as needed

FOR GARNISH:

Paprika

Ground black pepper

SPECIAL EQUIPMENT:
Extra-large stockpot (14+ quarts)

1. Rinse the meat and place it in an extra-large stockpot. Add 2 gallons of water, cover with the lid, and set over high heat. When the water has come to a boil, crack the lid and turn the heat to low. Allow to simmer, with the lid ajar, for 5 to 6 hours, until all of the meat has fallen off the bones.
2. After about 4 hours, add up to another 2 quarts of water, making sure that the bones and meat are completely submerged. Don't add any more water in the last 1 to 2 hours of cooking.
3. Once all of the meat has fallen off the bones, turn off the heat. Set a colander over a large bowl, then pour the contents of the pot through the colander. Dump the strained meat and bones into a large dish. Pour the cooking liquid through a fine-mesh strainer into a clean bowl. Set the bowl of strained cooking liquid and the dish of meat/bones aside to cool.
4. When the meat is cool to the touch, go through and remove all of the bones and large pieces of skin. Then chop or tear the meat into small pieces and mix in the garlic.
5. Evenly divide the meat and garlic mixture between two 13 by 9-inch dishes, spreading it out into an even layer. (See the note below for other dish size options.)
6. Return to the cooled liquid. Skim off the liquid fat on top and discard. Then taste the liquid and add salt to taste. Ham hocks are typically salted, so you probably won't need to add much salt, if any.

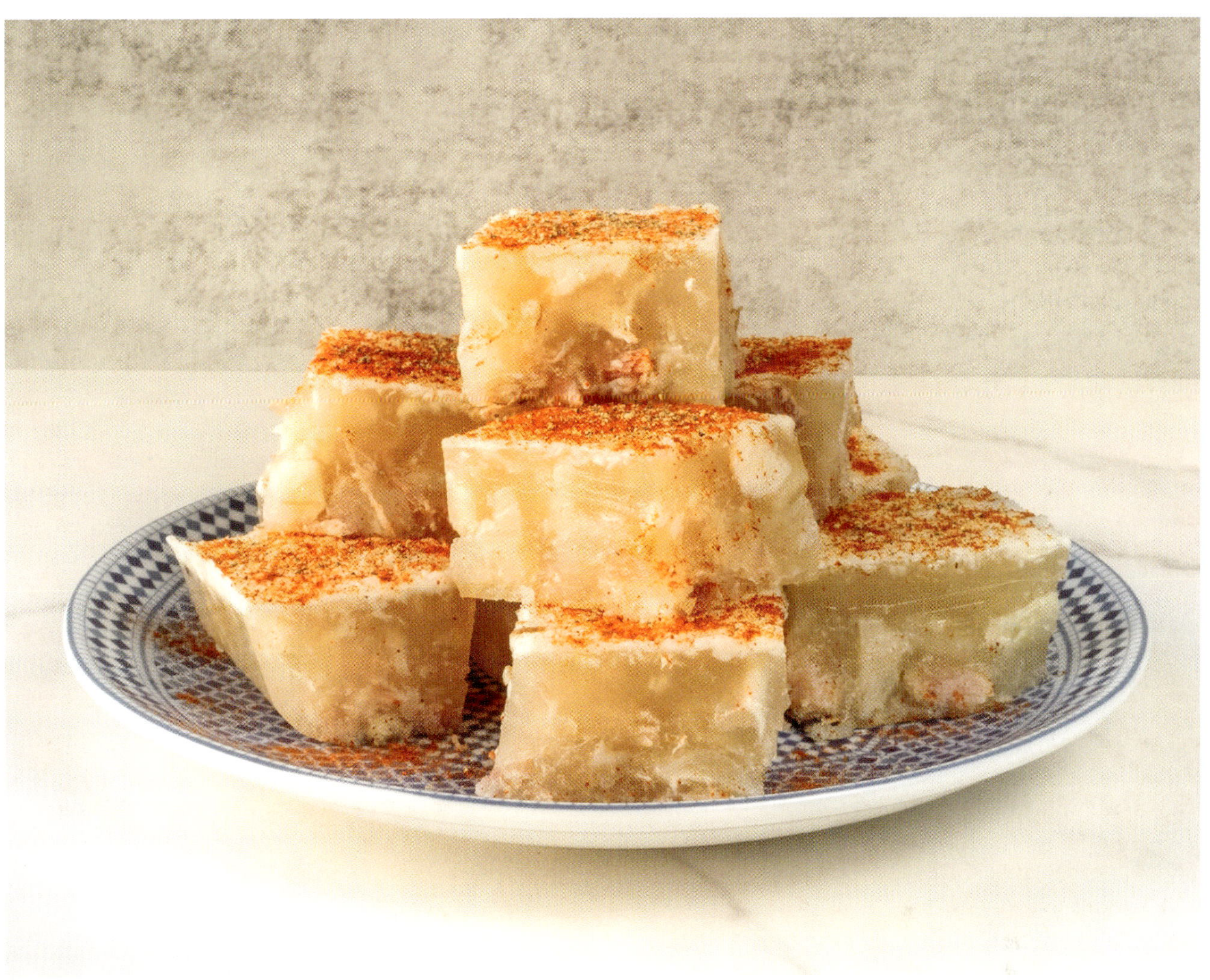

7 Ladle 1½ inches of the cooking liquid into each dish and place in the refrigerator to cool overnight. It will solidify into gelatin.

8 Cut into 1-inch squares and sprinkle with paprika and black pepper. This dish is served cold. It will keep in the refrigerator for a couple of weeks, and I do not advise freezing it.

Note:

If you don't have two 13 by 9-inch dishes, you can use three 11 by 7½-inch dishes or five or six smaller storage containers. The key is for the meat to be distributed in a single layer and for the sides of the dishes or containers to be at least 2 inches high to allow for the cooking liquid.

PER SERVING

calories: **278** | fat: **21g** | protein: **20g** | carbs: **1g** | macro split: **69/30/1**

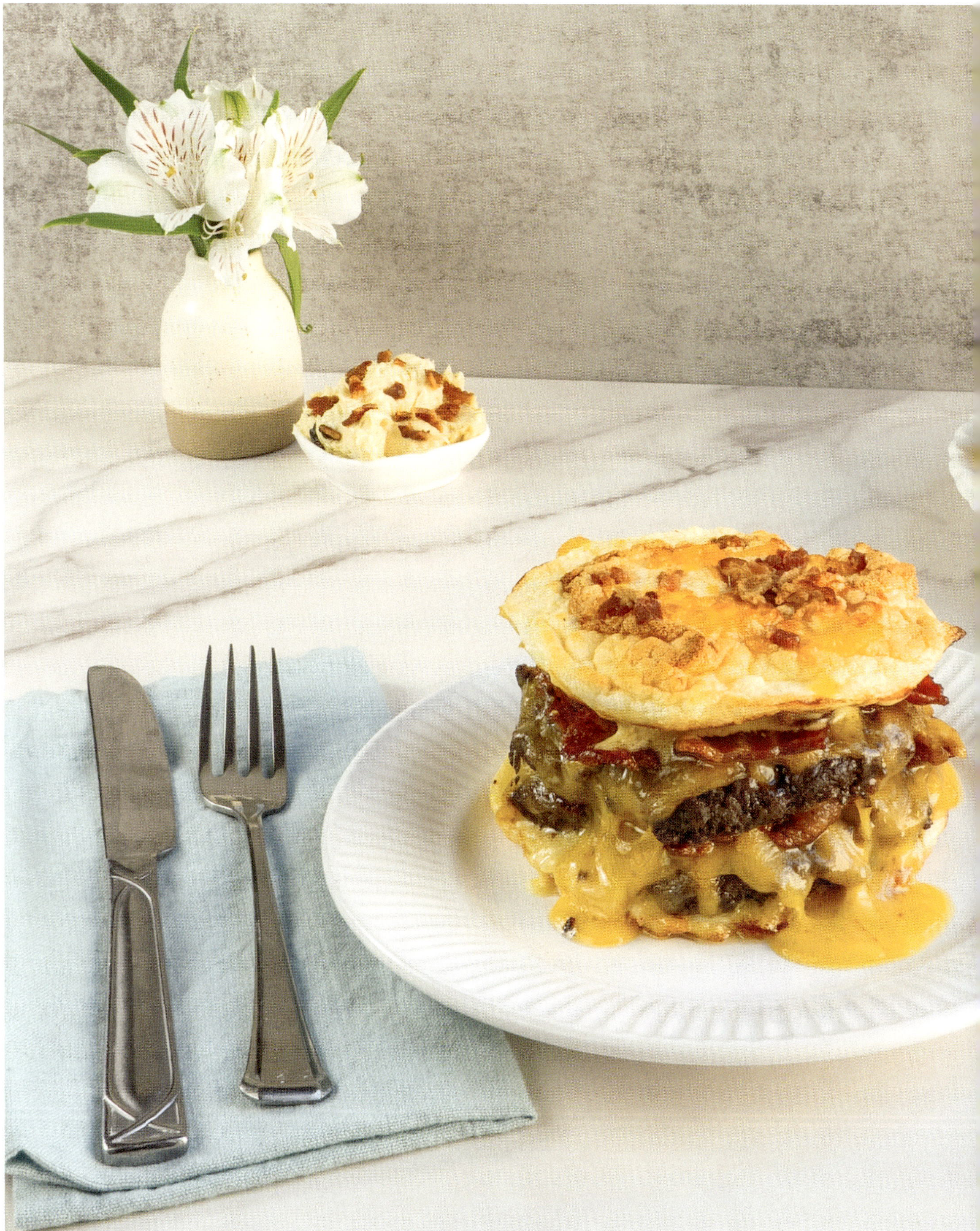

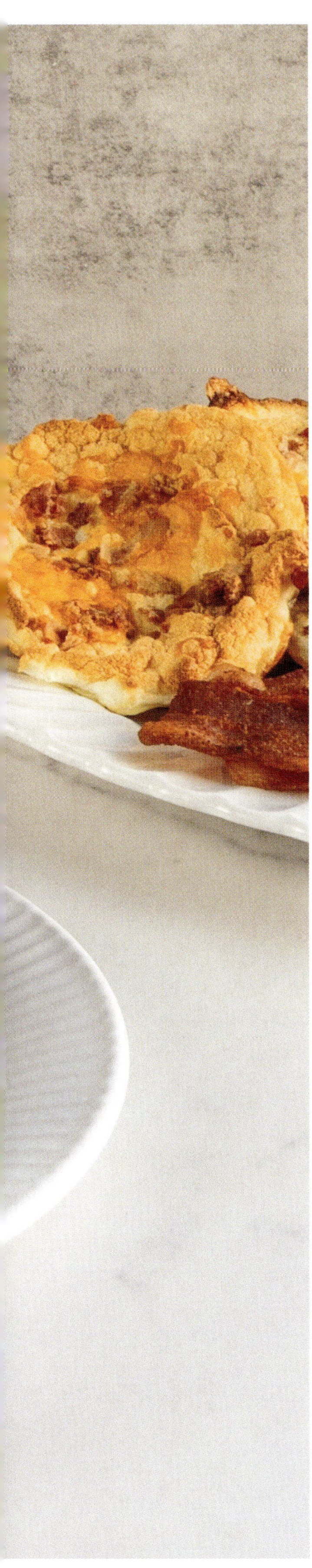

CHAPTER 12
SOUPS AND SANDWICHES

262 Chicken Soup

265 Hearty Meat Soup

266 Fajita Wrap

269 Extreme Double Bacon Cheeseburger

270 Pot Roast Sandwich

273 Spicy Chicken Sandwiches

YIELD: 10 servings

PREP TIME: 5 minutes

COOK TIME: 6 hours 15 minutes

CHICKEN SOUP

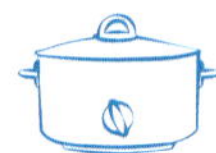
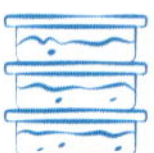

Nothing warms the soul like a bowl of chicken soup. This easy, hands-off recipe delivers rich, comforting flavor, as if you'd spent hours in the kitchen—yet it's surprisingly simple to make.

- 1 whole (4- to 5-pound) chicken
- 1½ quarts water
- 3 teaspoons salt, divided
- 1 teaspoon garlic powder
- 1 teaspoon onion powder
- ½ teaspoon ground white pepper
- 1 sprig fresh rosemary

1. Put the chicken, water, and 2 teaspoons of the salt in a slow cooker and cook on low until the meat is falling off the bones, 5 to 6 hours.
2. When the chicken is done, pour the contents of the slow cooker through a colander set over a large bowl or pot to capture the broth.
3. Pour the strained broth back into the slow cooker and stir in the remaining teaspoon of salt along with the spices and rosemary sprig. Let the rosemary steep for 30 minutes.
4. While the rosemary is steeping, clean the chicken: Remove the bones and skin and discard, then chop or tear the meat into small pieces.
5. When the rosemary is done steeping, remove the sprig and discard. Strain the broth one more time with a fine-mesh strainer and return it to the slow cooker.
6. Add the chicken to the broth and cook on low for 15 more minutes to warm through before serving.

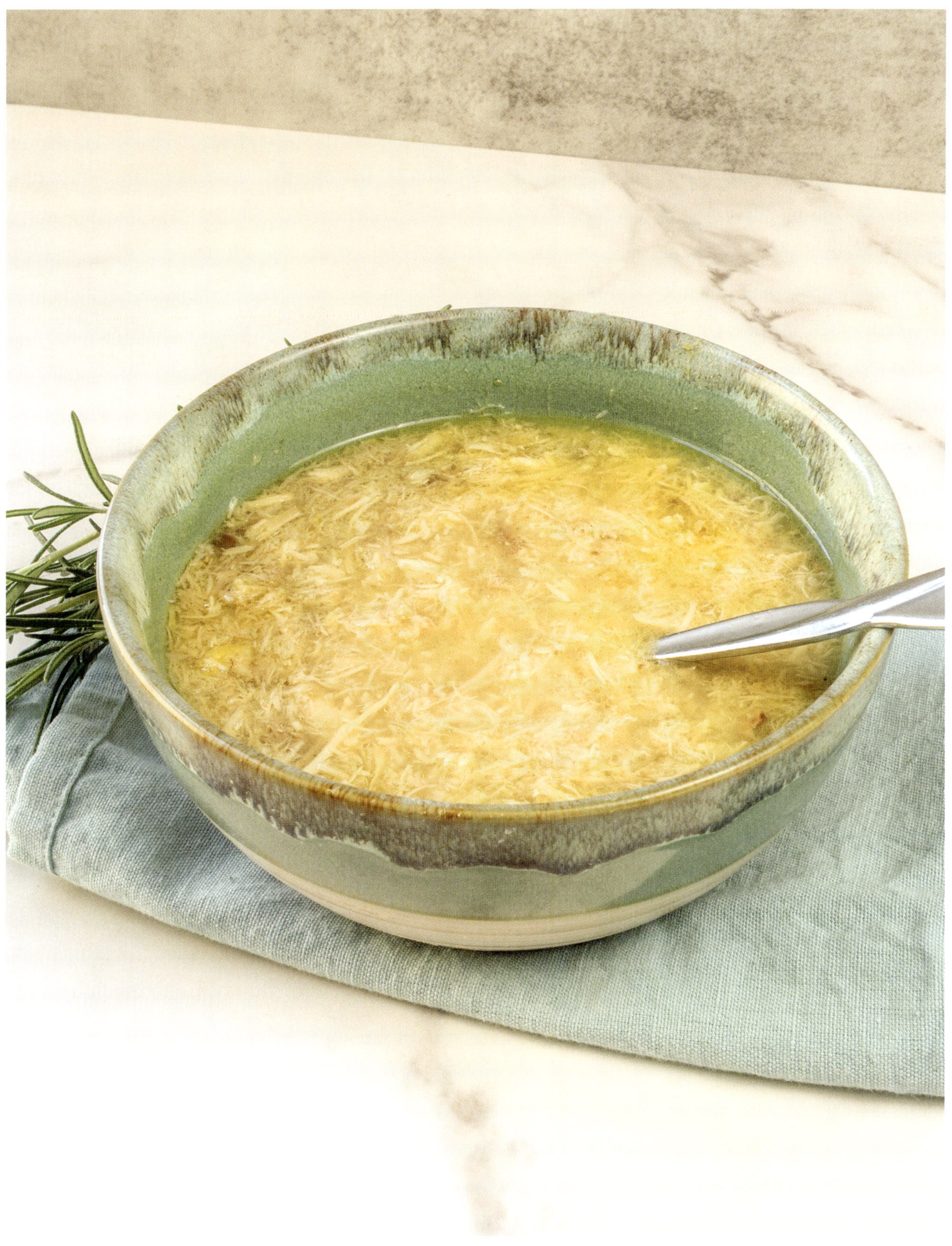

PER SERVING (1 cup)	calories: **288** | fat: **20g** | protein: **25g** | carbs: **0g** | macro split: **65/35/0**

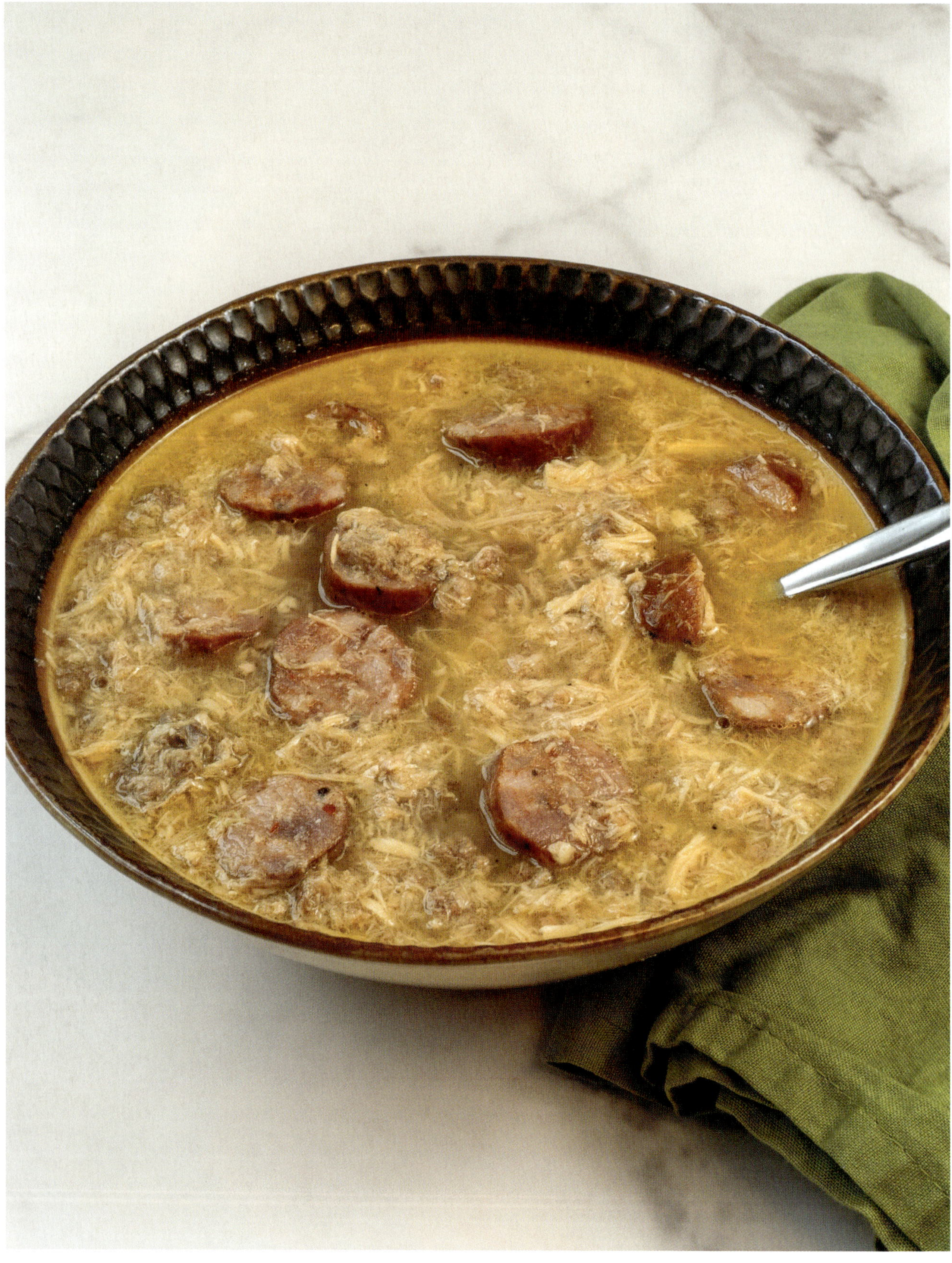

PER SERVING (1 cup)	calories: **639** | fat: **51g** | protein: **42g** | carbs: **2g** | macro split: **73/26/1**

YIELD: 10 servings

PREP TIME: 10 minutes

COOK TIME: 7 hours

HEARTY MEAT SOUP

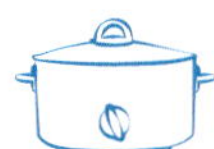
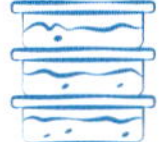

This filling soup combines tender chicken, savory ground beef, and spicy andouille sausage in a rich, flavorful broth. Perfect for a cozy meal, it's packed with protein and spices, making every spoonful warm, satisfying, and delicious.

- 1 whole (4- to 5-pound) chicken
- 1½ quarts water
- 4 teaspoons salt, divided
- 1 pound 80/20 ground beef
- 1 teaspoon onion powder
- 1 teaspoon garlic powder
- ½ teaspoon ground white pepper
- 1 sprig fresh rosemary
- 2 pounds andouille sausage, sliced

1. Put the chicken, water, and 2 teaspoons of the salt in a slow cooker and cook on low until the meat is falling off the bones, 5 to 6 hours.
2. When the chicken is almost done, brown the ground beef in a large frying pan over medium heat, crumbling it as it cooks.
3. Once the chicken is fully done, turn off the slow cooker and pour the contents through a colander set over a large bowl or pot to capture the broth. Pour the strained broth back into the slow cooker and stir in the remaining 2 teaspoons of salt along with the spices and sprig of rosemary. Let the rosemary steep for 30 minutes.
4. While the rosemary is steeping, clean the chicken: Remove the bones and skin and discard, then chop or tear the meat into small pieces.
5. When the rosemary is done steeping, remove the sprig and discard. Strain the broth one more time with a fine-mesh strainer and return it to the slow cooker. Return the chicken to the broth along with the cooked ground beef and sliced sausage. Cook on low for another hour before serving.

YIELD: 2 wraps

PREP TIME: 15 to 20 minutes (not including time to make flatbread batter)

COOK TIME: 25 minutes

FAJITA WRAP

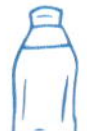
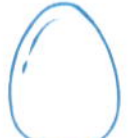

This quick and delicious wrap is easy to make and endlessly customizable. While this recipe uses steak, you can also try it with chicken, pork, lamb, shrimp, or a combination of meats. The spicy sour cream adds a flavorful kick that brings it all together. You can also add some fajita vegetables if you are doing keto or a keto cheat meal. If you choose to include vegetables, you can use red, green, yellow, and/or orange bell peppers, cut into strips, and a medium-size white onion, cut into slices.

1 batch Cottage Cheese Flatbread batter (page 371)

1 teaspoon Cajun Seasoning (page 346)

1 pound thinly sliced strip steak or marbled fajita meat

½ teaspoon salt

½ teaspoon garlic powder

1 pound sliced fajita vegetables (optional, for keto version)

FOR THE SPICY SOUR CREAM:

½ cup full-fat sour cream

2 teaspoons hot sauce

⅛ teaspoon salt

1. Preheat the oven to 360°F. Line a sheet pan with parchment paper.
2. Pour the flatbread batter into two even-sized rounds on the prepared pan. Evenly sprinkle the rounds of batter with the Cajun seasoning. Bake until golden brownish and cooked through, 30 to 35 minutes. While the flatbreads are in the oven, prepare the fillings for the fajitas.
3. Place the steak in a large frying pan over medium-high heat and season with the salt and garlic powder. Cook until the meat is browned on all sides and cooked medium-rare to medium, 5 to 7 minutes. Transfer the meat to a bowl and set aside.
4. If using fajita vegetables, cook them in the same pan you used to cook the steak, in the fat left over from cooking the meat, over medium heat until tender. If needed, add butter, beef tallow, or bacon grease to the pan to keep the vegetables from sticking.
5. Make the spicy sour cream: Stir together the sour cream, hot sauce, and salt in a small bowl and set aside.
6. Once the flatbreads are ready, slather them with the spicy sour cream, using about ¼ cup per flatbread, then top with the meat and, if doing the keto version, the fajita veggies.

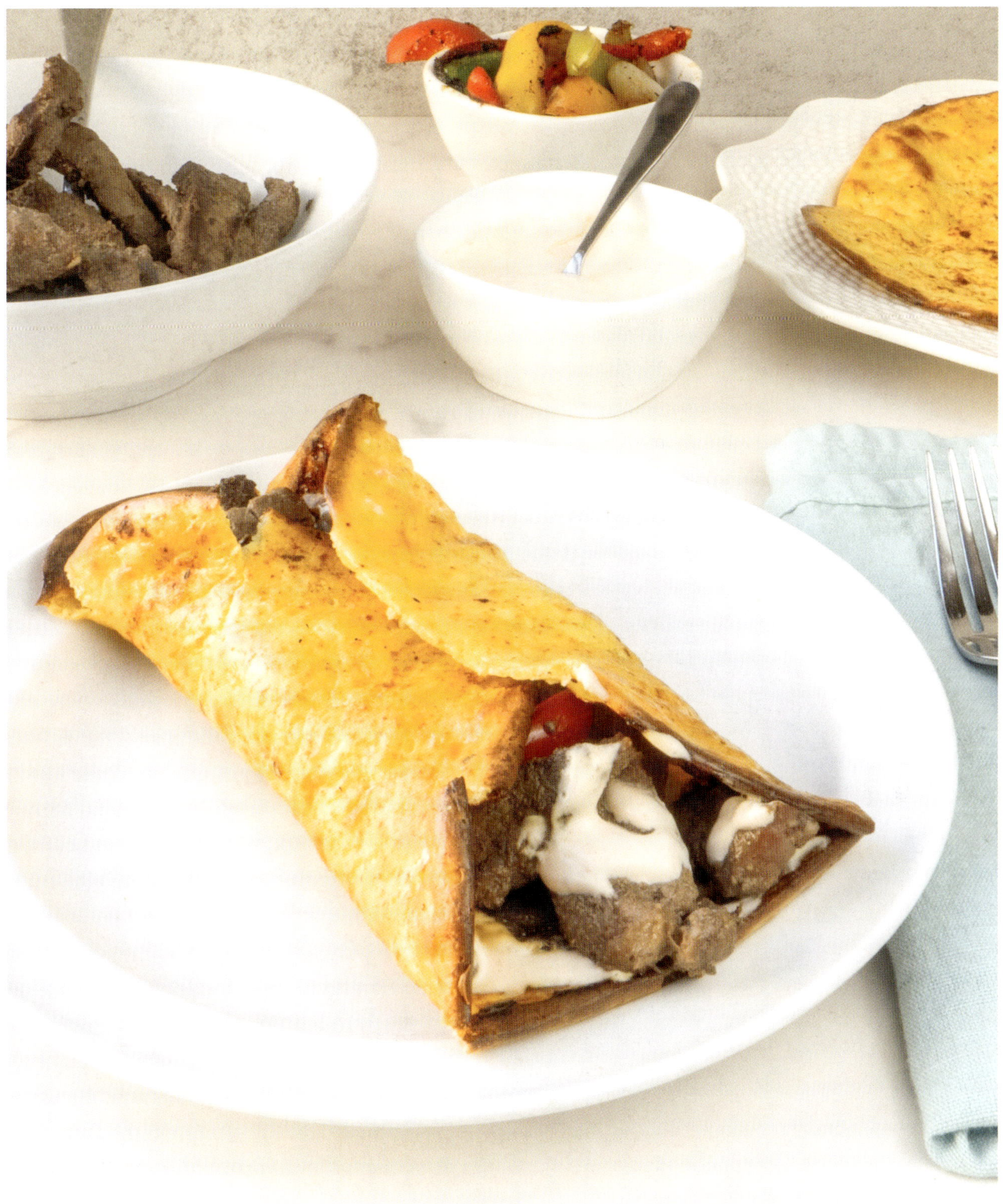

PER WRAP (carnivore version)	calories: **398** | fat: **24g** | protein: **37g** | carbs: **6g** | macro split: **55/38/7**
PER WRAP (keto version)	calories: **430** | fat: **24g** | protein: **38g** | carbs: **13g** | macro split: **52/36/12**

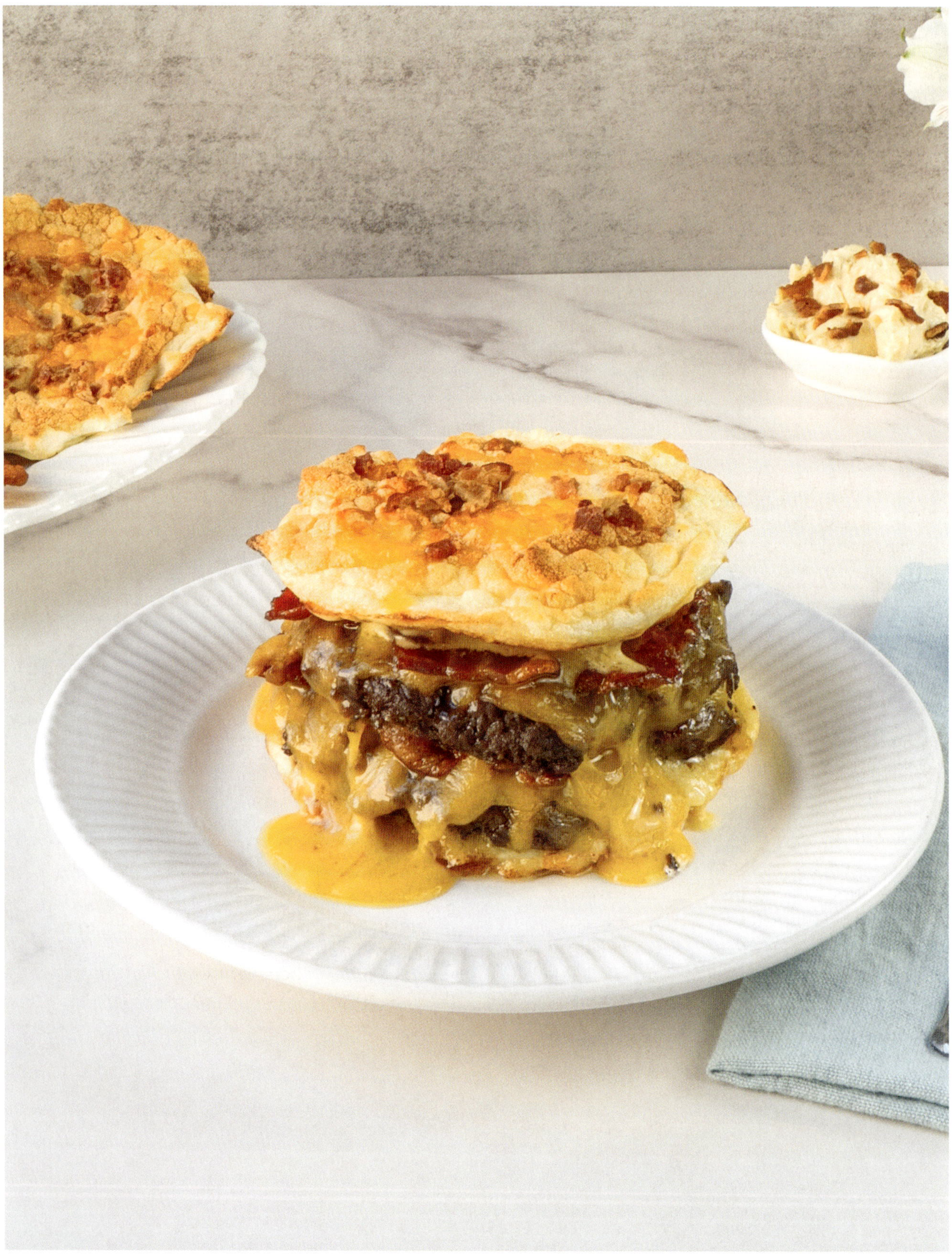

PER DOUBLE BURGER

calories: **1104** | fat: **85g** | protein: **78g** | carbs: **2g** | macro split: **68/31/1**

YIELD: 4 double burgers

PREP TIME: 5 minutes (not including time to cook bacon or make buns or mayo)

COOK TIME: 25 minutes

EXTREME DOUBLE BACON CHEESEBURGER

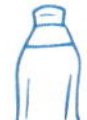
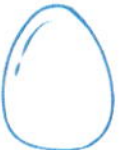

I set out to re-create a classic double bacon cheeseburger from a popular fast-food chain, but in a fully carnivore-friendly way. My version is loaded with extra cheese and bacon, and it has just 2 grams of carbs! The result is a bacon-packed delight, and I couldn't be happier with how it turned out.

2 pounds 80/20 ground beef

2 teaspoons salt

1 teaspoon garlic powder

1 teaspoon onion powder

2 tablespoons bacon grease or salted butter, for the pan

8 slices cheddar or American cheese

8 tablespoons Bacon Mayonnaise (page 352) or store-bought avocado oil mayonnaise

8 Bacon & Cheese Cloud Buns (page 373)

8 strips bacon, cooked and cut in half crosswise

SPECIAL EQUIPMENT:
Burger press

1. Put the ground beef in a large mixing bowl and add the salt and spices. Using your hands, mix thoroughly. Divide into eight 4-ounce portions and roll each into a ball.
2. Put the bacon grease in a large frying pan and set over medium-high heat. Allow the fat to heat up, then add two or three of the ground beef balls, leaving 2 to 3 inches of space between them.
3. Allow the balls to cook for 1 minute, then smash them flat with the burger press until they are about ½ inch thick. Cook for another 2 to 3 minutes, then flip and cook for 2 to 3 minutes on the other side. Top each patty with a slice of cheese. Once the cheese is melted, remove the patties from the pan and set aside on a plate.
4. Repeat this process with the rest of the ground beef balls and cheese slices until all of the patties are cooked and topped with cheese.
5. To assemble the burgers, spread 1 tablespoon of mayo on the cut sides of each bun. Then, on each bottom bun, layer a cheeseburger patty, two half slices of bacon, another cheeseburger patty, two more half slices of bacon, and then the top bun, mayo side down.

YIELD: 1 sandwich

PREP TIME: 5 minutes (not including time to cook pot roast or make mayo or bread)

POT ROAST SANDWICH

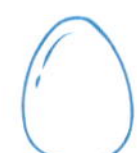

Pot roast is a fuss-free, set-it-and-forget-it recipe that's perfect for meal prep. It's also fantastic in sandwiches, especially when paired with bacon mayo and a touch of hot sauce for extra flavor. Cloud bread creates the perfect base for this delicious sandwich.

2 tablespoons Bacon Mayonnaise (page 352) or store-bought avocado oil mayonnaise

2 slices Cloud Bread Loaf (page 372)

6 ounces cooked pot roast (page 219), freshly made or rewarmed

1 teaspoon hot sauce (optional)

1. Spread 1 tablespoon of mayo on each slice of bread.
2. Lay the pot roast on one of the mayo-slathered slices of bread.
3. Top with the hot sauce, if using, and then the second slice of bread, mayo side down. Enjoy!

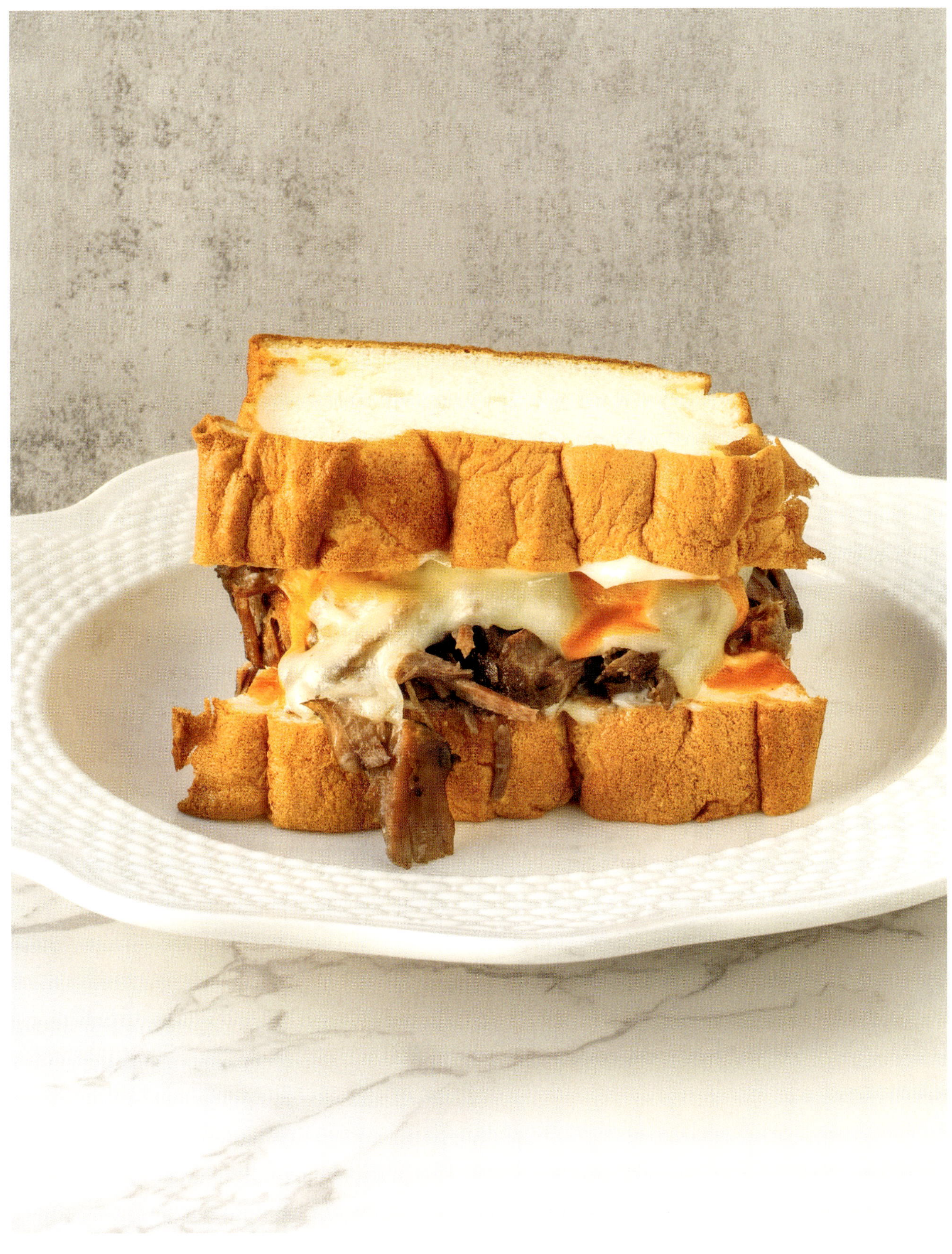

PER SANDWICH	calories: **670** | fat: **53g** | protein: **42g** | carbs: **1g** | macro split: **74/26/0**

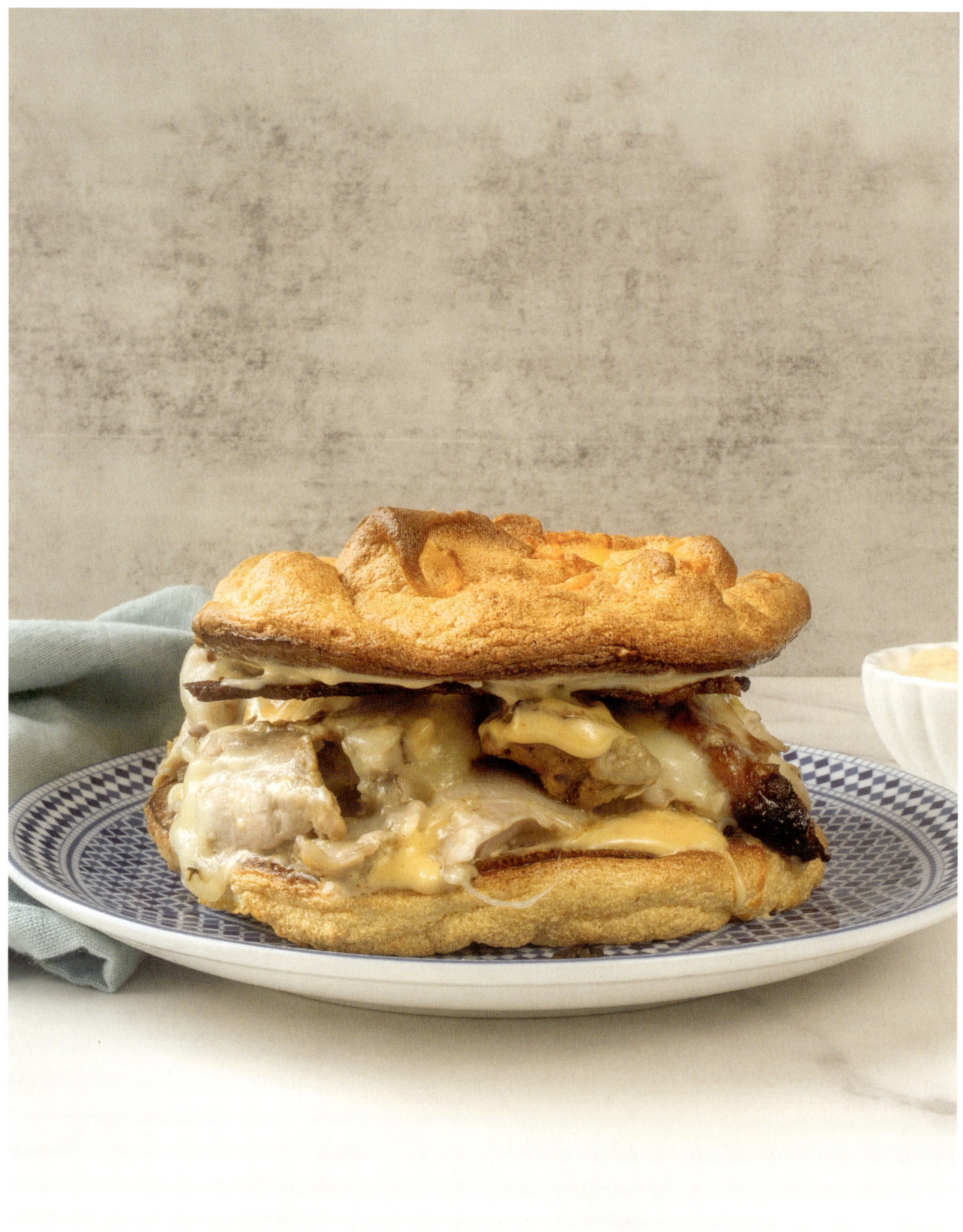

PER SANDWICH	calories: **811** | fat: **65g** | protein: **48g** | carbs: **1g** | macro split: **74/25/1**

YIELD: 6 sandwiches

PREP TIME: 20 minutes, plus time to marinate chicken if desired (not including time to make seasoning, mayo, or buns or cook bacon)

COOK TIME: 40 minutes

SPICY CHICKEN SANDWICHES

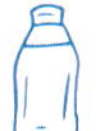 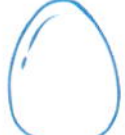

A few years back, my sister-in-law couldn't stop raving about Popeye's new spicy chicken sandwich—and for good reason. It was delicious! I created this recipe to capture that same amazing flavor but without the carbs and seed oils. Give it a try and see if you agree—I think I nailed it! Try marinating the chicken in dill pickle juice; this step is optional but gives the thighs an undertone of flavor that you can't beat.

2 pounds bone-in, skin-on chicken thighs

2 cups dill pickle juice (optional)

1 tablespoon avocado oil

¼ cup Chicken & Pork Seasoning (page 348)

½ cup medium-hot hot sauce, such as Cholula

TO BUILD THE SANDWICHES:

6 slices pepper Jack cheese

12 strips bacon, cooked and cut in half crosswise

12 tablespoons Spicy Mayonnaise (page 356)

6 Cloud Buns (page 372), split

Sliced dill pickles (optional, for keto version)

1. If desired, marinate the chicken thighs in the pickle juice for at least 12 or up to 24 hours.
2. Set an oven rack in the top position and preheat the oven to 425°F. Fit a sheet pan with a wire rack and set aside.
3. Put the chicken thighs in a large mixing bowl; if you've marinated them, discard the pickle juice after removing the thighs. Pour in the avocado oil and toss, then sprinkle with the seasoning mix and toss until evenly coated.
4. Pour the hot sauce onto a small plate. Dip each thigh into the hot sauce, then flip and dip the other side.
5. Lay the hot sauce-covered thighs on the wire rack and insert a meat thermometer into one of them. Bake on the top rack of the oven for 30 to 35 minutes, until the chicken reaches an internal temperature of 150°F. Turn the oven to broil and allow the skin to crisp up. Pull the chicken out of the oven once the internal temperature reaches 160°F.
6. Using your fingers, remove the bone from each thigh by pulling gently and discard; leave the skin intact. Arrange the meat into six portions that fit on a cloud bun.
7. Place a slice of cheese over each portion of chicken, then top each with four half-slices of bacon.
8. Spread 1 tablespoon of spicy mayo on the cut sides of each bun.
9. Use a spatula to pick up a chicken, cheese, and bacon portion and place it on the bottom half of one of the buns. Add pickle slices, if using, then put the top bun on the sandwich. Repeat with the remaining buns and fixings to make a total of six sandwiches.

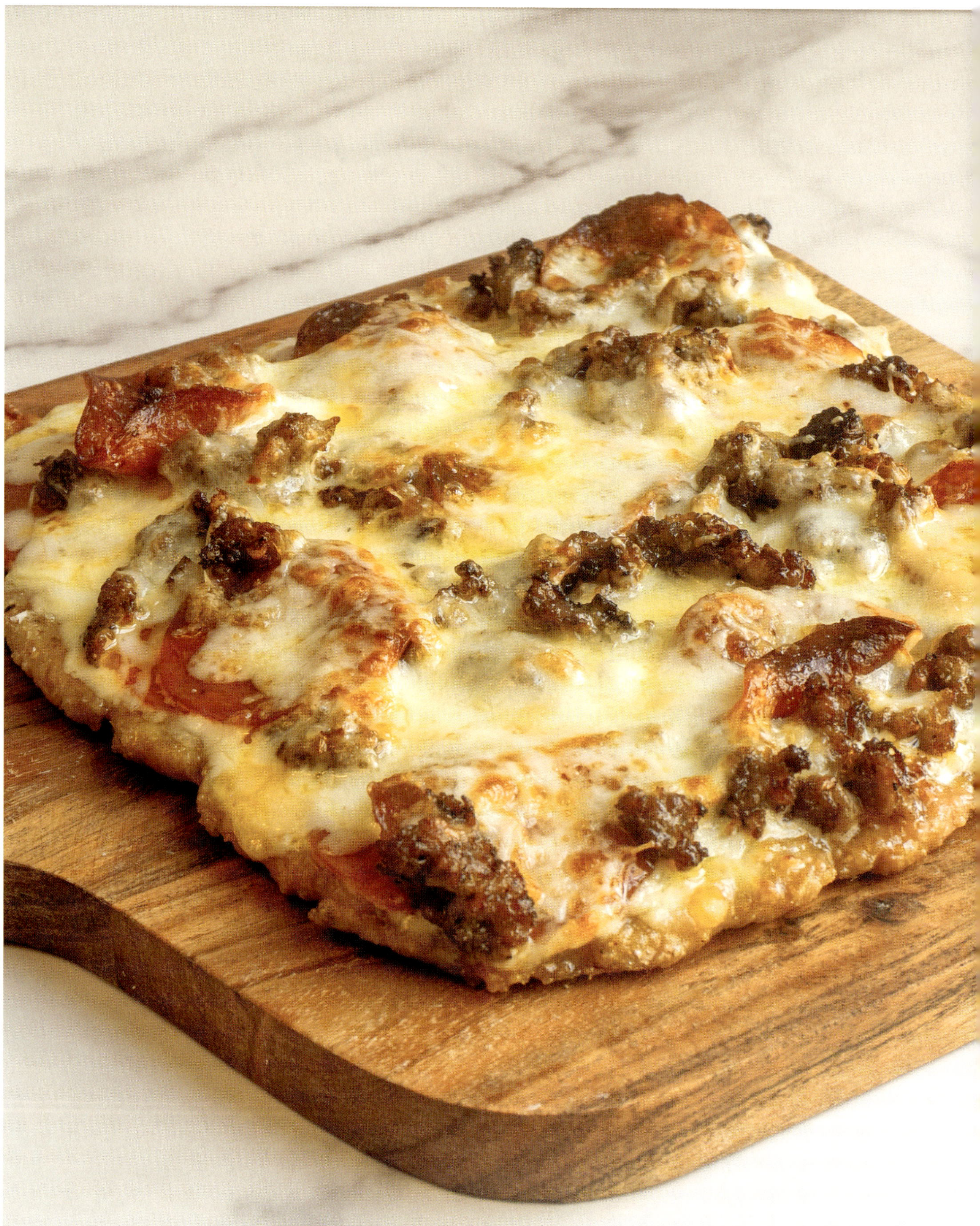

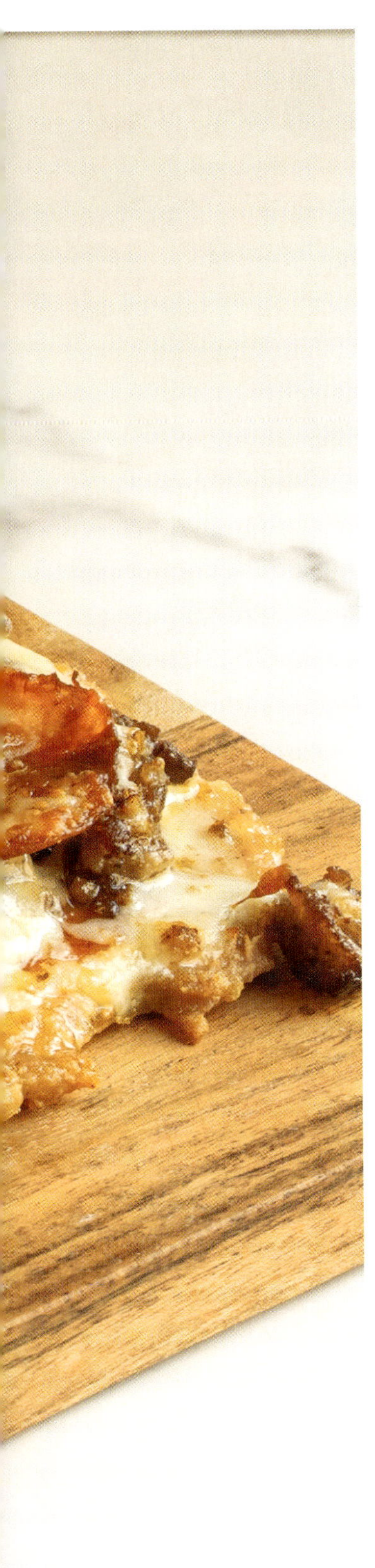

CHAPTER 13
REPLACEMENT RECIPES

276 Beef Stroganoff

278 Carnivore Mac & Cheese Casserole

283 Carnivore White Pizza

286 Spicy Bacon-Wrapped Chorizo Dogs

289 Carnivore Tacos

290 Chili Cheese Dog Meatballs

293 Crab Cakes with Rémoulade

294 Taco Balls

297 Carnivore Quesadilla

YIELD: 2 servings

PREP TIME: 10 minutes (not including time to make noodles)

COOK TIME: 30 minutes

BEEF STROGANOFF

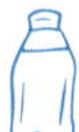 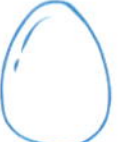

If you've been longing for a warm, comforting noodle dish, look no further—this recipe has you covered. This creamy beef stroganoff is a delicious carnivore twist on the classic that's every bit as satisfying as the original. Packed with rich, savory flavors and a velvety sauce, it's not only tastier than the high-carb version but also incredibly easy to make. Perfect for a cozy weeknight dinner, it comes together effortlessly and disappears even faster!

1 pound 80/20 ground beef

1 cup beef bone broth

1 teaspoon salt

1 teaspoon garlic powder (optional)

4 ounces (½ cup) full-fat cream cheese

1 batch Carnivore Noodles (page 364), for serving

1. Cook the ground beef in a medium frying pan over medium heat until no pink remains, about 10 minutes. As the meat cooks, break it up with a spatula. Do not drain the fat.
2. Reduce the heat to medium-low and pour in the broth; let it simmer for a few minutes. Stir in the salt and garlic powder, if using.
3. Cut the cream cheese into chunks and add them to the beef mixture, stirring until fully melted. Simmer over low heat until it reduces by half to three-quarters, about 10 minutes. It will look way too liquid-y at first, but trust me, it will reduce down and become thick and smooth, with the consistency of a thick gravy. Season with salt to taste.
4. Divide the noodles between two shallow bowls and ladle half of the beef stroganoff into each bowl.

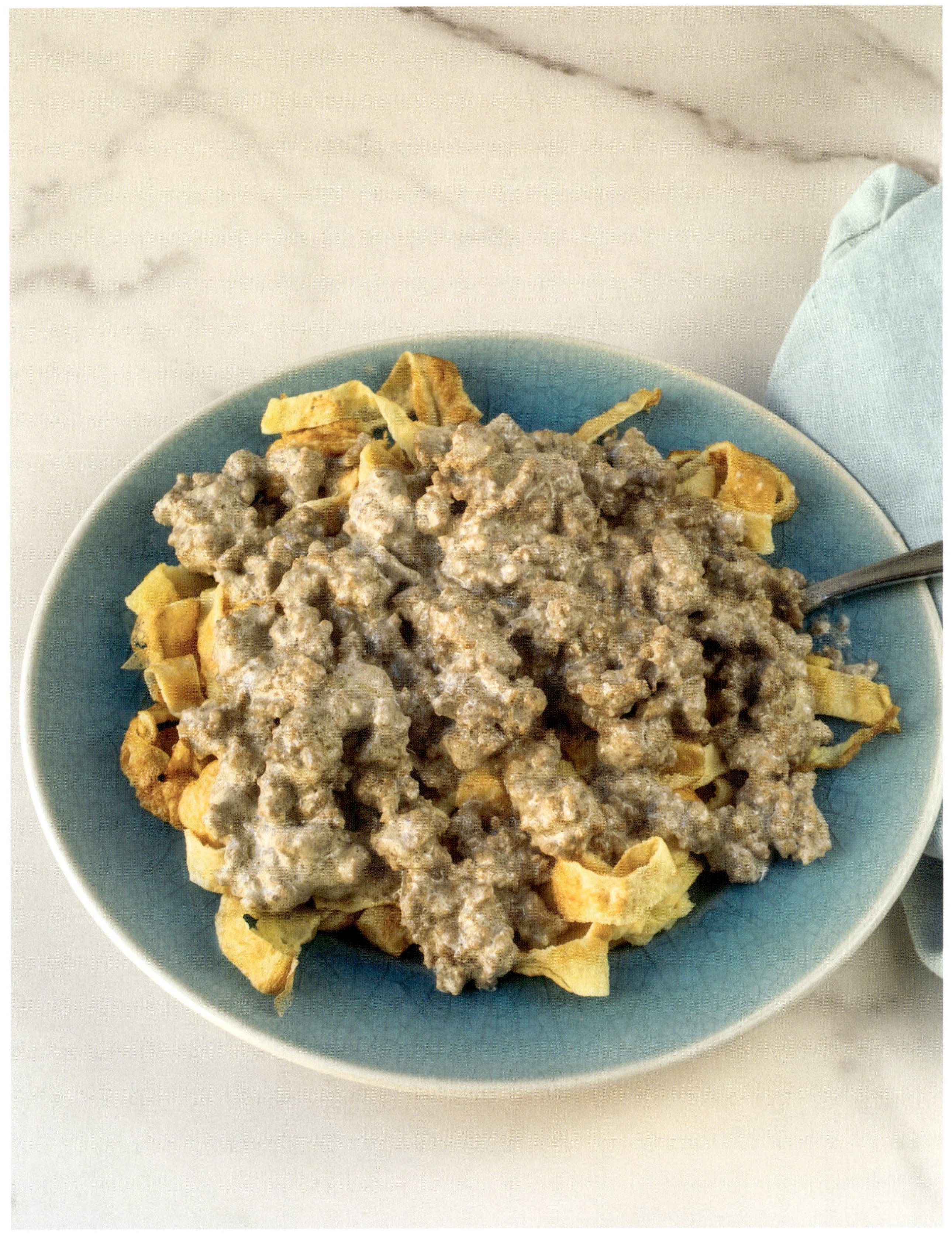

PER SERVING calories: **925** | fat: **65g** | protein: **45g** | carbs: **3g** | macro split: **69/29/2**

YIELD: 6 servings

PREP TIME: 45 minutes (not including time to cook bacon)

COOK TIME: 35 minutes

CARNIVORE MAC & CHEESE CASSEROLE

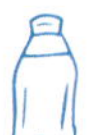
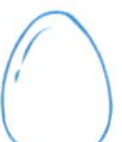

I discovered the base recipe for this mac and cheese on AshEats.com and adapted it to make it more carnivore-friendly. Of course, I couldn't resist adding a generous amount of extra cheese—because more cheese is always a good idea! This dish is best enjoyed fresh, but if you happen to have any leftovers (which is unlikely because it's such a hit), you can store them for up to a couple of days and reheat the leftovers in the microwave. Trust me, this recipe is a crowd-pleaser!

FOR THE BREADCRUMBS:

1 cup plain pork rinds

½ cup grated Parmesan cheese

½ cup grated Cotija or other hard white cheese, such as feta

FOR THE "MACARONI":

2 tablespoons salted butter or ghee, for the pan

2 pounds ground chicken

4 large eggs

Pinch of salt

FOR THE CHEESE SAUCE:

½ cup whole milk

½ cup heavy cream

1 cup grated Parmesan cheese

½ cup grated Cotija or other hard white cheese, such as feta

2 teaspoons prepared yellow mustard

1 tablespoon freshly squeezed lemon juice (optional)

Salt, if needed

FOR THE TOPPING:

½ cup chopped cooked bacon

½ cup shredded mozzarella cheese

½ cup shredded sharp yellow cheddar cheese

½ cup shredded white cheddar cheese

MAKE THE BREADCRUMBS:

1. Put the pork rinds in a blender or food processor and blend to a fine powder. Pour the powder into a medium bowl. (Do not clean the blender or food processor; you will use it to make the "macaroni.")
2. Add the cheeses to the powdered pork rinds and mix with a spoon or your hands to combine. Set aside.

MAKE THE "MACARONI":

1. Melt the butter in a medium frying pan over medium-high heat.
2. Meanwhile, using the blender or food processor, blend the ground chicken with the eggs and salt until it becomes a paste.

(recipe continues)

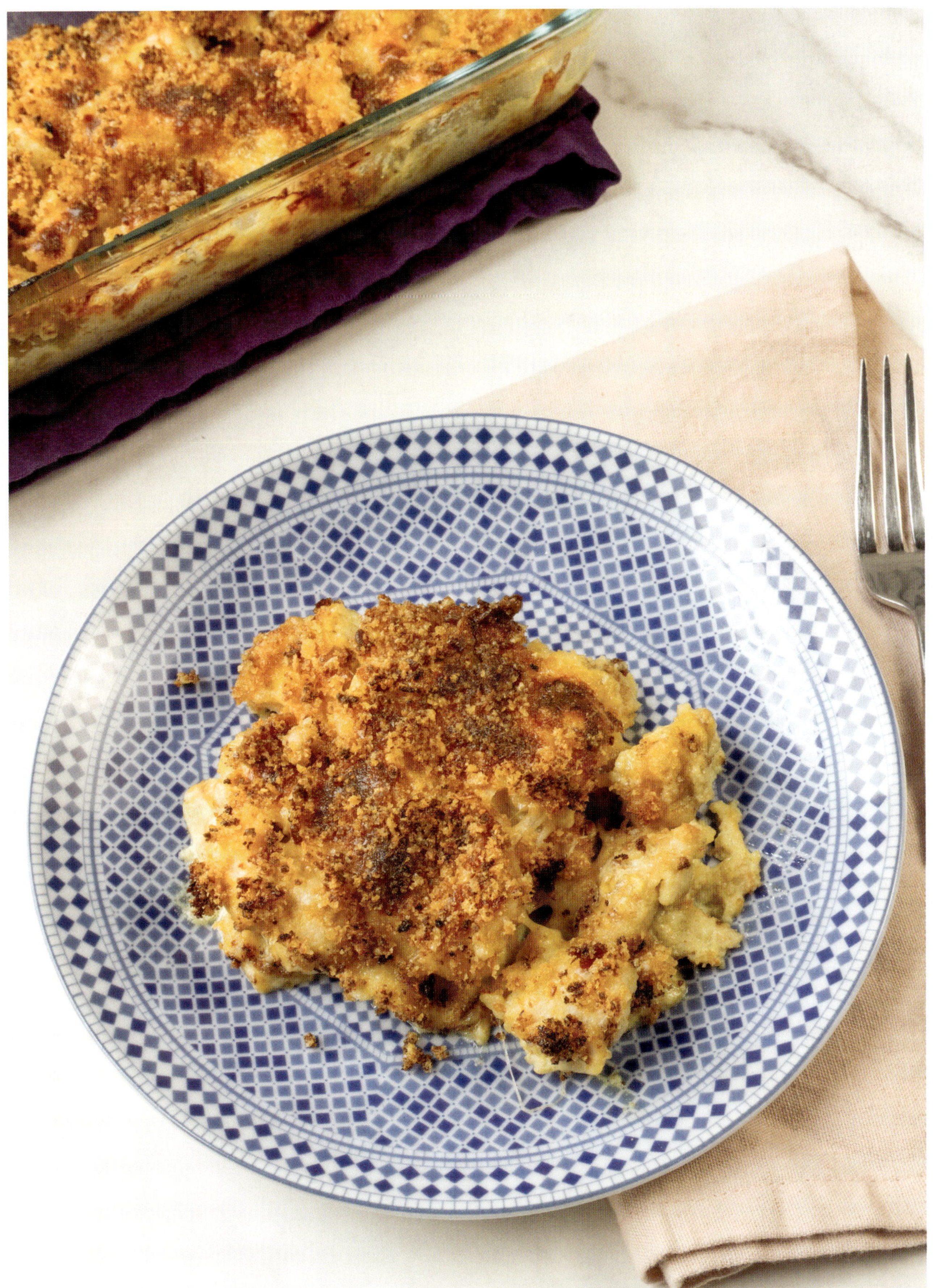

3. Scoop the paste into a gallon-sized plastic bag, push the chicken mixture down into one corner, and then snip off that corner of the bag.
4. Pipe several long tubes of the chicken mixture into the hot pan and pan-fry them until golden brown. Flip the tubes over and cut them into 1-inch-long "nuggets" with the edge of your spatula.
5. Once the nuggets are golden brown on both sides, remove them from the pan and place them in an 11 by 7½-inch casserole dish. Preheat the oven to 400°F.

MAKE THE CHEESE SAUCE:

1. Pour the milk and cream into a medium saucepan and bring to a boil over medium heat while stirring. Once boiling, turn down the heat to medium-low and slowly stir in the cheeses.
2. Add the mustard and lemon juice, if using, to the sauce while stirring. Taste and add salt if needed. Keep stirring until the sauce is smooth, then remove the pan from the heat.

BUILD THE CASSEROLE:

1. Cover the chicken nuggets with the cheese sauce, stirring to ensure the "macaroni" is evenly coated.
2. Sprinkle the bacon and mozzarella and cheddar cheeses over the chicken pieces and sauce, then sprinkle the breadcrumbs on top.
3. Bake for 15 to 20 minutes, until the cheese on top is melted and bubbly. Then turn the oven to broil and let the top crisp up for 3 to 5 minutes, until the cheese and breadcrumbs are browned a bit. Be sure to watch carefully during the broiling process so that the top of the mac and cheese doesn't burn.
4. Let cool for 10 to 15 minutes, then enjoy!

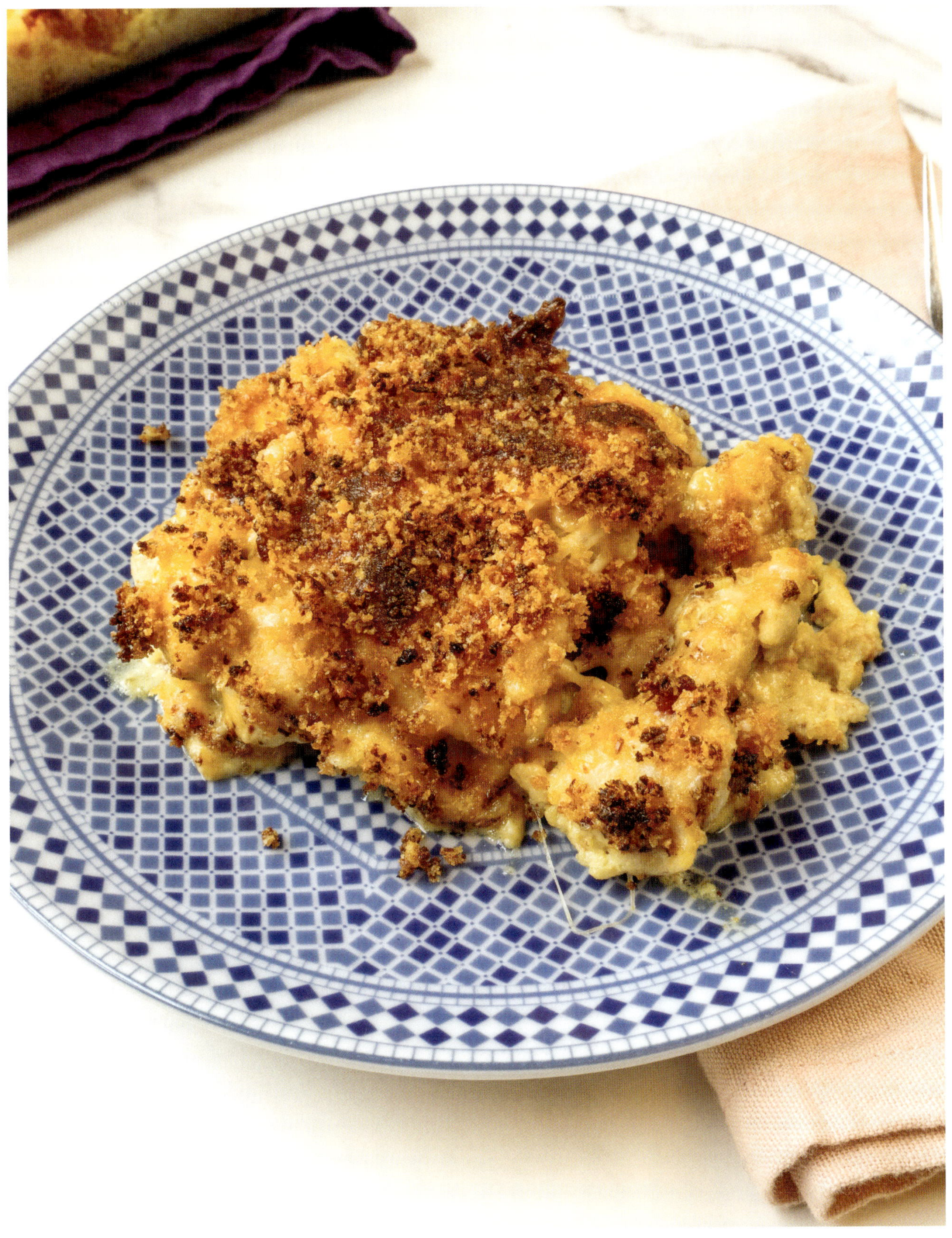

PER SERVING | calories: **885** | fat: **66g** | protein: **67g** | carbs: **3.3g** | macro split: **68/31/1**

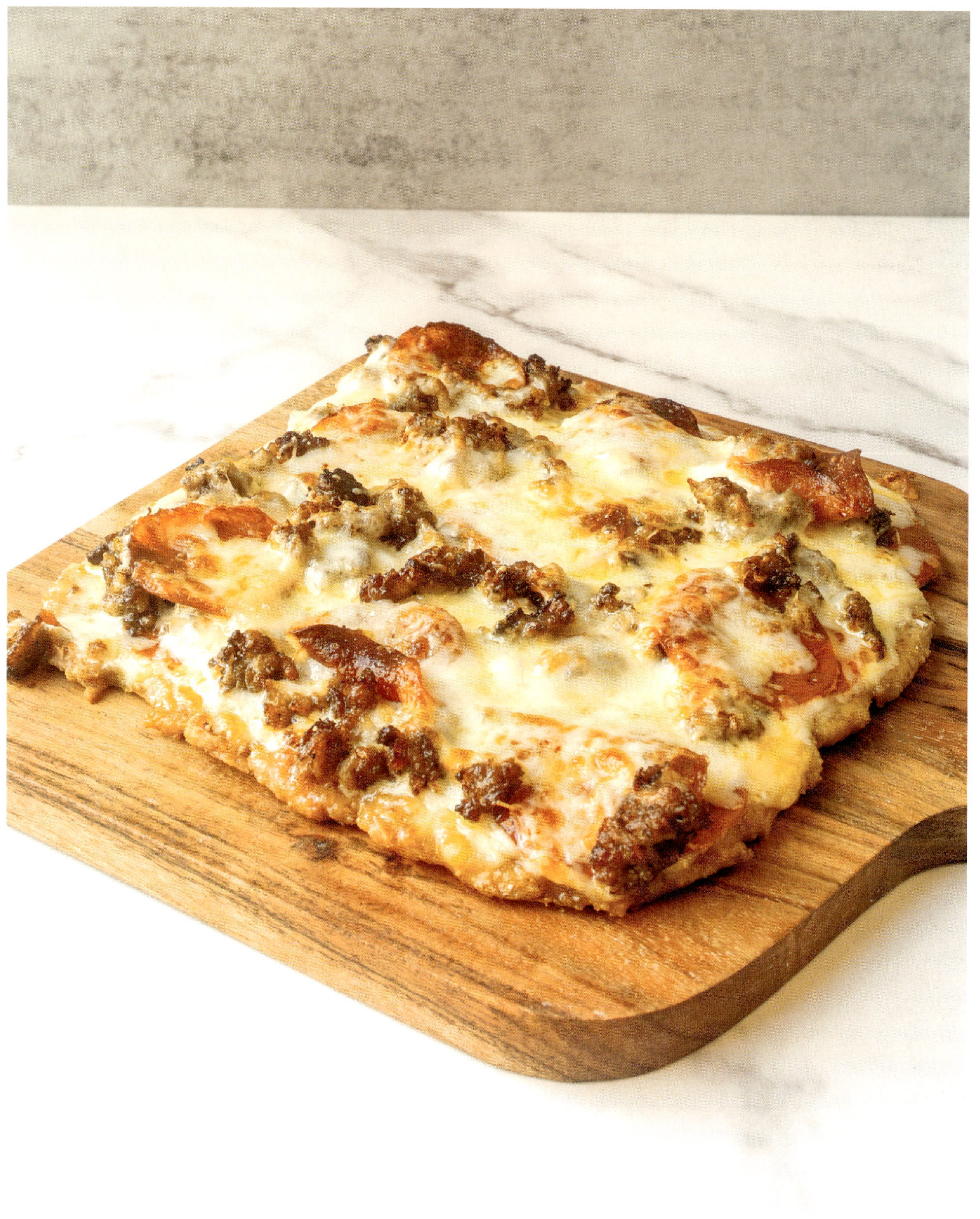

YIELD: 2 individual pizzas

PREP TIME: 25 minutes (not including time to cook chicken breast)

COOK TIME: 35 to 55 minutes, depending on method

CARNIVORE WHITE PIZZA

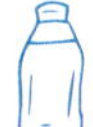
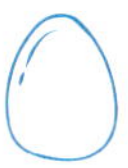
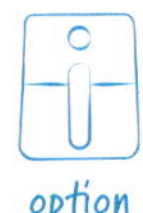

These white pizzas are delicious and filling. They may look small, but I can only eat three-quarters of one before I am stuffed. They can be prepared in the oven or the air fryer if you prefer. This may be better than a real pizza!

FOR THE CRUST:

½ cup plain pork rinds

1 pound ground chicken

1 large egg

½ cup grated Parmesan cheese

½ teaspoon salt

½ teaspoon garlic powder (optional)

½ teaspoon Italian seasoning, plus extra for garnish (optional)

FOR THE SAUCE AND TOPPINGS:

1 batch Alfredo Sauce (page 351)

9 slices high-quality pepperoni (see note)

½ cup shredded mozzarella cheese

¼ cup grated Parmesan cheese

½ cup shredded cooked chicken breast

MAKE THE CRUST:

1. If using the oven, preheat it to 400°F. Fit a sheet pan with a wire rack.
2. In a blender or small food processor, grind the pork rinds to a coarse powder. Transfer the ground pork rinds to a large mixing bowl and add the ground chicken, egg, Parmesan cheese, salt, and, if using, garlic powder and Italian seasoning. Mix the crust ingredients together until well combined.
3. Take a sheet of parchment paper and press half of the chicken mixture into a ½-inch-thick pizza crust shape of your choice. (If using an air fryer for this recipe, use the air fryer tray as a template for the shape of your crust.) Form a second crust with the remaining chicken mixture on a separate piece of parchment paper.
4. If using an air fryer, use the parchment paper to flip the chicken crust onto the air fryer tray, then put the tray in the air fryer. Set the air fryer to air-fry mode at 400°F and cook for 15 minutes, flipping the crust over at the halfway mark. When the first crust is done, remove it from the air fryer and repeat with the second crust.

   If using the oven, use the parchment paper to flip both chicken crusts onto the wire rack, leaving some space between them. Bake for 20 minutes.
5. Keep an eye on the crust as it cooks. You will know it is done when it has shrunk a little bit and is white in color.
6. While the crusts are cooking, prepare the Alfredo sauce, following the instructions on page 351.

(recipe continues)

BUILD THE PIZZAS:

1 If using the oven, preheat it to 350°F. Fit a sheet pan with a wire rack and set aside.

2 Evenly spread one-third of the Alfredo sauce on top of each baked chicken crust, depending on how much sauce you like on your pizza. I cover the entire crust in a thick layer of sauce.

3 Evenly layer on the pepperoni slices, followed by a thin layer of mozzarella, using about 2 tablespoons of cheese on each pizza. Sprinkle half of the Parmesan cheese on the pizzas as well, using about 1 tablespoon on each.

4 Add a layer of shredded chicken, dividing it equally between the pizzas, then add a bit more Alfredo sauce to the top (saving a little to garnish the baked pizzas). Top the pizzas with the rest of the mozzarella and Parmesan.

5 If using an air fryer, set it to 350°F and cook each pizza in the air fryer tray for 10 to 13 minutes, until the cheese is melted.

If using the oven, bake both pizzas on the wire rack for 15 minutes, or until the cheese is melted.

6 After removing the pizzas from the air fryer or oven, drizzle with the reserved Alfredo sauce and, if desired, a bit of Italian seasoning.

7 Cut into slices and enjoy!

Note:

When buying pepperoni, be sure to read the ingredient label. I try to avoid anything with a ton of preservatives, sugar, and/or vegetable seed oils. I also look for pepperoni with less than 1 gram of carbs per serving.

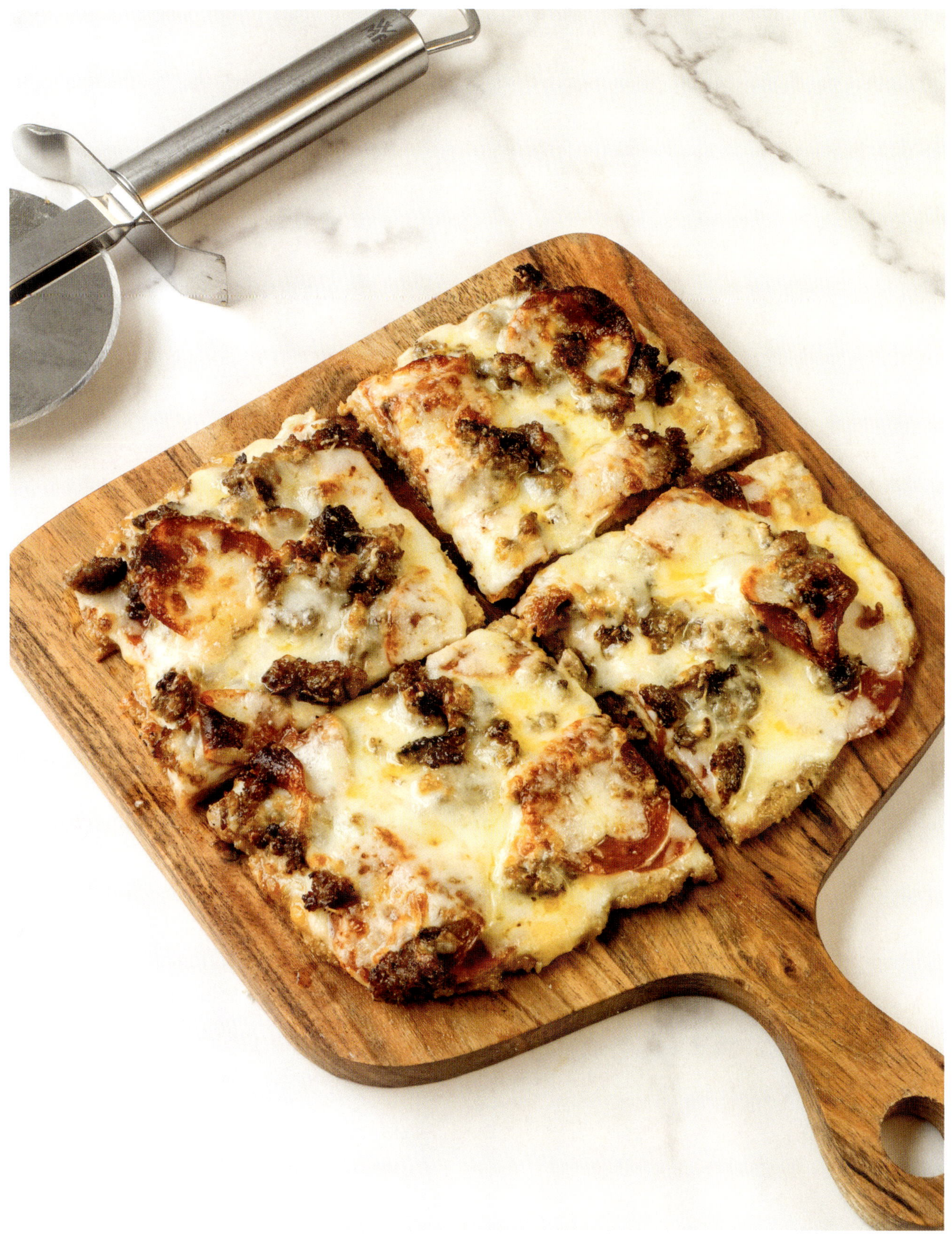

PER PIZZA | calories: **1265** | fat: **88g** | protein: **108g** | carbs: **11g** | macro split: **62/34/3**

YIELD: 6 servings

PREP TIME: 15 minutes

COOK TIME: 16 to 20 minutes, depending on method

SPICY BACON-WRAPPED CHORIZO DOGS

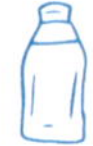

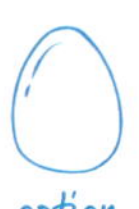

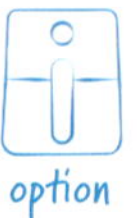

I first saw versions of this recipe on Instagram and had to try it. Chorizo adds a bold, smoky kick that takes these loaded dogs to the next level. You could put them into a Cottage Cheese Flatbread (page 371) or Carnivore Flatbread (page 367) or just eat them with a fork and knife.

- 8 ounces fresh (raw) chorizo
- 8 ounces 80/20 ground beef
- ½ teaspoon salt
- 1 (3-ounce) block spicy cheese, such as pepper Jack or spicy Gouda
- 3 all-beef hot dogs
- 6 strips bacon
- 6 tablespoons Spicy Mayonnaise (page 356), for serving (optional)

1. If using the oven, preheat it to 425°F and line a sheet pan with parchment paper.
2. Put the chorizo, ground beef, and salt in a large bowl and mix thoroughly.
3. Cut the cheese into six equal-sized sticks.
4. Cut the hot dogs in half crosswise and pair one cheese stick with each half dog.
5. Completely wrap each cheese stick/hot dog in one-sixth of the meat mixture to make a "dog." Then wrap each dog with a strip of bacon. You can use a toothpick to secure the bacon strip in place.
6. If using the oven, place the wrapped dogs on the prepared pan and bake for 13 to 15 minutes, until the bacon has cooked through and chorizo/beef mixture is brown. Turn the oven to the broil setting and cook for another 3 to 5 minutes to crisp up the bacon.

   If using an air fryer, place the wrapped dogs in the air fryer basket and set to air-fry mode at 400°F for 16 minutes, flipping once. The dogs are done when the bacon is crispy and the chorizo/beef mixture is browned and cooked through.
7. Allow to cool for 10 minutes, then top with the spicy mayo, if desired, and enjoy!

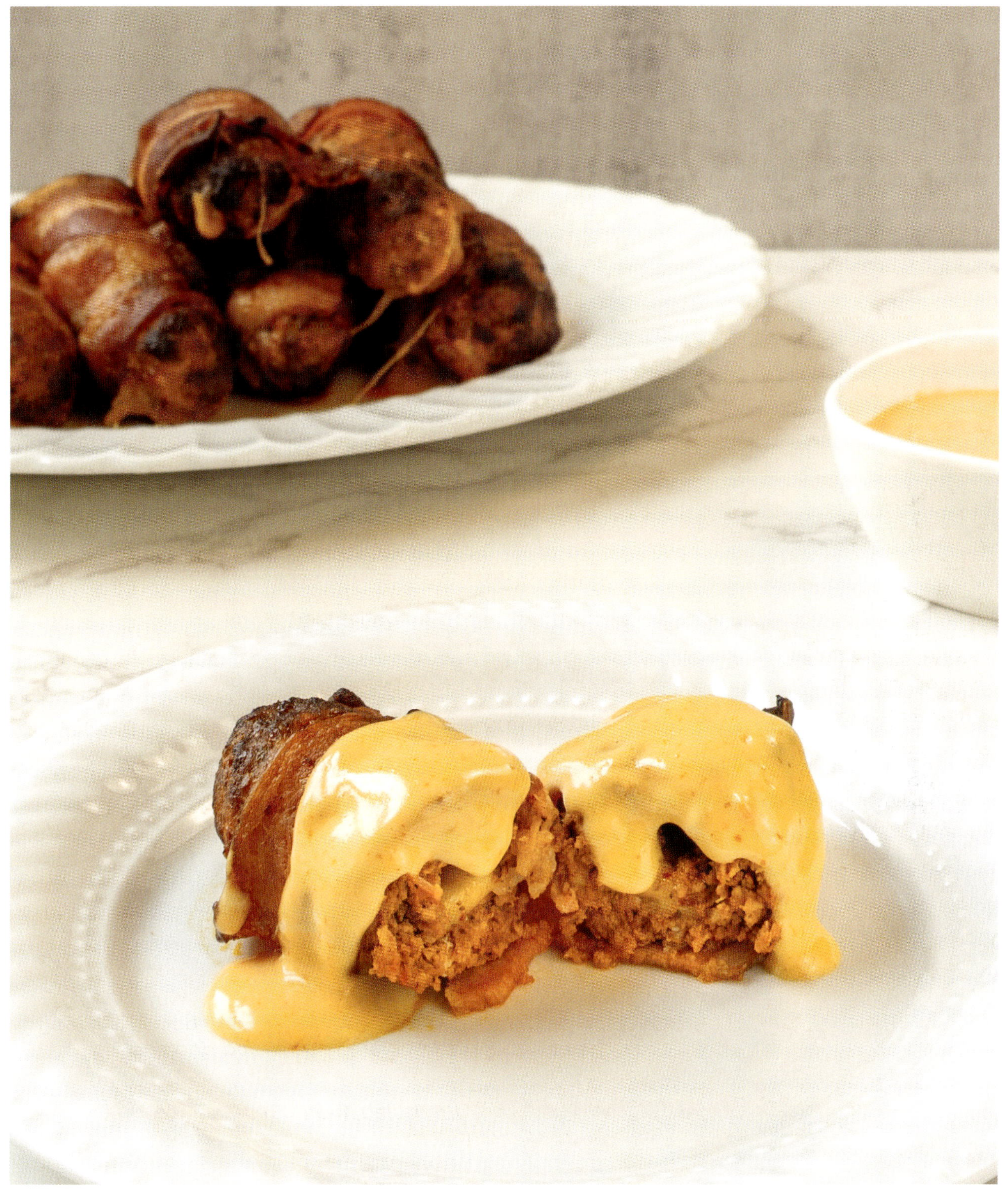

PER SERVING (with spicy mayo)	calories: **561** | fat: **49g** | protein: **26.5g** | carbs: **3.2g** | macro split: **79/19/2**
PER SERVING (without spicy mayo)	calories: **425** | fat: **31g** | protein: **22.5g** | carbs: **1.5g** | macro split: **74/24/2**

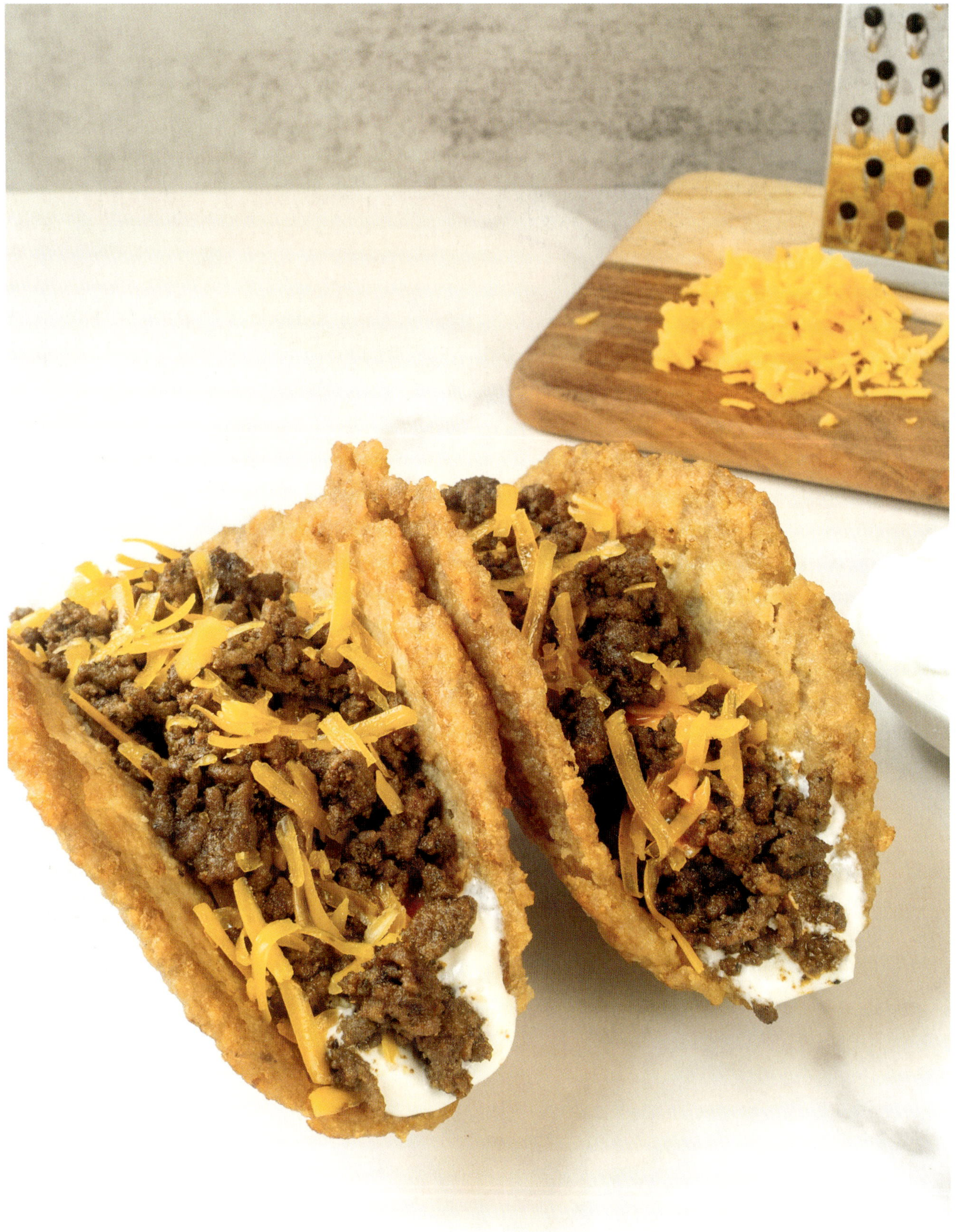

PER TACO	calories: **607** | fat: **41g** | protein: **58g** | carbs: **2g** | macro split: **61/38/1**

YIELD: 4 tacos
PREP TIME: 15 minutes
COOK TIME: 25 minutes

CARNIVORE TACOS

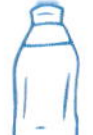 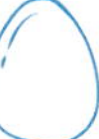

Tacos are one of my all-time favorite foods, so finding a way to enjoy them while staying carnivore was a top priority. This chicken-based taco shell is juicy and protein-packed and lets me savor tacos without the drawbacks of a flour or corn shell.

FOR THE TORTILLAS:

1 cup plain pork rinds

1 pound ground chicken

2 large eggs

½ cup grated Parmesan cheese

1 teaspoon salt

2 teaspoons bacon grease or salted butter, for the pan

FOR THE FILLING:

1 pound 80/20 ground beef

2 to 3 tablespoons Taco Seasoning (page 350)

2 tablespoons water

TOPPINGS (OPTIONAL):

4 tablespoons full-fat sour cream

4 tablespoons shredded cheddar cheese

Hot sauce

SPECIAL EQUIPMENT:
Burger or tortilla press (optional)

1 Start by making the "batter" for the chicken tortillas. Put the pork rinds in a blender or food processor and grind to a fine powder. Transfer the powder to a large bowl. Add the ground chicken, eggs, Parmesan, and salt and mix thoroughly with your hands.

2 Divide the chicken mixture into four equal portions and roll each into a ball. Lay a sheet of parchment paper on the counter or a cutting board, then place a chicken ball in the center of the paper and lay a second piece of parchment paper on top. Press the ball flat with a burger or tortilla press (or use a rolling pin or a flat plate) until it is ¼ inch thick. Repeat with the remaining balls to make a total of four tortillas.

3 Heat the bacon grease in a medium frying pan over medium heat until it is bubbling slightly. Then fry each chicken tortilla individually for 3 to 4 minutes per side, until golden brown. When done, remove the tortillas from the heat and set aside on a plate. If the frying pan is dry, you can add more bacon grease or butter before cooking the next tortilla.

4 While the tortillas are cooking, prepare the taco meat. In another medium frying pan over medium heat, cook the ground beef until it is no longer pink, about 10 minutes. As the meat cooks, break it up with a spatula. Then sprinkle with 2 to 3 tablespoons of taco seasoning, depending on how much taco flavor you want. Add the water and stir until the beef is evenly coated with the spices.

5 Build your tacos! I like to put some sour cream on the tortillas before adding the meat, which I top off with some shredded cheddar and hot sauce. Make them your own with whatever toppings you enjoy!

YIELD: 8 meatballs (4 per serving)

PREP TIME: 10 minutes

COOK TIME: 24 minutes

CHILI CHEESE DOG MEATBALLS

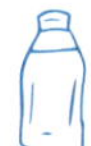

I wanted to re-create a dish that would bring back memories of the last days of summer. The first thing that came to mind was the chili cheese dogs I used to enjoy as a kid at the Winnebago County Fair. Since a bun wasn't an option, I got creative and turned them into meatballs!

1 pound 80/20 ground beef

4 all-beef hot dogs, diced

¾ cup shredded cheddar cheese, divided

2 tablespoons Chili Spice Seasoning (page 349)

1. Preheat the oven to 400°F and place a wire rack in a 13 by 9-inch sheet pan (aka quarter sheet pan).
2. Put the ground beef, diced hot dogs, ½ cup of the cheddar, and the seasoning mix in a medium bowl and mix thoroughly with your hands.
3. Divide the mixture into eight equal portions (2½ to 3 ounces each) and roll each into a ball. Arrange the balls on the wire rack.
4. Bake for 22 minutes, or until the meatballs are browned and have shrunk in size by about a third. Evenly top the meatballs with the remaining ¼ cup of cheese and bake for another 2 minutes to melt the cheese.
5. Allow the meatballs to cool for 5 to 7 minutes, then enjoy!

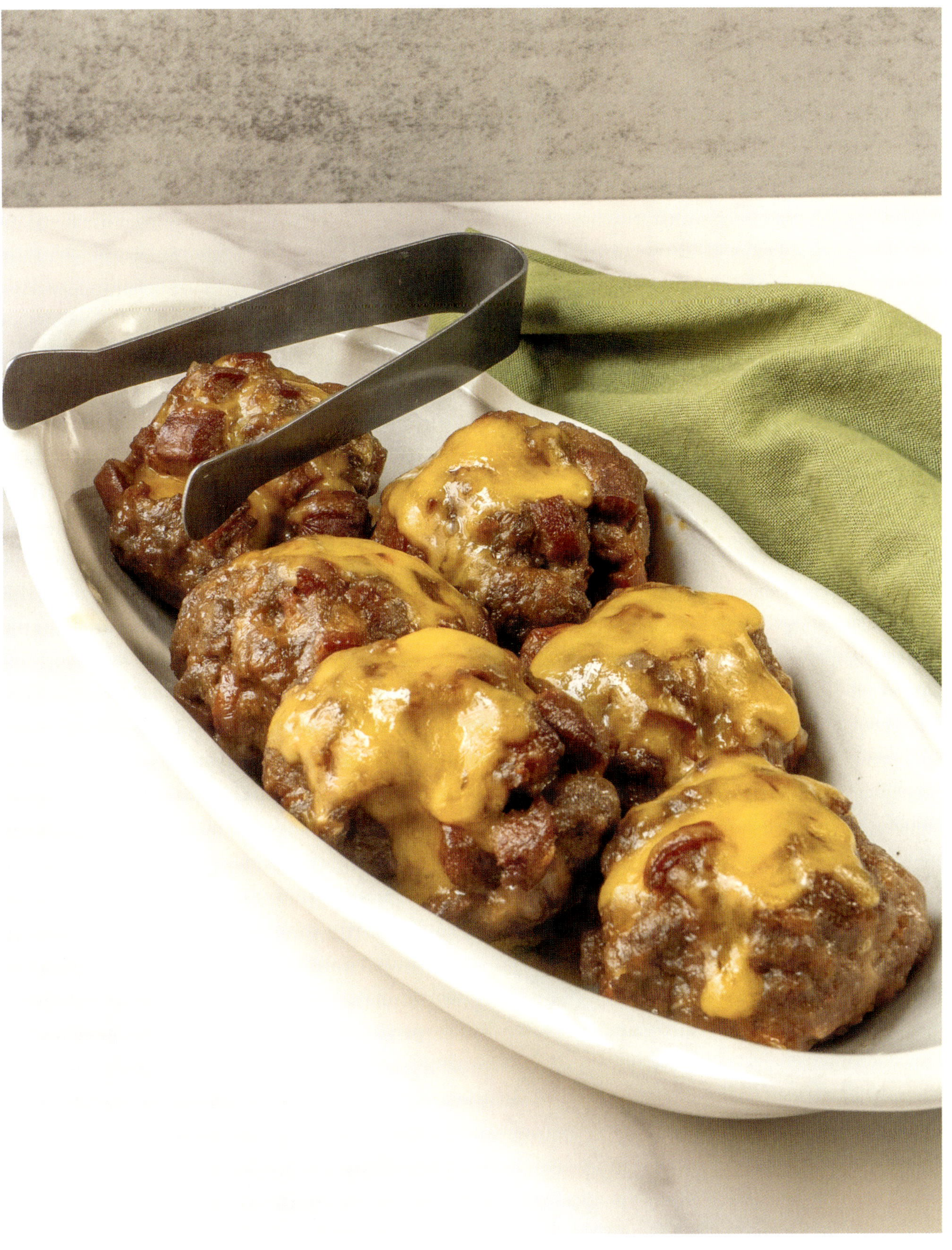

PER SERVING	calories: **1124** | fat: **83g** | protein: **84g** | carbs: **5g** | macro split: **68/31/1**

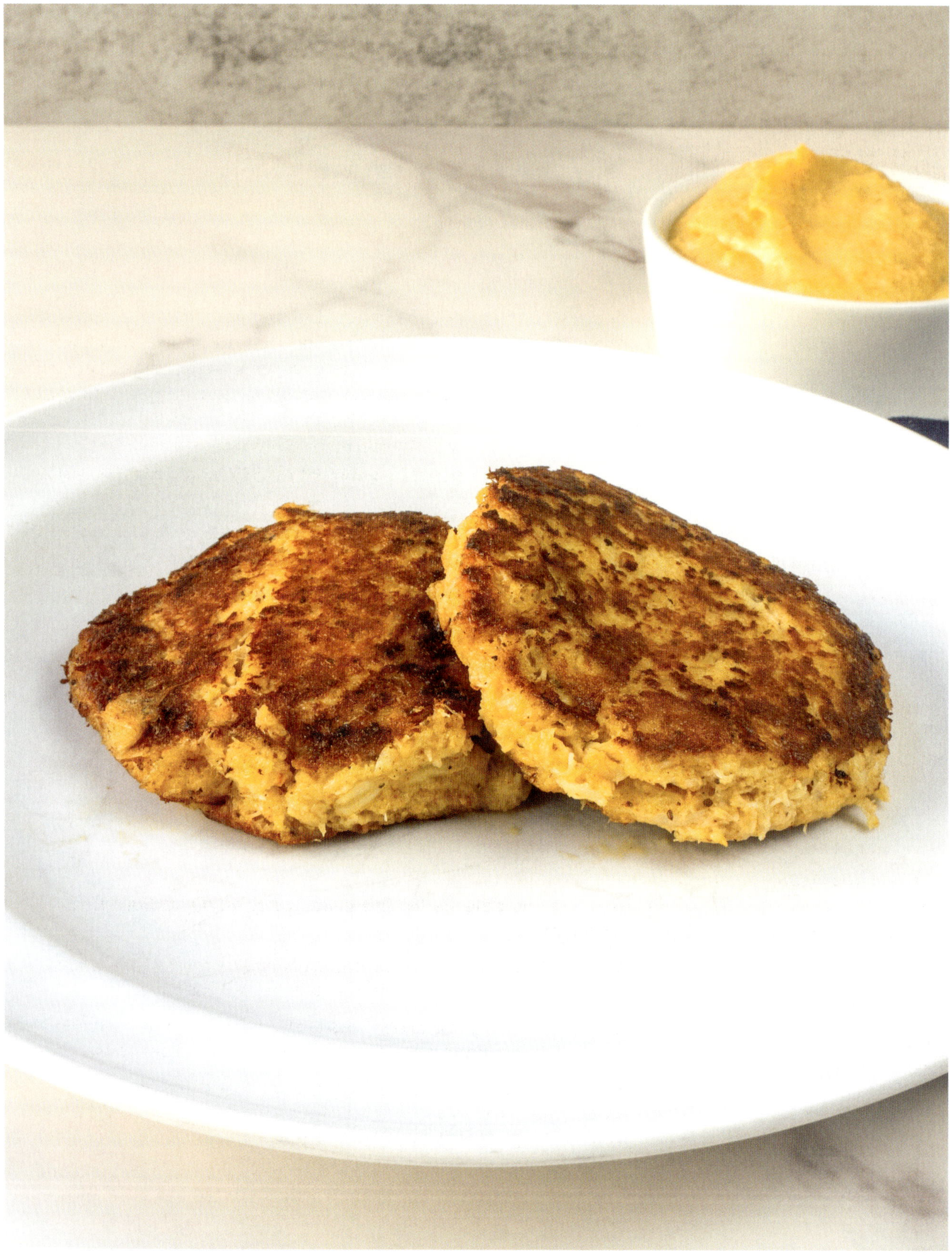

PER SERVING	calories: **471** | fat: **33g** | protein: **46g** | carbs: **1g** | macro split: **61/37/1**

YIELD: 4 crab cakes (2 per serving)

PREP TIME: 15 minutes (not including time to make mayo)

COOK TIME: 12 minutes

CRAB CAKES WITH RÉMOULADE

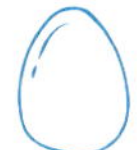

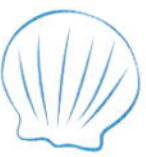

Sometimes I need a break from beef, butter, bacon, and eggs and crave something entirely different. That's when I turn to these savory crab cakes. They're versatile enough to serve as an appetizer, side dish, or main course. Paired with a zesty rémoulade sauce, they pack a flavorful punch, and the omega-3s from the crab are a welcome bonus! The beef gelatin in this recipe helps the cakes hold together, since we are not using any crackers or pork rinds. No need to dissolve the gelatin; just add it straight to the mix!

FOR THE CRAB CAKES:

12 ounces canned or fresh lump crab meat

1 large egg

1 tablespoon freshly squeezed lemon juice (optional)

1 tablespoon Bacon Mayonnaise (page 352), Marrownaise (page 355), or store-bought avocado oil mayonnaise

2 teaspoons Dijon mustard

1 teaspoon Old Bay seasoning

1 teaspoon Worcestershire sauce

1 teaspoon unflavored beef gelatin powder

1 tablespoon salted butter, for the pan

FOR THE RÉMOULADE SAUCE:

¼ cup Bacon Mayonnaise (page 352), Marrownaise (page 355), or store-bought avocado oil mayonnaise

1½ teaspoons Dijon mustard

1½ teaspoons minced dill pickles (optional, for keto version)

1 teaspoon medium-hot hot sauce, such as Cholula

½ teaspoon Cajun Seasoning (page 346)

½ teaspoon prepared horseradish (optional, for keto version)

½ teaspoon freshly squeezed lemon juice (optional)

1. Put the ingredients for the crab cakes in a medium bowl and mix well.
2. Using your hands, divide the crab mixture into four equal portions and shape each into a ½-inch-thick patty.
3. Before cooking the crab cakes, mix together the ingredients for the rémoulade sauce in a small dish and set to the side.
4. Melt the butter in a large frying pan over medium heat. Then place the crab cakes in the pan and cook for 5 to 6 minutes per side, until golden brown.
5. Remove the crab cakes from the pan and place on a plate. Top each with a heaping tablespoon of the rémoulade sauce and serve.

YIELD: 16 taco balls (4 per serving)

PREP TIME: 10 minutes

COOK TIME: 15 to 22 minutes, depending on method

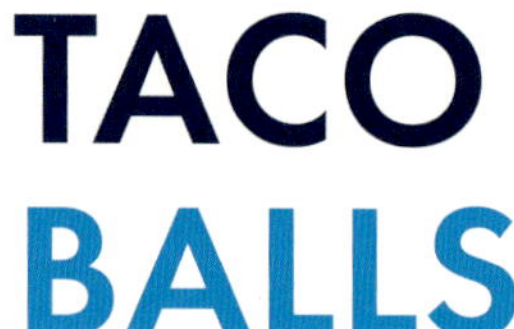

TACO BALLS

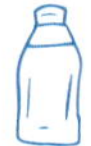

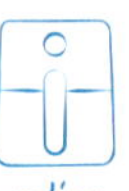

This recipe began as an experiment—I wanted to create something taco inspired using the air fryer. That's how these taco balls came to be, and they've quickly become one of my all-time favorites. You'll find both air fryer and oven instructions below.

- 2 pounds 80/20 ground beef
- 3 to 5 tablespoons Taco Seasoning (page 350), divided
- ½ cup grated Cotija cheese
- ½ cup shredded sharp cheddar cheese, plus 2 tablespoons for garnish
- 1 ounce (2 tablespoons) full-fat cream cheese, at room temperature
- Full-fat sour cream, for garnish (optional)

1. If using the oven, preheat it to 400°F. Fit a sheet pan with a wire rack and set aside.
2. Put the ground beef in a large mixing bowl and add 2 to 3 tablespoons of taco seasoning, depending on how taco-y you want the beef to taste. I use 3 tablespoons for a strong taco flavor. Using your hands, mix thoroughly and set aside.
3. In another bowl, combine the Cotija and cheddar cheeses and 1 to 2 tablespoons of taco seasoning, depending on how strong of a taco taste you want. I use 2 tablespoons. Add the cream cheese and mix until well incorporated. Roll the cheese mixture into sixteen balls, about 1 inch in diameter.
4. Take a small amount (about 2 ounces) of the seasoned ground beef, roll it into a ball, and then flatten it into a little pancake, about 3 inches in diameter. Place a cheese ball in the center and fold the beef around it, pinching it together at the top and rolling to seal. Repeat with the remaining beef and cheese balls.
5. If using an air fryer, set as many taco balls as will fit comfortably on the air fryer tray with a bit of space between them. You may need to cook them in two batches. Set to air-fry mode at 400°F and cook for 15 to 17 minutes, until browned and the cheese is melty. Turn the balls several times throughout the cooking process.

   If using the oven, set the taco balls on the pan fitted with the wire rack and bake for 22 minutes, turning once at the 11-minute mark, until the balls are browned and the cheese is melty.
6. If using sour cream, place 2 to 3 tablespoons in each serving bowl. Add four taco balls to each bowl and top the balls with a sprinkle of cheddar cheese. Enjoy!

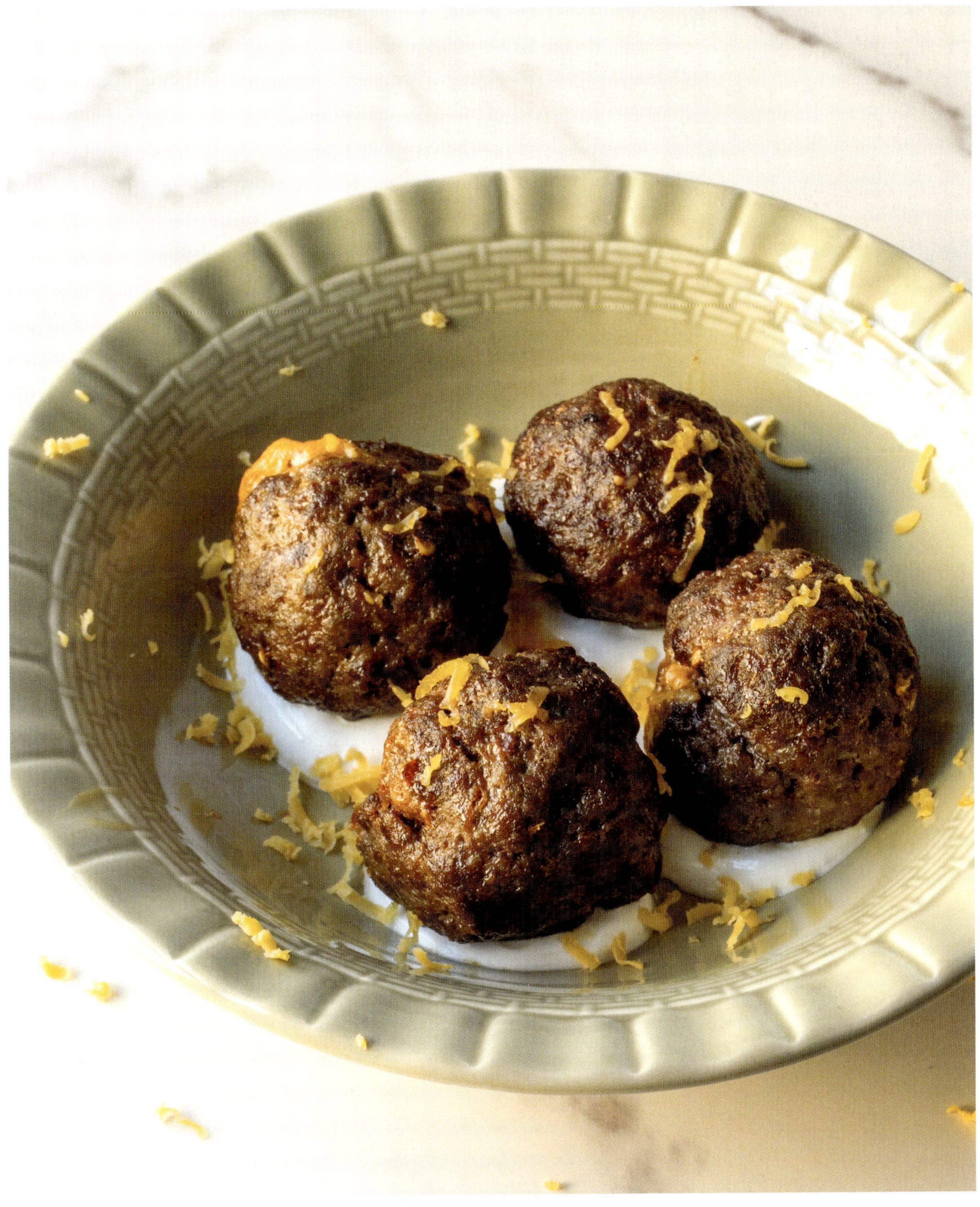

PER SERVING (without sour cream)	calories: **781** | fat: **63g** | protein: **50g** | carbs: **2g** | macro split: **73/26/1**
PER SERVING (with 3 tablespoons sour cream)	calories: **856** | fat: **70g** | protein: **50g** | carbs: **4g** | macro split: **74/24/2**

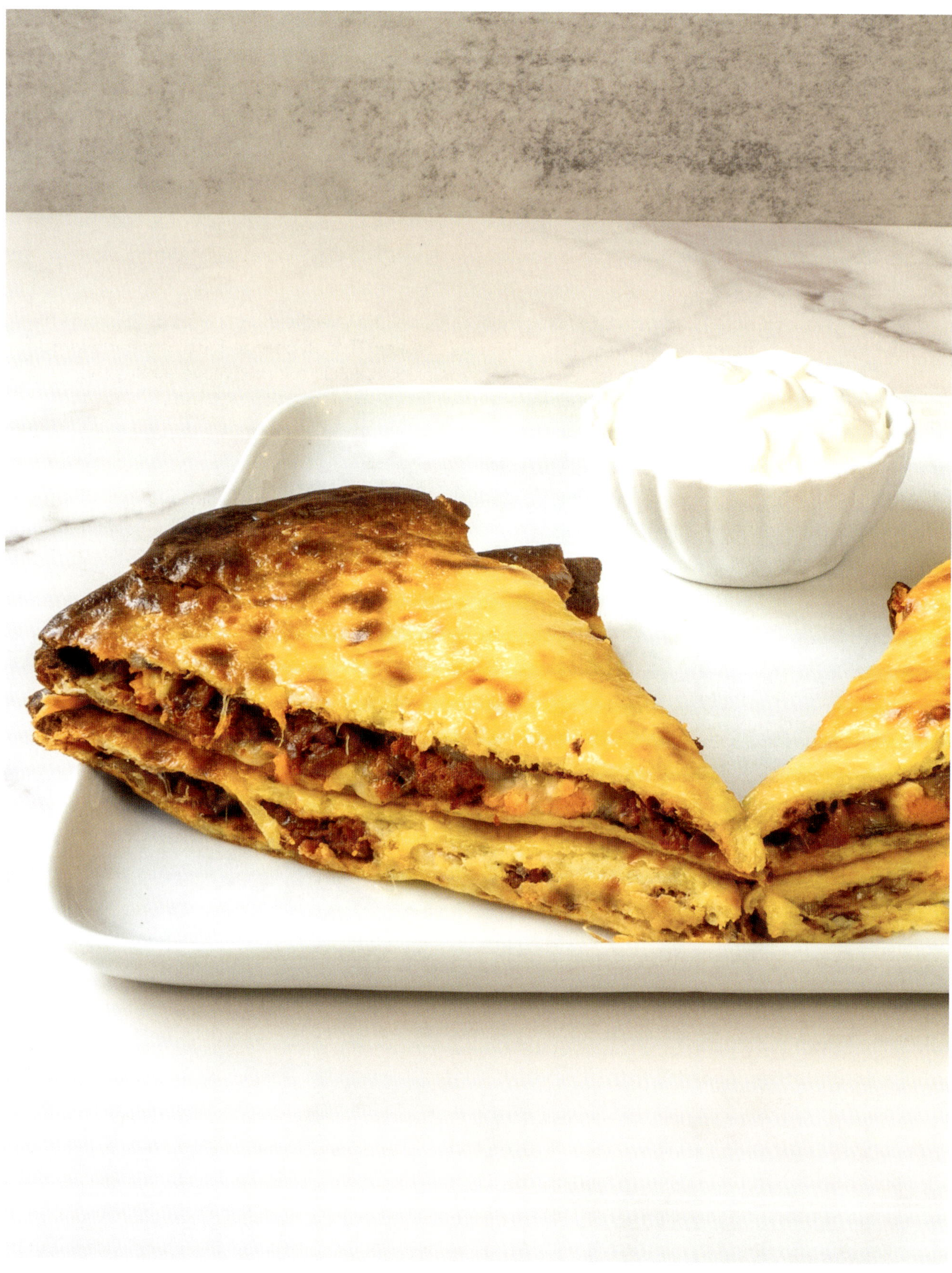

PER SERVING	calories: **1099** | fat: **85g** | protein: **75g** | carbs: **13g** | macro split: **68/27/5**

YIELD: 2 servings

PREP TIME: 10 minutes (not including time to make flatbread or cook chorizo)

COOK TIME: 15 minutes

CARNIVORE QUESADILLA

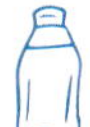
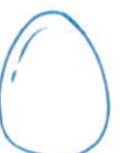

Who doesn't love a quesadilla? For a while, they were off the table for me because of the flour tortillas. That all changed with my Carnivore Flatbread—now, quesadillas are back in the mix! I love serving them with a side of sour cream for the perfect finishing touch.

1 Carnivore Flatbread (page 367) or Cottage Cheese Flatbread made without everything bagel seasoning (page 371)

8 ounces cooked crumbled fresh (raw) chorizo

½ cup shredded rotisserie chicken (white meat)

1 cup shredded mozzarella cheese

3 tablespoons full-fat sour cream, for dipping

1. Preheat the oven to 350°F.
2. Place the baked flatbread on a sheet pan with the underside facing up. Evenly sprinkle the chorizo, chicken, and mozzarella across the bottom half. Then fold the other half of the flatbread over the fillings.
3. Bake until the cheese is melted, 10 to 15 minutes.
4. Cut into four wedges and serve with a side of sour cream.

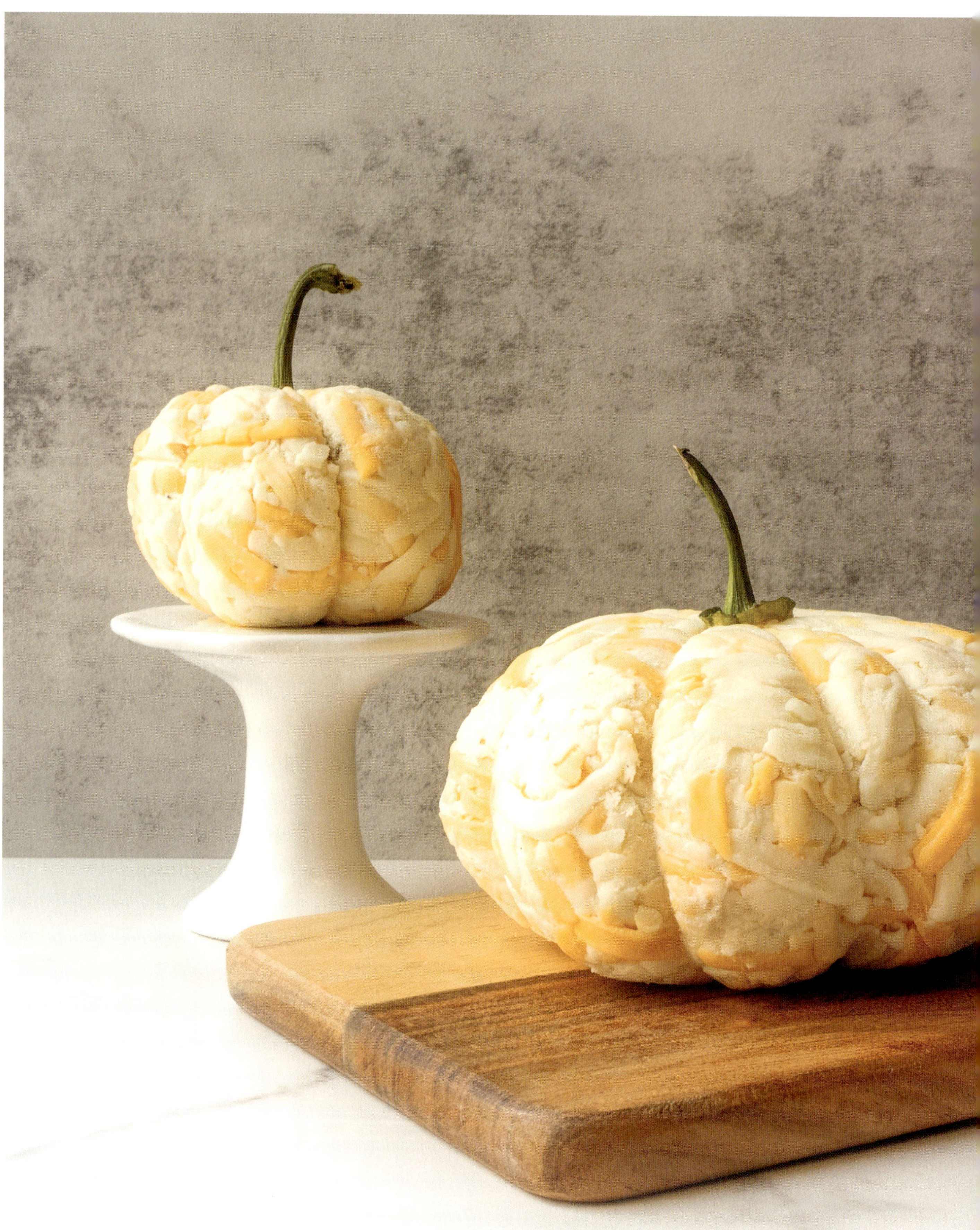

CHAPTER 14
HOLIDAY MEALS

300 Brined Spatchcocked Turkey

305 Spiced Pumpkin-Shaped Cheese Ball

306 Carnivore Gravy

309 Air Fryer Brined Turkey Breast

310 Turkey Alfredo

313 Turkey Sandwich

314 Pumpkin Spice Cheesecake

YIELD: 12 to 16 servings

PREP TIME: 30 minutes, plus 24 hours to brine and 12 hours to dry

COOK TIME: 1 hour 25 minutes to 1 hour 35 minutes, depending on size of bird

BRINED SPATCHCOCKED TURKEY

A few years ago, my husband started spatchcocking our turkeys, and the results were so incredible that now it's the only way we cook them! Spatchcocking involves removing the backbone and flattening the bird, which reduces the cooking time by more than half and ensures even roasting. We brine the turkey beforehand to make it juicier and more flavorful. We've found that a medium-sized turkey, between 12 and 16 pounds, works best for this method. It fits perfectly on a sheet pan fitted with a wire rack, making the process seamless. When hosting a larger group for Thanksgiving, we simply prepare two medium-sized turkeys instead of one extra-large one. A spatchcocked bird of this size typically cooks in about an hour and a half and is perfectly juicy and flavorful every time!

1 (12- to 16-pound) fresh whole turkey, thawed if frozen (see note, page 302)

FOR THE BRINE:

1 cup kosher salt

2 to 3 cups hot water

FOR THE HERB BUTTER:

1 cup (2 sticks) salted butter

1 tablespoon finely chopped fresh rosemary

1 tablespoon finely chopped fresh sage

1 tablespoon finely chopped fresh thyme

6 cloves garlic, minced

1 cup dry sherry, for the pan

SPECIAL EQUIPMENT: 5-gallon food-safe bucket, very sharp kitchen shears, baster, electric knife

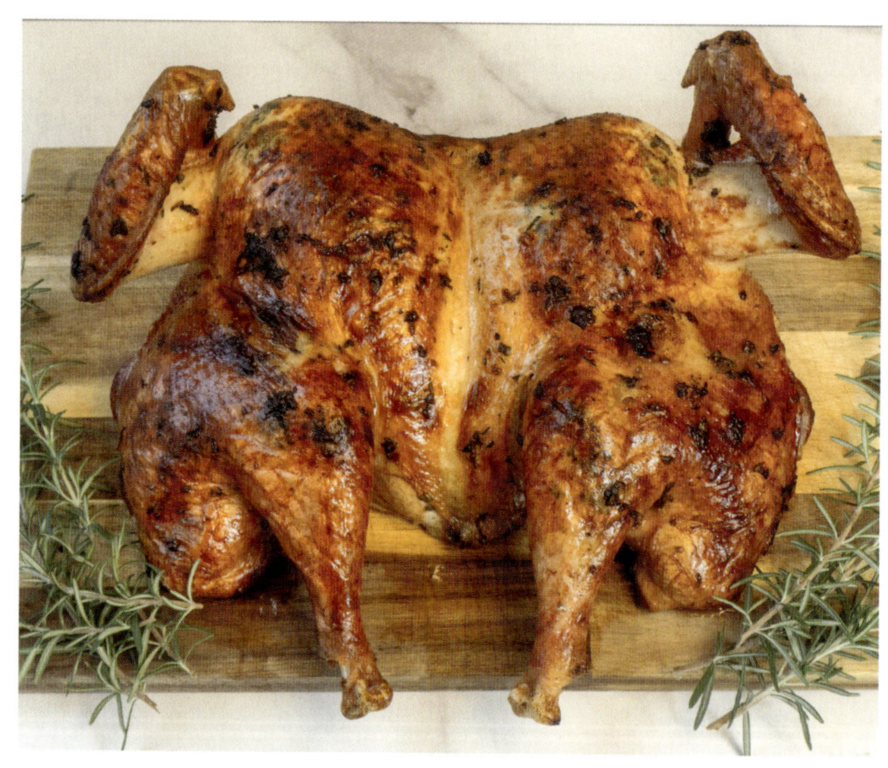

1 In a clean 5-gallon food-safe bucket, dissolve the kosher salt in the hot water. Allow the salted water to cool, then place the turkey in the bucket and fill with fresh cold water until the turkey is fully submerged, 2½ to 3 gallons. Place the bucket in the refrigerator and allow the turkey to brine for 24 hours.

2 Once brining is complete, remove the turkey from the bucket and rinse thoroughly. Then pat the skin dry and place the turkey on a sheet pan fitted with a wire rack. Put the turkey back in the fridge for 12 hours to allow the skin to dry out a bit (this will help you get crispy skin).

3 Remove the turkey from the refrigerator and place breast side down on a large wooden cutting board. Using sharp kitchen shears, cut the backbone out of the turkey. This can take some effort, but really sharp shears make quick work of this task.

4 Flip the bird breast side up and press down firmly on the breastbone. You will feel a little pop and then the bird will lie flat on the cutting board. Then turn the legs out and tuck in the wings.

5 Return the prepared turkey to the wire rack, laying it breast side up.

6 Preheat the oven to 350°F. While the oven preheats, make the herb butter.

7 Put the butter in a medium microwave-safe bowl and microwave on high for 30 seconds to soften it. Then add the herbs and garlic to the butter and stir well.

8 Put on some food-safe gloves and, using your hands, spread the herb butter all over the skin of the turkey, as well as the underside of the bird. I also like to spread some of the butter under the skin for extra flavor. I find the skin to be looser around the neck area, so I insert my gloved hands under the skin there and try to loosen the skin under the wings and legs and then add the herb butter. Retuck the wings if needed.

9 Place one meat thermometer in the breast and another in the leg. If you have only one thermometer, place it in the breast. You don't want the breast meat to overcook, and the leg and wing meat is more forgiving. Put the turkey in the oven and, before closing the door, pour in the dry sherry and then add water until the pan is halfway full.

An Animal-Based Thanksgiving

Here's a Thanksgiving menu that is sure to delight even non-carnivores! For Easter, just swap out the turkey and gravy for ham.

- Deviled Eggs (page 253)
- Brined Spatchcocked Turkey (page 300)
- Carnivore Gravy (page 306)
- Carnivore Mac & Cheese Casserole (page 278)
- Garlicky Smothered Brussels Sprouts (page 323) or Garlicky Smothered Green Beans (page 328)
- Pumpkin Spice Cheesecake (page 314)

(recipe continues)

10 Cook the bird until the temperature in the breast reaches 110°F, about 6 minutes per pound, basting with the liquid from the pan every 15 to 20 minutes. Add more water to the pan if the basting liquid starts getting low.

11 Once the breast hits 110°F, turn the oven up to 400°F and continue roasting and basting every 10 to 15 minutes now. The higher oven temperature will allow the skin to become golden brown and crispy. When the temperature of the breast hits 153°F, pull the turkey from the oven and place it on top of the stove, then wrap in aluminum foil and cover with a couple of dish towels. The bird will continue to cook, with the temperature of the breast eventually reaching 165°F. Once the breast temperature has reached 165°F, uncover the bird to keep it from cooking further.

12 When properly cooked, the final temperature of the rested leg meat should reach 180°F. Note that the leg meat thermometer will typically read higher than the breast, and that is okay. The rested leg meat can go as high as 190°F and still be moist. If, after the rested breast meat has reached 165°F on the counter, the temperature of the leg and thigh meat hasn't reached 180°F, you can always remove the legs and thighs and place them back in the oven to cook until they reach 170°F. Then pull them and wrap them like you did with the entire turkey and allow the temperature to rise to 180°F.

13 Save the pan drippings to make Carnivore Gravy (page 306), if desired.

14 Carve with an electric knife and spread the meat on an extra-large platter for serving.

Note

If you're planning to make gravy (see my recipe on page 306), be sure to reserve the neck and giblets found in a package inside the turkey cavity.

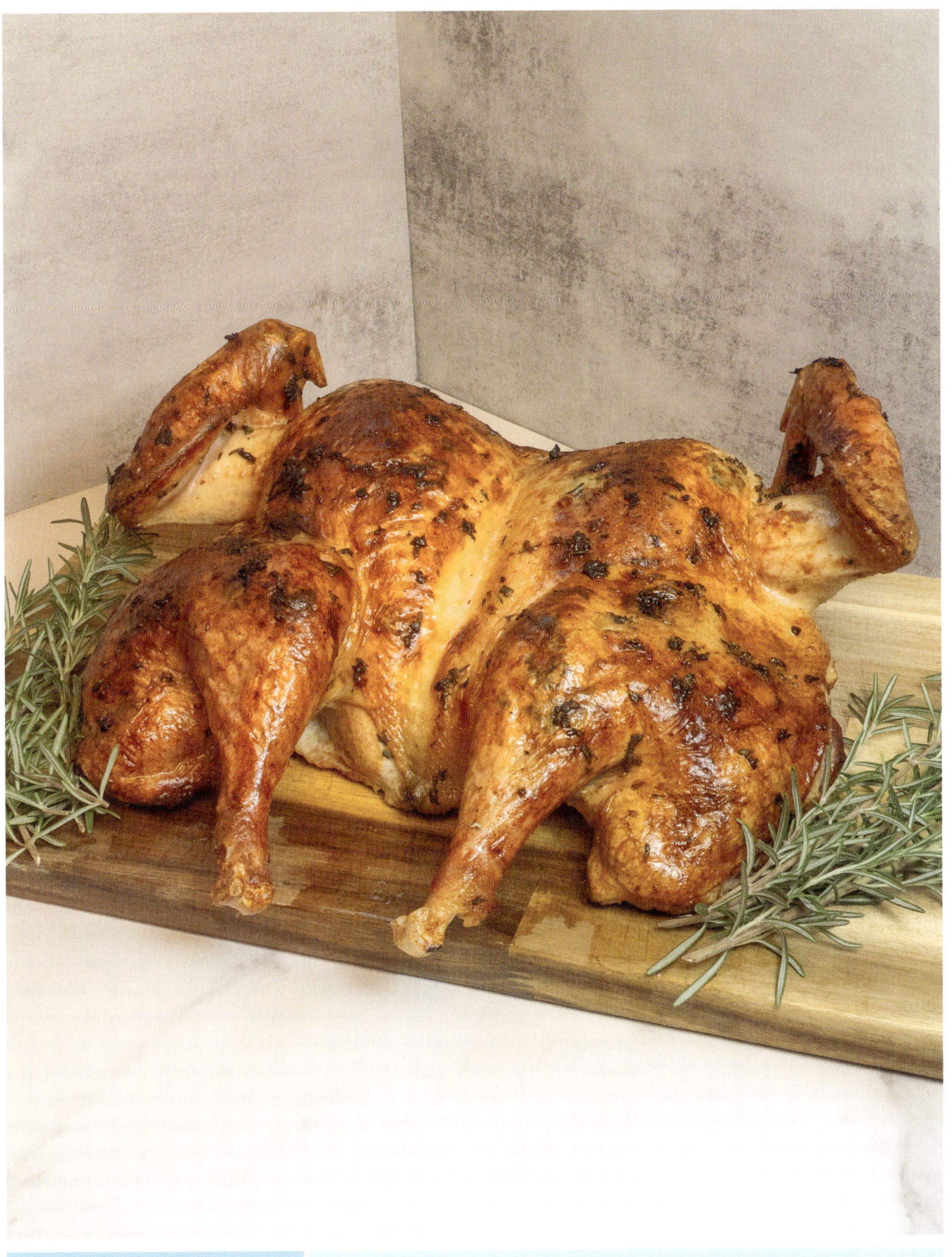

PER SERVING (1 pound, equal parts white and dark meat)

calories: **646** | fat: **18g** | protein: **120g** | carbs: **0g** | macro split: **25/75/0**

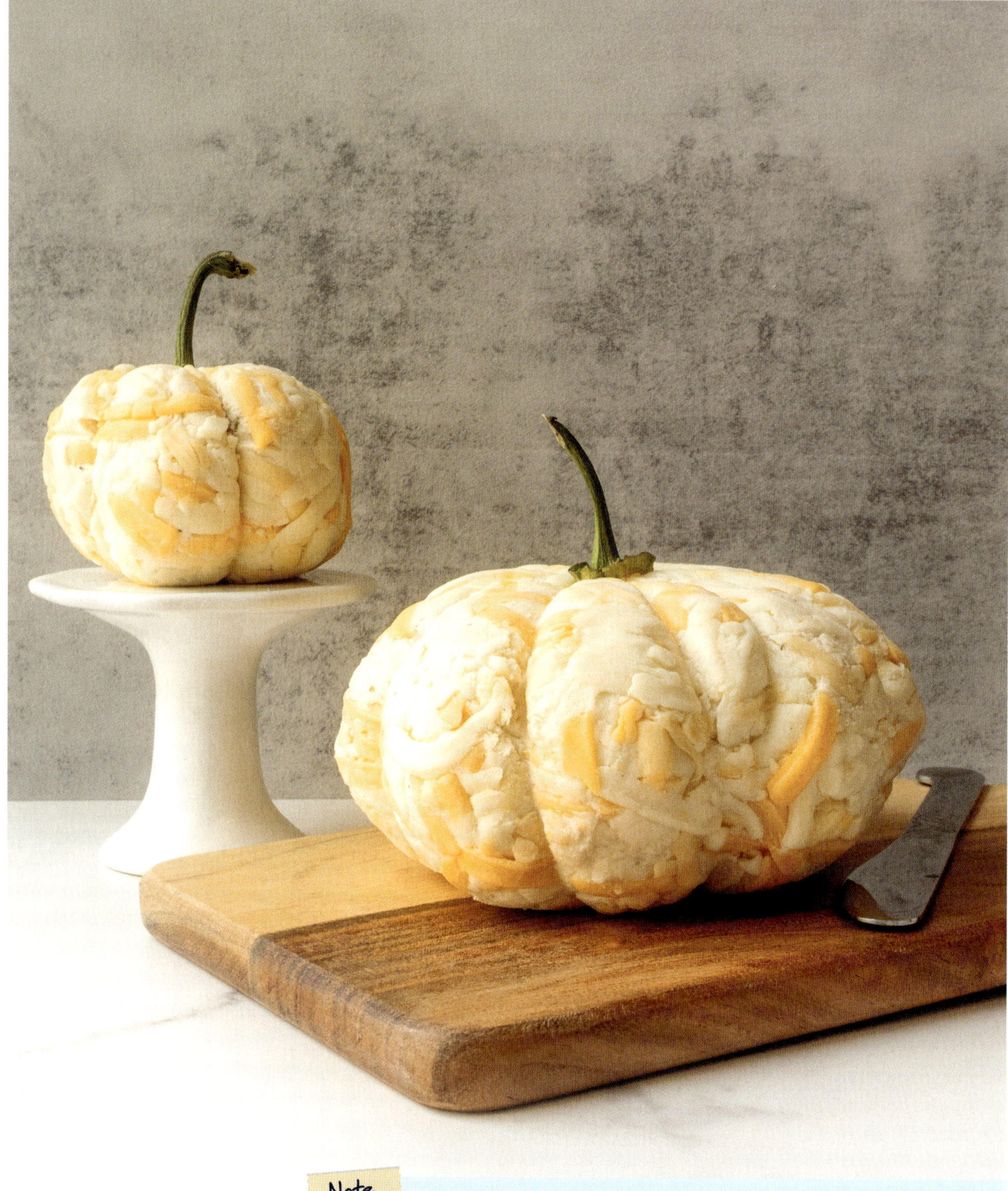

Note

For the spice/herb blend, I like to use Trader Joe's 21 Seasoning Salute or herbes de Provence.

PER SERVING	calories: **200** | fat: **21g** | protein: **2g** | carbs: **1g** | macro split: **94/4/2**

YIELD: 12 servings

PREP TIME: 15 minutes, plus 2½ hours to chill

SPICED PUMPKIN-SHAPED CHEESE BALL

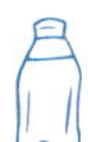

This spicy twist on my classic American Kajmak recipe (page 357) is not only packed with flavor but also doubles as a festive centerpiece! Shaped into a charming pumpkin, it's the perfect addition to your holiday tablescape, bringing both beauty and deliciousness to the table. The piquant spices in this version elevate the creamy kajmak, making it ideal for spreading, dipping, or serving alongside your favorite carnivore dishes. It's versatile, festive, and sure to impress your guests!

- 1 (8-ounce) package full-fat cream cheese, at room temperature
- 1 cup (2 sticks) salted butter, at room temperature
- 1 teaspoon minced garlic
- 1 teaspoon Worcestershire sauce
- 1 teaspoon Tabasco (optional)
- 1 teaspoon spice/herb blend of choice (optional; see note)
- ¼ teaspoon ground black pepper
- ¼ teaspoon Cajun Seasoning (page 346)
- ¼ teaspoon garlic powder
- ½ cup shredded yellow cheddar cheese

SPECIAL EQUIPMENT:
Butcher's twine

1. Put the cream cheese and butter in a large bowl or the bowl of a stand mixer. Using a hand mixer or the stand mixer, beat on medium speed until smooth. Add the garlic, Worcestershire sauce, Tabasco (if using), and spices and mix until fully combined. I recommend scraping the sides of the bowl with a silicone spatula and mixing once more to ensure everything is well combined.
2. Lay out a long sheet of plastic wrap and place the cream cheese mixture in the center. Wrap it up into a ball, twist at the top, and place in the refrigerator to firm up, at least 20 to 30 minutes.
3. Spread out the shredded cheese on a small plate.
4. Remove the plastic wrap from the chilled cheese ball and roll the ball in the shredded cheese, pressing it in lightly. Then rewrap in plastic wrap, twist the plastic wrap at the top, and finalize the shape of your ball to look like a rough pumpkin (round on the sides but flat on the top and bottom). Then cut off the excess plastic wrap at the top.
5. Cut a 3-foot length of butcher's twine and wrap it around the ball to form the ridges of the pumpkin, crisscrossing the twine in the back. Do this four times, then tie the twine into a bow on the top.
6. Place the pumpkin in the refrigerator to chill for at least 2 hours, or until ready to serve. It will remain spreadable even when chilled. Just before serving, cut off the twine and remove the plastic wrap. If you want it to look like a real pumpkin, top it with the stem of a bell pepper. Wrapped tightly in plastic wrap, this will keep in the fridge for up to 2 weeks.

YIELD: 2 cups (¼ cup per serving)

PREP TIME: 5 minutes

COOK TIME: 30 minutes

CARNIVORE GRAVY

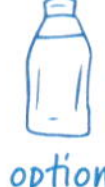

I discovered this recipe on AshEats.com, and it was an instant hit when we made it for Thanksgiving in 2023. Over time, we've made a few tweaks to make it our own, like incorporating chicken bone broth. I also love using turkey drippings for extra flavor—it takes the gravy to the next level. For the perfect pairing, check out my Brined Spatchcocked Turkey recipe (page 300).

½ cup (1 stick) salted butter

Giblets and neck reserved from whole turkey

2 cups chicken bone broth

2 to 2½ cups defatted turkey drippings (reserved from Brined Spatchcocked Turkey, page 300)

1 cup cold water

3 tablespoons unflavored beef gelatin powder

½ cup heavy cream (optional, for a creamy gravy)

1 to 2 tablespoons guar gum or xanthan gum (optional, for a thicker gravy)

Salt, if needed

1. Put the butter and turkey giblets and neck in a large frying pan or sauté pan. Cook the giblets and neck over medium heat for 8 to 10 minutes to allow the butter to become infused with their flavor.
2. Remove the giblets and neck from the pan and add the chicken broth and turkey drippings. Simmer over medium heat until reduced by about half, about 20 minutes.
3. While the broth and drippings are reducing, bloom the gelatin: Put the cold water in a bowl and stir in the gelatin 1 tablespoon at a time, then continue stirring slowly for about 1 minute.
4. Once the broth and drippings have reduced by half, turn off the heat and stir in the bloomed gelatin.
5. If you want a creamy gravy, add the cream and stir thoroughly. If you want a thicker gravy, add the thickener and stir until fully dissolved.
6. Taste the gravy and season to taste with salt, if needed. (We find the gravy plenty salty as is, thanks to the salt in the broth and turkey drippings.) This gravy will become gelatinous once cooled, but it turns back into liquid once reheated. It will keep in the refrigerator for up to 1 week.

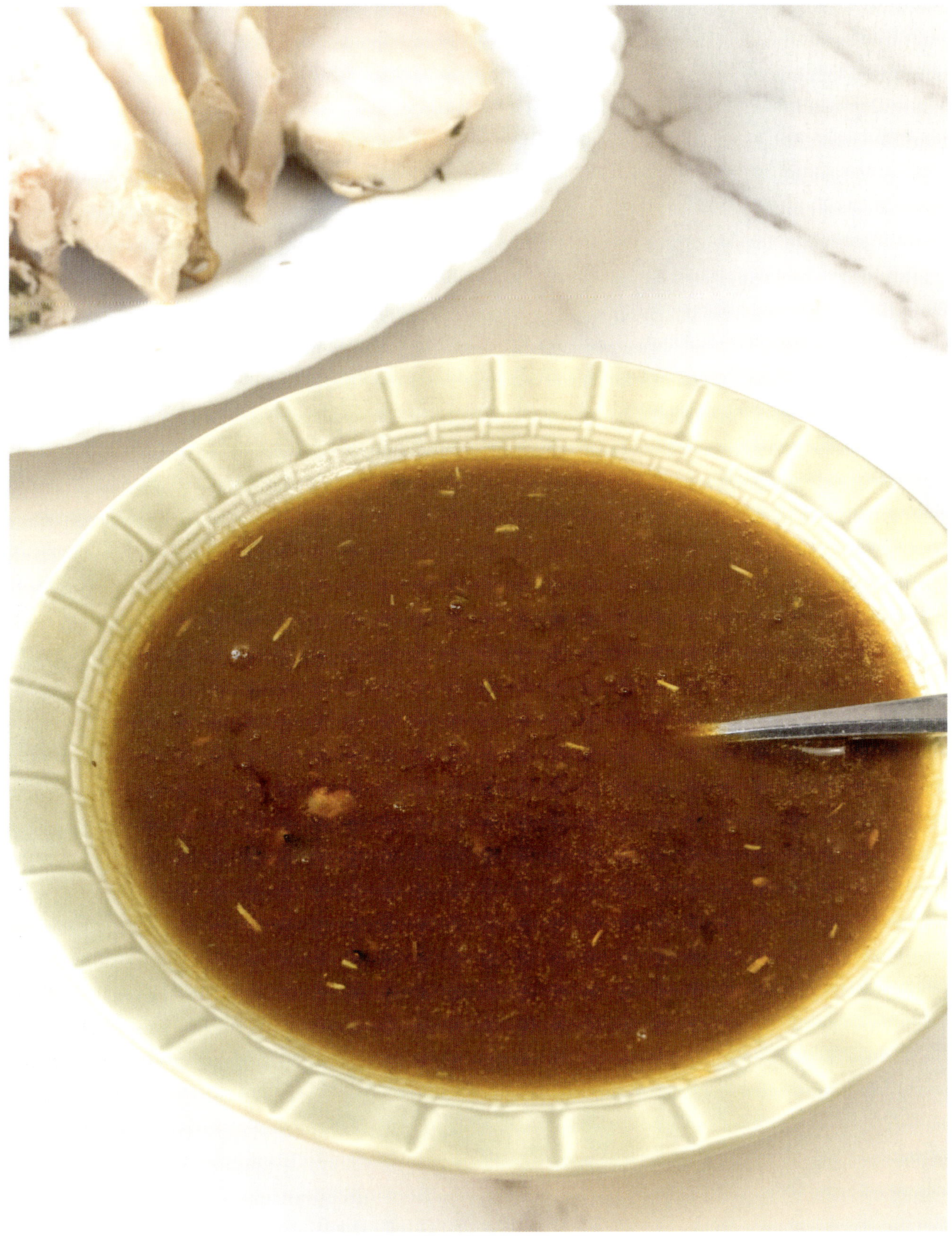

PER SERVING

calories: **572** | fat: **56g** | protein: **9g** | carbs: **0g** | macro split: **93/7/0**

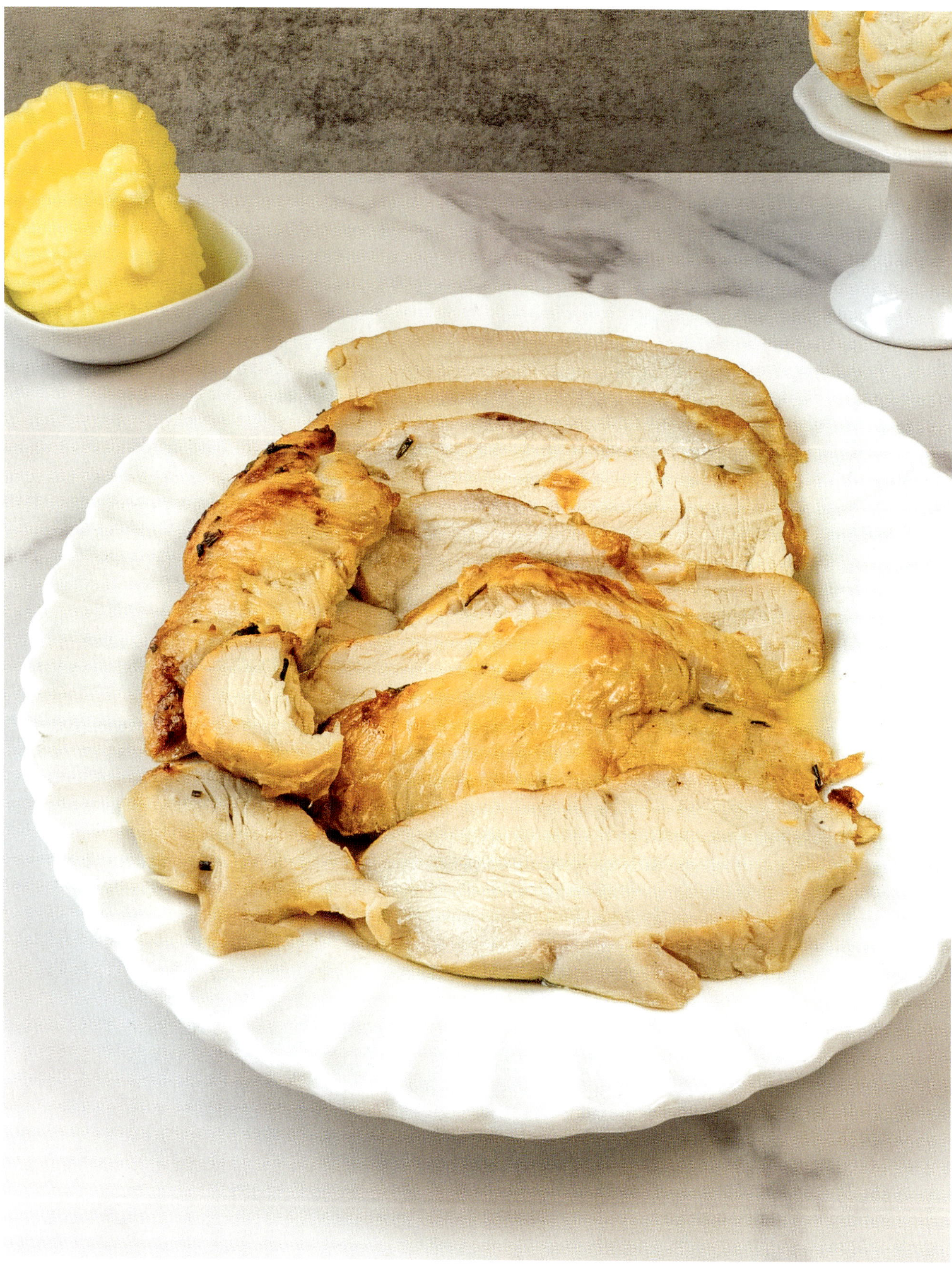

PER SERVING (8 ounces)	calories: **300** | fat: **8g** | protein: **48g** | carbs: **0g** | macro split: **27/73/0**

YIELD: 6 servings

PREP TIME: 15 minutes, plus 12 hours to brine and 12 hours to dry

COOK TIME: 40 minutes

AIR FRYER BRINED TURKEY BREAST

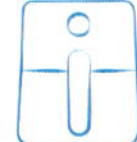

If a whole turkey seems like too much, a small turkey breast might be just right! A three-pound turkey breast fits perfectly in the air fryer, making both cooking and cleanup a breeze. It provides enough meat for your holiday meal, plus some extra for turkey sandwiches.

½ cup kosher salt, for the brine

1 to 2 cups hot water, for the brine

1 (3-pound) boneless, skin-on turkey breast

½ cup (1 stick) salted butter

2 tablespoons fresh rosemary needles

1. Dissolve the salt in the hot water and set aside to cool.
2. Put the turkey breast in a large bowl and cover with cold water. Pour the cooled salted water into the bowl with the turkey. Place the bowl in the refrigerator and allow the turkey to brine for 12 hours.
3. Remove the turkey breast from the brine and thoroughly rinse with fresh cold water. Then pat it dry. Place on a sheet pan fitted with a wire rack and put back in the refrigerator, uncovered, for 12 hours, or until the outside is dry.
4. Remove the turkey from the refrigerator. Put the butter in a small glass bowl and microwave for 30 seconds to soften. Mix the butter and rosemary until blended, then slather the herbed butter all over the turkey. Insert a temperature probe, then wrap the turkey in aluminum foil.
5. Place the wrapped turkey in an air fryer and set to slow-cook mode (or air-fry mode if your air fryer doesn't have a slow-cook mode) at 230°F for 25 minutes. Check the internal temperature of the turkey; when done, it should be 150°F. If needed, continue cooking the turkey for up to an additional 10 minutes, until the temperature reaches 150°F.
6. Take the turkey breast out of the air fryer and remove it from the foil wrapping. Put the turkey back in the air fryer, pour the melted butter from the foil over it, and air-fry at 450°F until the turkey reaches an internal temperature of 158°F. This step will crisp up the skin.
7. Pull the turkey breast from the air fryer and allow it to rest for 10 minutes before slicing and serving. The final temperature will go up a few degrees more, to between 160°F and 164°F.

YIELD: 2 servings

PREP TIME: 5 minutes (not including time to make noodles or sauce)

COOK TIME: 3 minutes

TURKEY ALFREDO

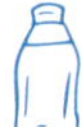
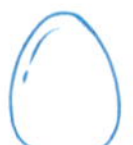

I'm always on the lookout for creative ways to use up leftover turkey, especially since we typically roast two or three turkeys during the holiday season. One of my favorite dishes to make is this rich and creamy turkey Alfredo. It's so flavorful and satisfying, you'd never guess it's fully carnivore! The "noodles" are made from Carnivore Crepes sliced into strips, giving it the perfect pasta-like texture. This dish is a great way to transform leftovers into a comforting, restaurant-quality meal that everyone will love. Plus, it's quick and easy, making it perfect for busy weeknights! Once the noodles and sauce are made, this dish comes together in no time.

- 1 batch Carnivore Noodles (page 364)
- 1 batch Alfredo Sauce (page 351)
- 1 cup diced leftover turkey
- 1 tablespoon salted butter

1. Divide the noodles evenly between two dinner plates.
2. After preparing the Alfredo sauce, allow it to cool for 5 minutes. While the sauce is cooling, warm the turkey with the butter in a medium frying pan over medium heat, moving the pieces of turkey around in the pan often. This will take 2 to 3 minutes.
3. Distribute the turkey evenly between the plates of noodles. Then top with the Alfredo sauce and enjoy!

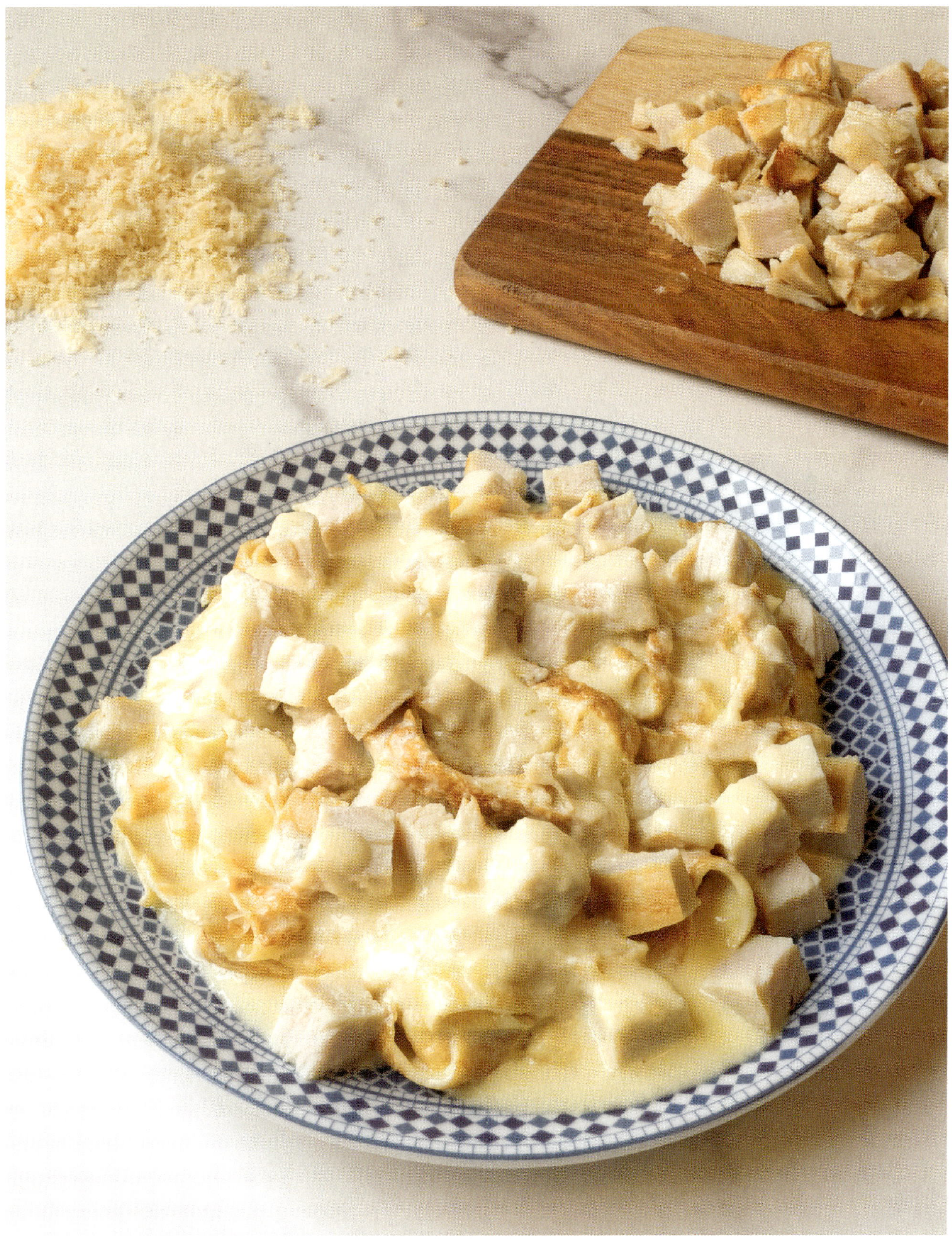

PER SERVING | calories: **734** | fat: **49g** | protein: **64g** | carbs: **6g** | macro split: **61/35/6**

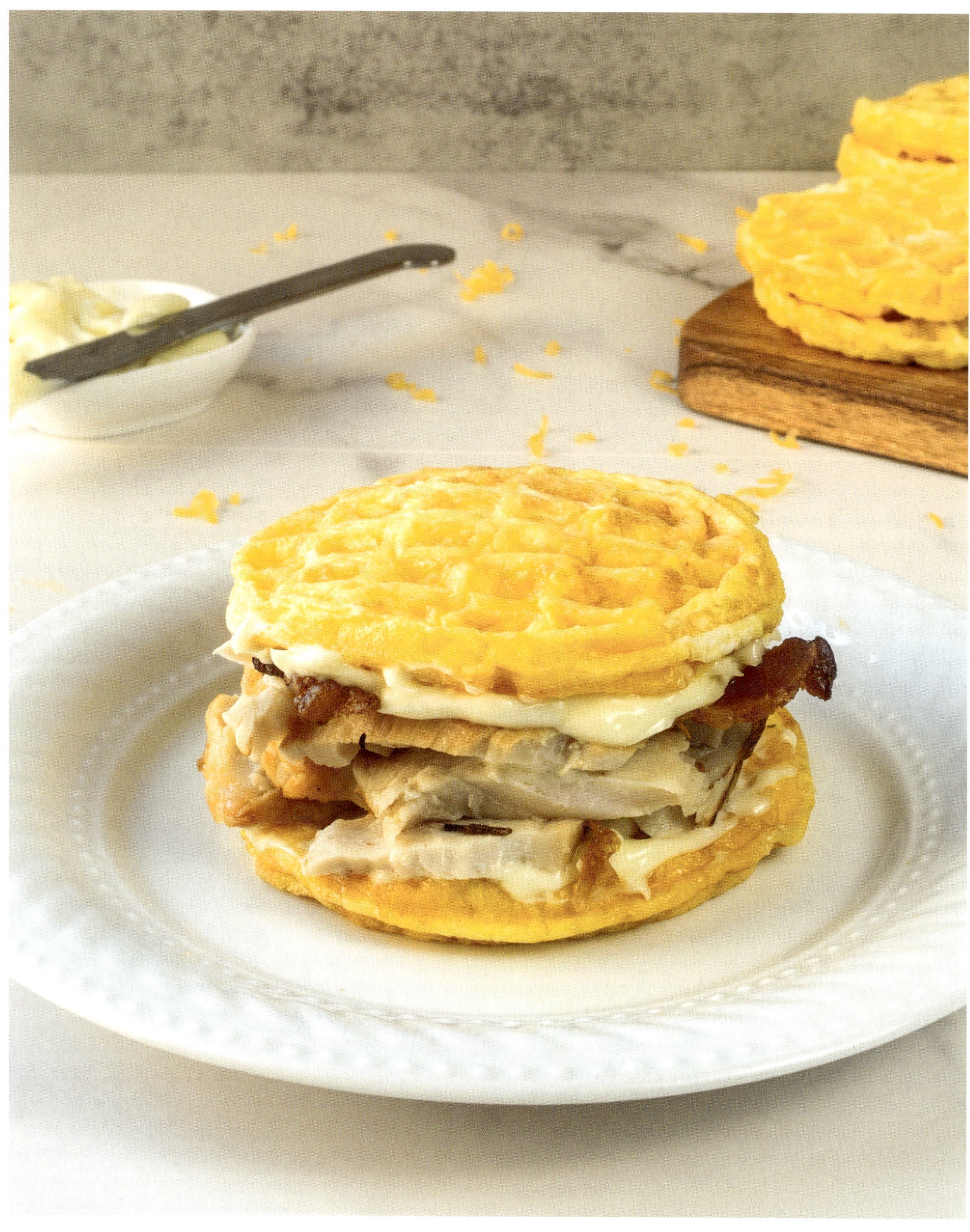

PER SANDWICH (with cloud bread)	calories: **588** | fat: **36g** | protein: **57g** | carbs: **1g** | macro split: **58/41/1**
PER SANDWICH (with chaffles)	calories: **748** | fat: **51g** | protein: **62g** | carbs: **1g** | macro split: **65/34/1**

YIELD: 1 sandwich

PREP TIME: 5 minutes (not including time to make bread or mayo or cook bacon)

TURKEY SANDWICH

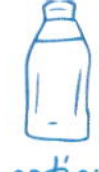

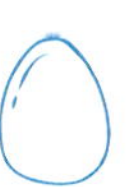

Growing up, my favorite part of Thanksgiving wasn't just the big meal—it was the turkey sandwiches we made later in the evening! There was something so comforting about piling leftover turkey onto soft bread for a second helping of holiday deliciousness. Now, I love that I can still enjoy this tradition while staying true to my carnivore lifestyle. Using my cloud bread or chaffles as the base, I can re-create those nostalgic sandwiches with a carnivore twist. Add a little mayo, some bacon, or even some leftover gravy, and it feels just like the classic I grew up loving—only better!

2 slices Cloud Bread Loaf (page 372) or 2 Chaffles (page 368)

2 tablespoons Bacon Mayonnaise (page 352) or store-bought avocado oil mayonnaise

8 ounces sliced turkey breast and/or leg meat (2 to 3 slices)

2 strips bacon, cooked

Put the bread or chaffles on a plate and slather 1 tablespoon of mayo on each piece. Layer the turkey slices and bacon strips on one of the mayo-slathered pieces of bread (or chaffles) and top with the other piece of bread (or chaffle), mayo side down. Enjoy!

YIELD: 8 servings

PREP TIME: 15 minutes, plus 4 hours to cool/chill

COOK TIME: 55 minutes

PUMPKIN SPICE CHEESECAKE

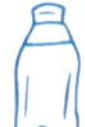
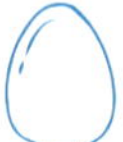

I found the original of this pumpkin spice cheesecake recipe on the Carnivorous Chef's YouTube channel and absolutely loved it! To make it even more carnivore-friendly, I've made a few adjustments. If you'd rather skip the pumpkin pie spice and sweetener, you'll have a classic plain (but not sweet) cheesecake. For an extra indulgence, try topping it with some freshly whipped heavy cream or, better yet, Whipped Cream & Mascarpone (page 341)—it's the perfect finishing touch!

- 2 (8-ounce) packages full-fat cream cheese, at room temperature
- ¾ cup full-fat sour cream
- 3 large eggs
- ¾ cup powdered allulose or other sugar substitute, such as stevia or monkfruit (optional)
- 1 teaspoon vanilla extract (optional)
- 2 tablespoons melted salted butter
- 2 teaspoons pumpkin pie spice, plus extra for sprinkling on top before baking (optional)

SPECIAL EQUIPMENT:

9-inch springform pan (optional)

1. Preheat the oven to 350°F. Grease a 9-inch springform pan or standard-depth pie pan with butter.
2. Put the cream cheese and sour cream in a large bowl or the bowl of a stand mixer fitted with the whisk attachment. Using a hand mixer or the stand mixer, mix on medium speed until well blended. Then slowly add the other ingredients one at a time: the eggs one by one, then the allulose (if using), vanilla (if using), butter, and pumpkin spice (if using), mixing to incorporate after each addition.
3. Pour the mixture into the prepared pan. If using a springform, wrap the bottom in foil to keep water from seeping in during baking.
4. Set the pan in a deep baking dish and pour hot water into the dish until it comes halfway up the side of the springform (or pie) pan.
5. Place the baking dish with the pan and water in the oven and bake for 50 to 55 minutes, until the cheesecake only slightly jiggles when you shake it.
6. Turn off the oven, crack open the oven door, and allow the cheesecake to cool in the oven for 30 minutes. Then pull the baking dish from the oven, remove the pan from the baking dish, and let it cool on top of the stove (or on the countertop on a cooling rack) for another 30 minutes. Finally, put the cheesecake in the refrigerator to chill for at least 3 hours before serving.

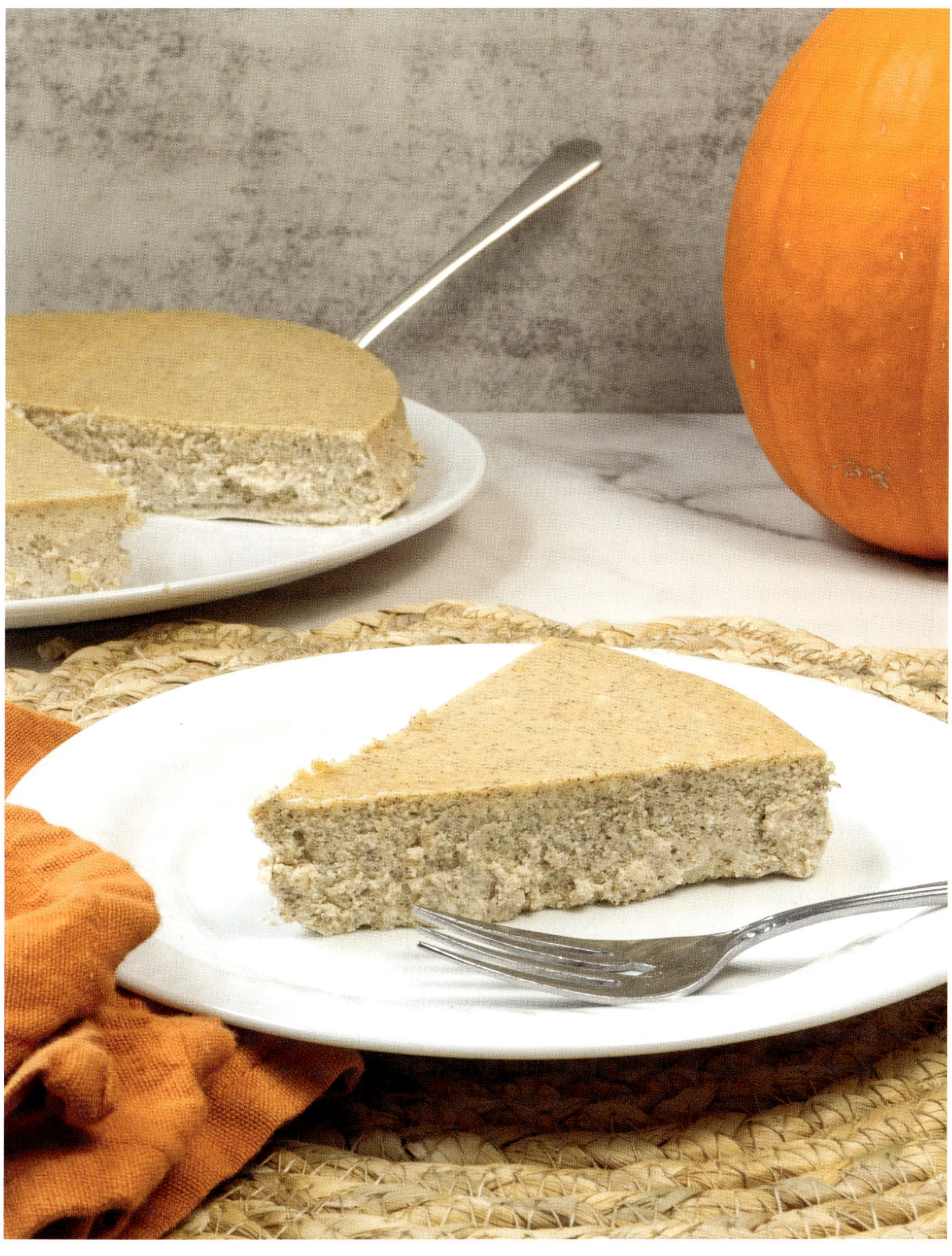

PER SERVING	calories: **299** | fat: **29g** | protein: **7g** | carbs: **3g** | macro split: **87/9/4**

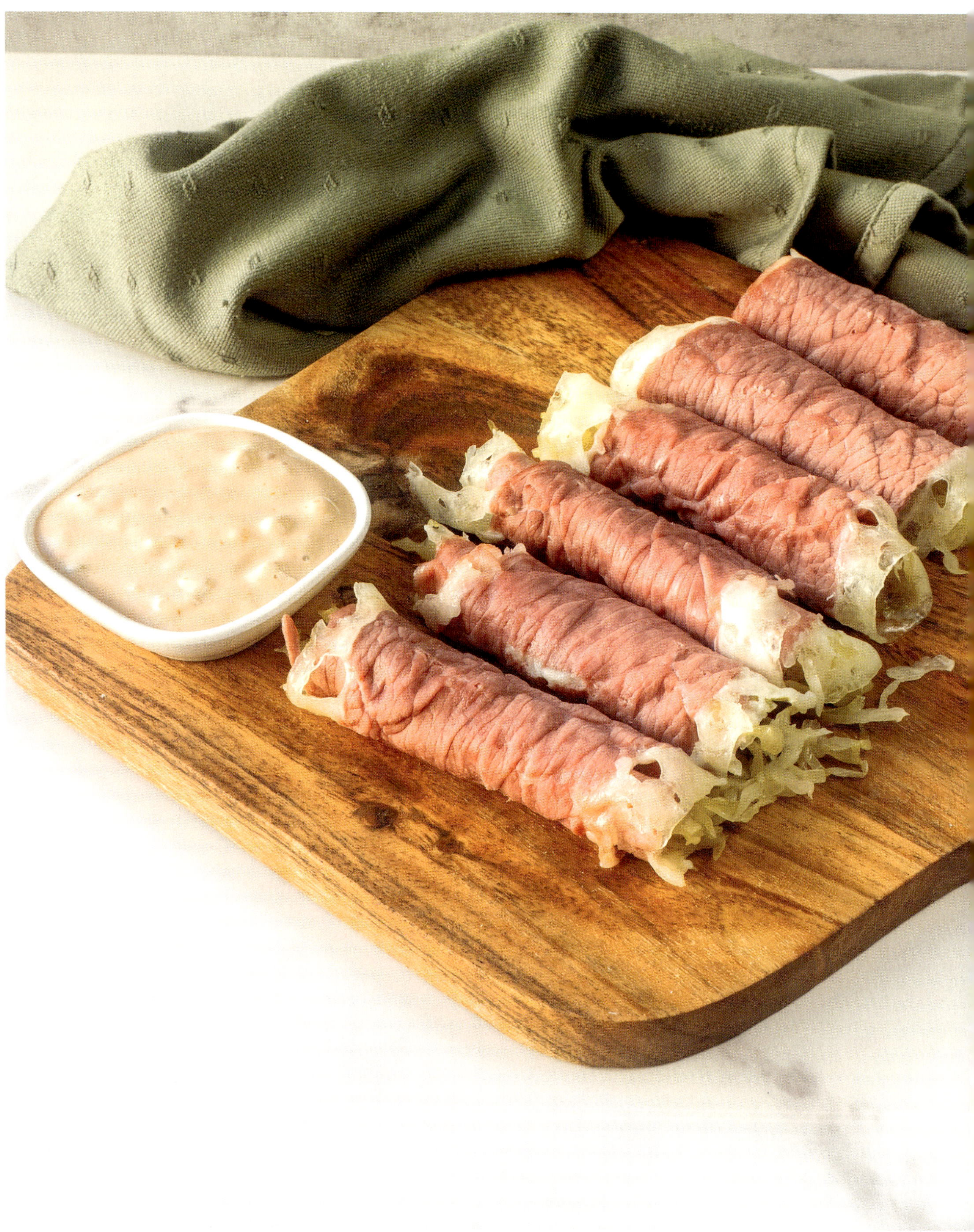

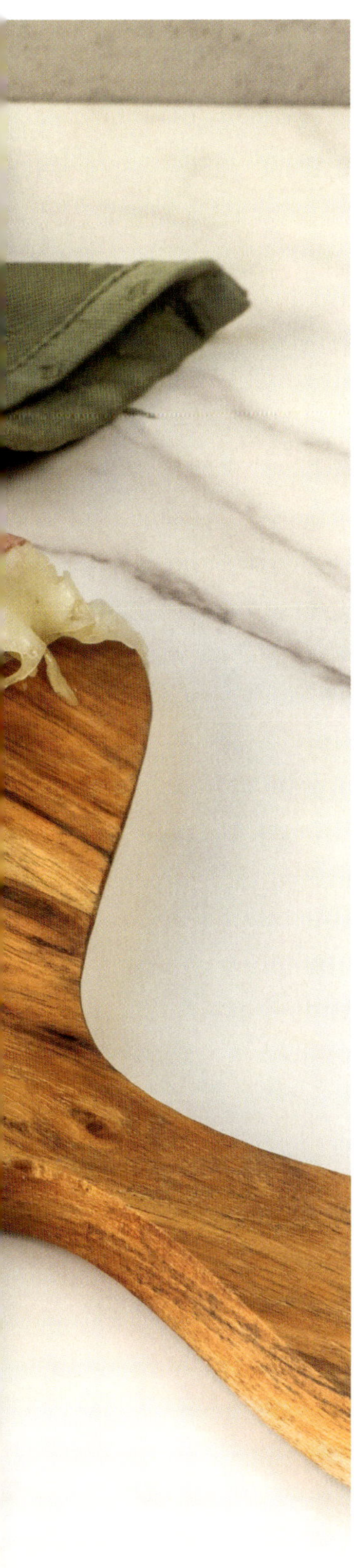

CHAPTER 15
KETO CHEAT MEALS

319 Jalapeño Poppers

320 Beefy Bacon-Wrapped Stuffed Onion Rings

323 Garlicky Smothered Brussels Sprouts

324 Wedge Salad

327 Reuben Roll-Ups

328 Garlicky Smothered Green Beans

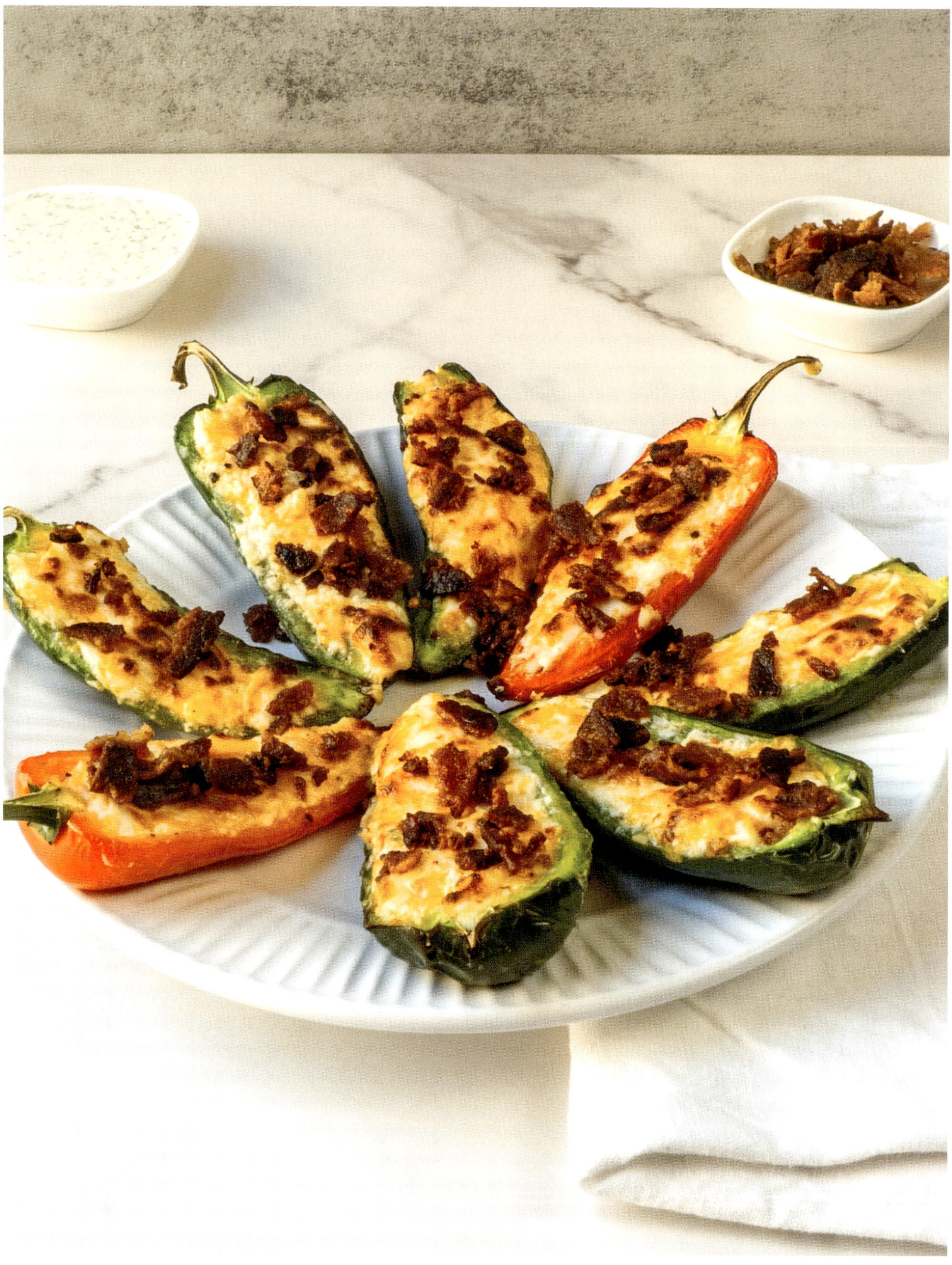

PER SERVING | calories: **373** | fat: **33g** | protein: **15g** | carbs: **5g** | macro split: **78/16/6**

YIELD: 16 poppers (4 per serving)

PREP TIME: 25 minutes (not including time to cook bacon)

COOK TIME: 20 to 32 minutes, depending on method

JALAPEÑO POPPERS

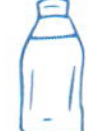

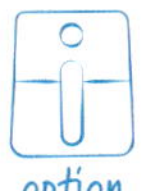

Every year, I make it a tradition to grow jalapeño peppers in my garden just for this recipe. It's a staple that never disappoints! These poppers are an incredibly flavorful and satisfying side dish or snack, packed with bold flavors and a touch of heat. They're low in carbs, making them a perfect addition to a monthly keto cheat meal. When you grow your own jalapeños, you can allow some to ripen on the plant until red before picking them; it makes for a pretty presentation to have a mix of green and red poppers. For this recipe, you have the option to cook the poppers in the oven or in an air fryer.

- 8 jalapeño peppers
- 1 (8-ounce) package full-fat cream cheese, at room temperature
- 1 cup shredded sharp cheddar cheese
- Pinch of salt
- Pinch of ground white pepper
- 4 strips bacon, cooked and crumbled

1. Cut the jalapeños in half lengthwise and clean out the seeds. Leave the membranes if you want the poppers to be a bit spicier.
2. Mix the cream cheese, cheddar, salt, and pepper in a large bowl until fully incorporated.
3. Spoon the cheese mixture into each half jalapeño, distributing the mixture evenly among the sixteen halves.
4. If cooking the poppers in the oven, preheat the oven to 400°F using the convection mode (on my oven, this is called "Quick Bake" mode). If your oven does not have a convection setting, set the temperature to 425°F. Arrange the stuffed jalapeños on a sheet pan and bake for 20 to 25 minutes, until the cheese is melty and the jalapeños are soft but still holding their shape.

   If cooking the poppers in an air fryer, working in batches, place the stuffed jalapeños in the air fryer basket, making sure not to crowd them, and air-fry at 400°F for 16 minutes, or until the cheese is melty and the jalapeños are soft but still holding their shape.
5. Remove from the oven or air fryer and sprinkle with the bacon. Allow to cool for 10 minutes before serving.

YIELD: 16 onion rings (4 per serving)

PREP TIME: 20 minutes

COOK TIME: 35 minutes

BEEFY BACON-WRAPPED STUFFED ONION RINGS

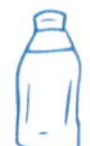
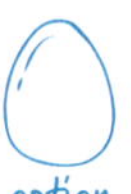
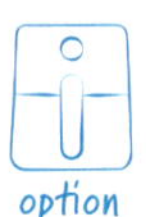

These beefy onion rings hardly qualify as a keto cheat meal since they're mostly meat. Pair them with creamy ranch dressing for a mouthwatering keto-friendly treat.

- 2 large white onions
- 1 pound 80/20 ground beef
- 1 cup shredded pepper Jack cheese
- ½ teaspoon salt
- ½ teaspoon garlic powder
- ½ teaspoon smoked paprika
- ¼ teaspoon ground white pepper
- 32 strips bacon
- Buttermilk Ranch Dressing (page 361), for dipping (optional)

1. Cut each onion into eight ½-inch-thick discs, making a total of sixteen discs. Take one of the discs and break it apart into rings. Take the largest ring and the next smaller ring that nestles nicely inside of the larger one. Pair them together and place on a sheet pan. Repeat with the other onion discs to make sixteen pairs and set aside. Reserve the remaining onion discs for another use.
2. Put the ground beef, cheese, salt, and spices in a medium bowl and mix well until combined.
3. Fill the inside of the larger onion ring with the meat mixture. Then place the smaller onion ring inside of it (see photo), pressing it against the meat to secure it in place.
4. Wrap each stuffed onion ring with two strips of bacon.
5. Preheat the oven to 400°F.
6. Arrange the bacon-wrapped onion rings on the sheet pan and bake for 25 to 35 minutes, until the bacon is crispy and browned. Let cool for 10 minutes before serving with ranch dressing, if desired.

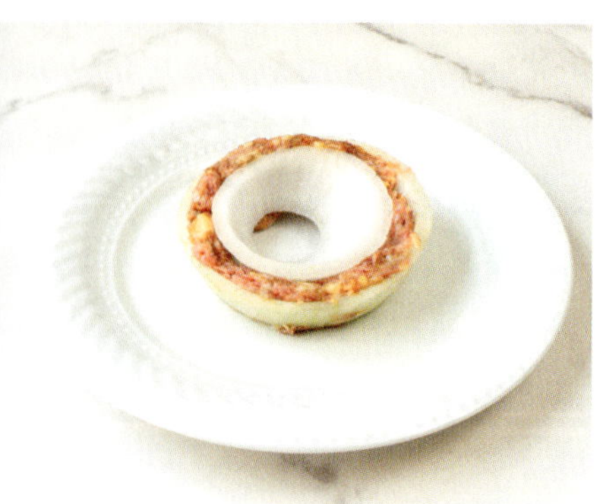

Note

Alternatively, you can batch-cook these in an air fryer. Put three or four bacon-wrapped onion rings in the air fryer basket, leaving a little space between them, and air-fry at 350°F for 20 minutes, flipping once, until the bacon is crispy and browned.

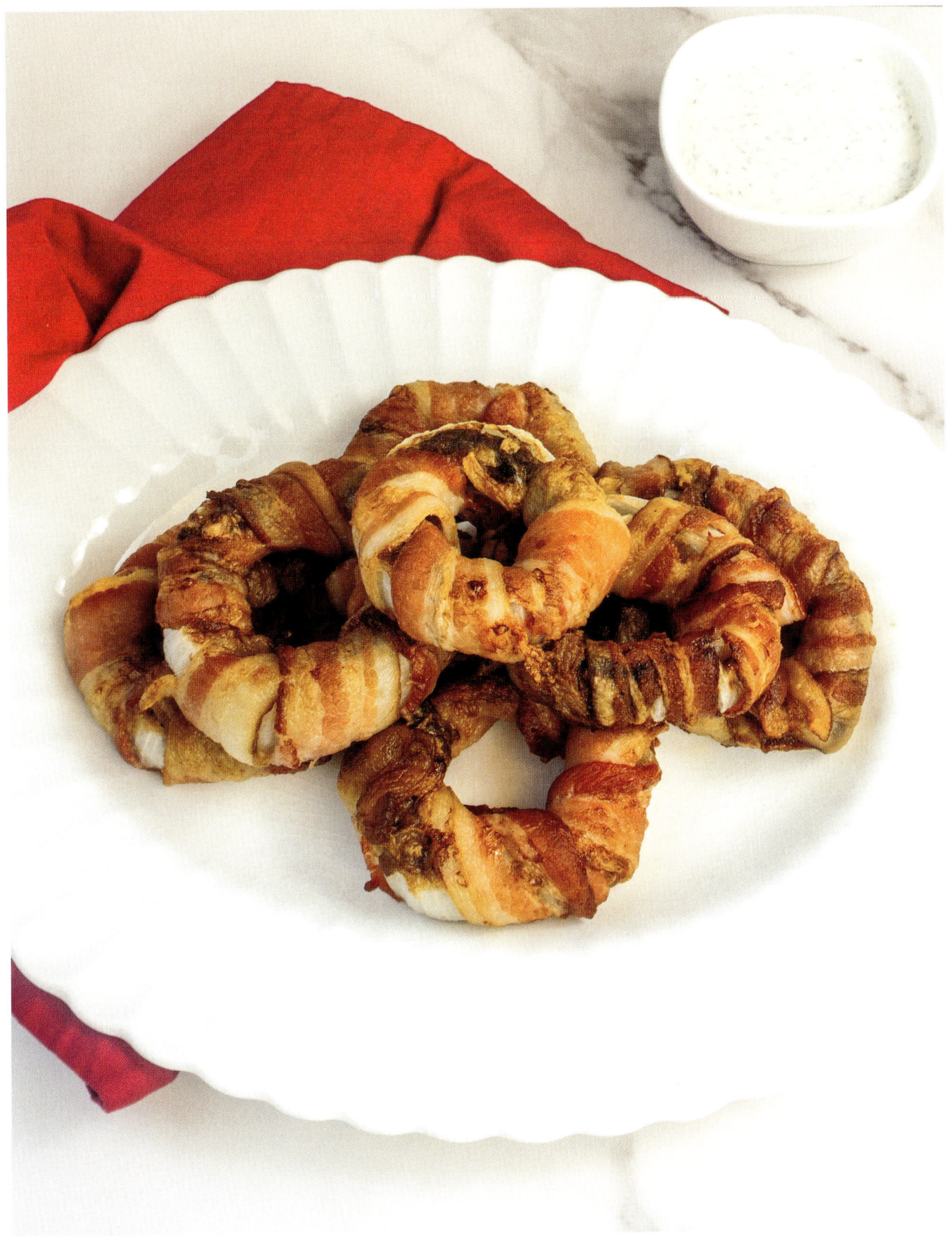

PER SERVING calories: **1062** | fat: **79g** | protein: **64g** | carbs: **6g** | macro split: **72/26/5**

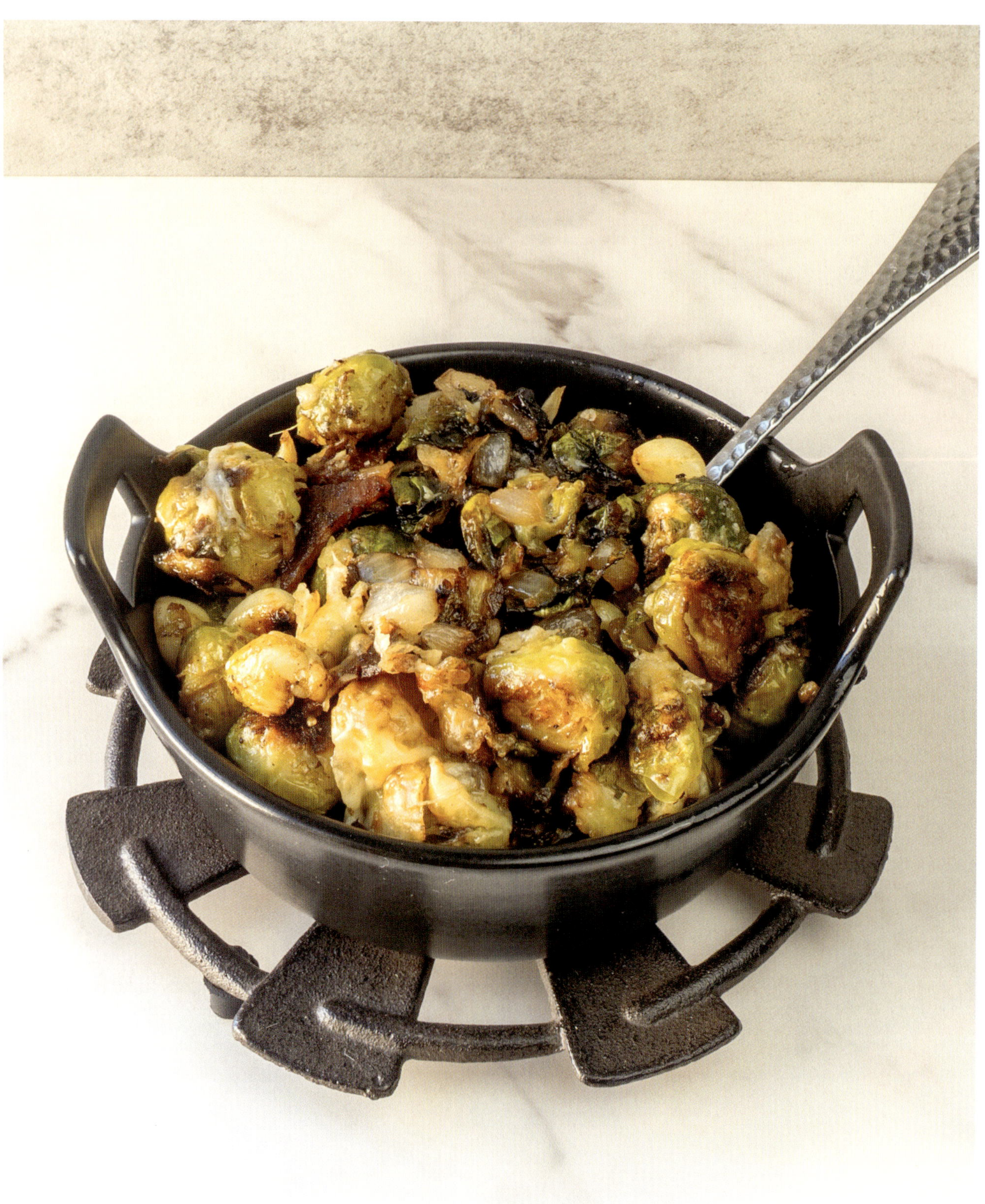

PER SERVING (½ cup) calories: **430** | fat: **31g** | protein: **12g** | carbs: **31g** | macro split: **62/10/28**

YIELD: 4 servings

PREP TIME: 10 minutes (not including time to cook bacon)

COOK TIME: 35 minutes

GARLICKY SMOTHERED BRUSSELS SPROUTS

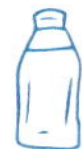

Brussels sprouts are my favorite choice for a keto cheat meal. Adding cheese and bacon takes them to the next level, making these veggies so delicious that you'll actually look forward to finishing them!

½ cup bacon grease

2 pounds Brussels sprouts, halved

12 cloves garlic, peeled, divided

1 tablespoon garlic powder

1 tablespoon onion powder

Salt and pepper

½ cup crumbled cooked bacon

½ cup shaved Asiago, Parmesan, and/or Romano cheese (see note)

1. Melt the bacon grease in a large frying pan, preferably ceramic or seasoned cast iron, over medium heat. Put the Brussels sprouts and six of the garlic cloves in the pan, then cover the pan with a lid or a piece of aluminum foil. Allow the Brussels sprouts to slowly steam and brown until they are cooked down and soft, stirring occasionally. This will take 20 to 30 minutes.
2. Using a garlic press, press the remaining six garlic cloves into the pan, then add the garlic powder, onion powder, and salt and pepper to taste. (When adding salt, keep in mind that the bacon and shaved cheese will add a salty element.) Stir to combine, cover, and cook for another 5 to 7 minutes, until the sprouts are fork-tender but not mushy.
3. Add the crumbled bacon and stir to combine, then top with the cheese. When the cheese starts to look melty, it is ready to serve.

Note

For convenience, I use BelGioiso's salad blend of shaved Italian hard cheeses, featuring Asiago, Parmesan, and Romano.

YIELD: 4 servings

PREP TIME: 10 minutes (not including time to make dressing or cook bacon and eggs)

WEDGE SALAD

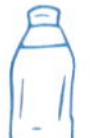 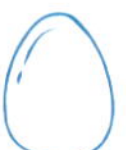 

Whenever my husband and I indulge in a steakhouse-style cheat meal, a wedge salad is always a must. This classic dish is surprisingly easy to re-create at home, and the key to perfection is keeping the lettuce ice-cold and serving it immediately for maximum freshness. Pair this crisp and flavorful salad with a perfectly grilled ribeye steak and a side of Garlicky Smothered Brussels Sprouts (page 323) for a keto cheat meal that's fit for royalty.

- 1 large head iceberg lettuce
- ½ cup Buttermilk Ranch Dressing (page 361)
- 16 cherry tomatoes, halved
- 4 strips bacon, cooked and crumbled
- 4 large hard-boiled eggs (see page 236), chopped
- ¾ cup blue cheese crumbles
- ¼ cup sliced green onions

1. Cut the head of lettuce into four wedges. Peel off any leaves that are wilted or brown.
2. Lay one wedge on a plate and spoon 2 tablespoons of the dressing on top. Then sprinkle one-quarter of each of the remaining ingredients on top of the wedge, letting them cascade down and around it. Repeat with the remaining lettuce wedges, dressing, and toppings. Serve immediately.

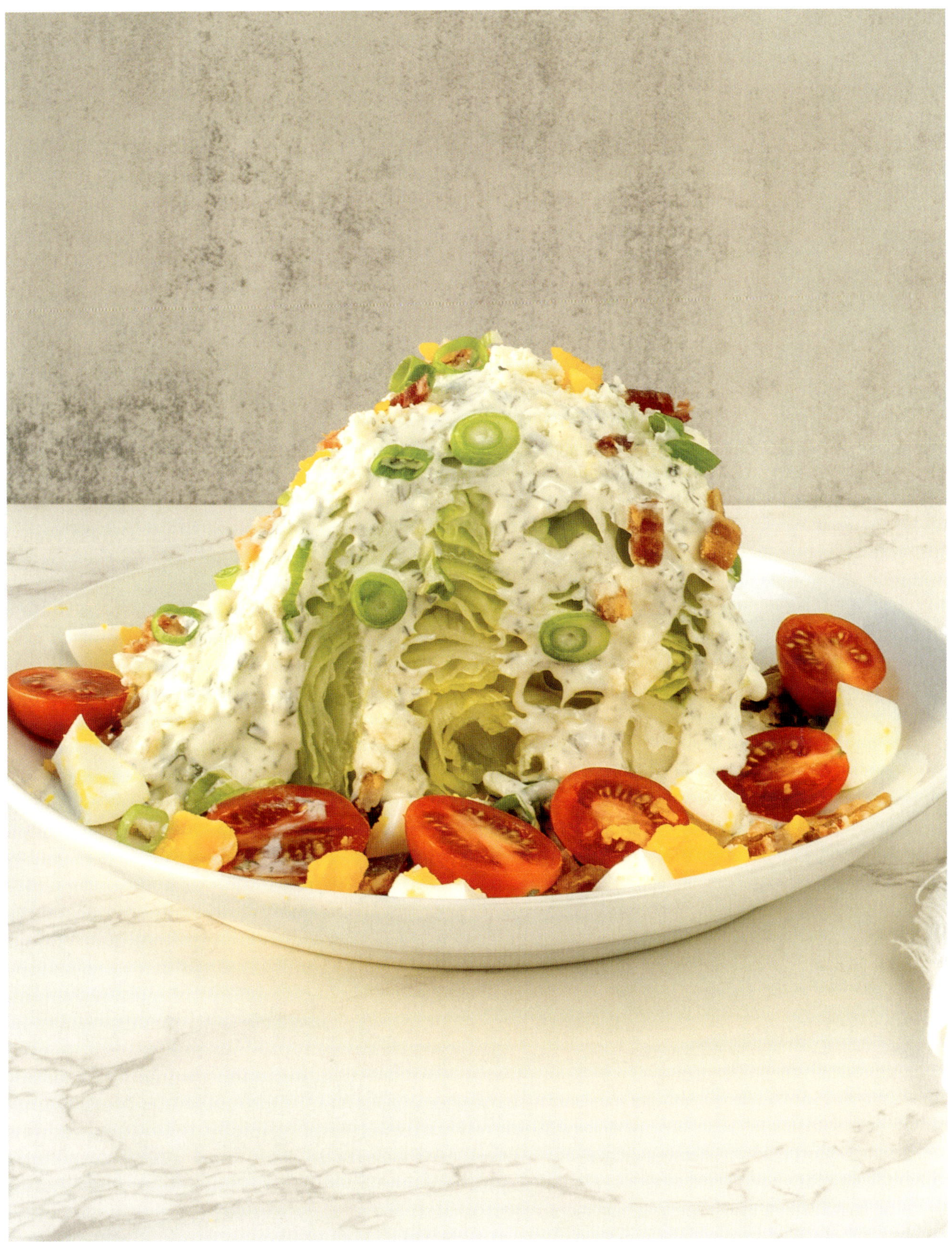

PER SERVING	calories: **381** | fat: **28g** | protein: **21g** | carbs: **9g** | macro split: **67/22/10**

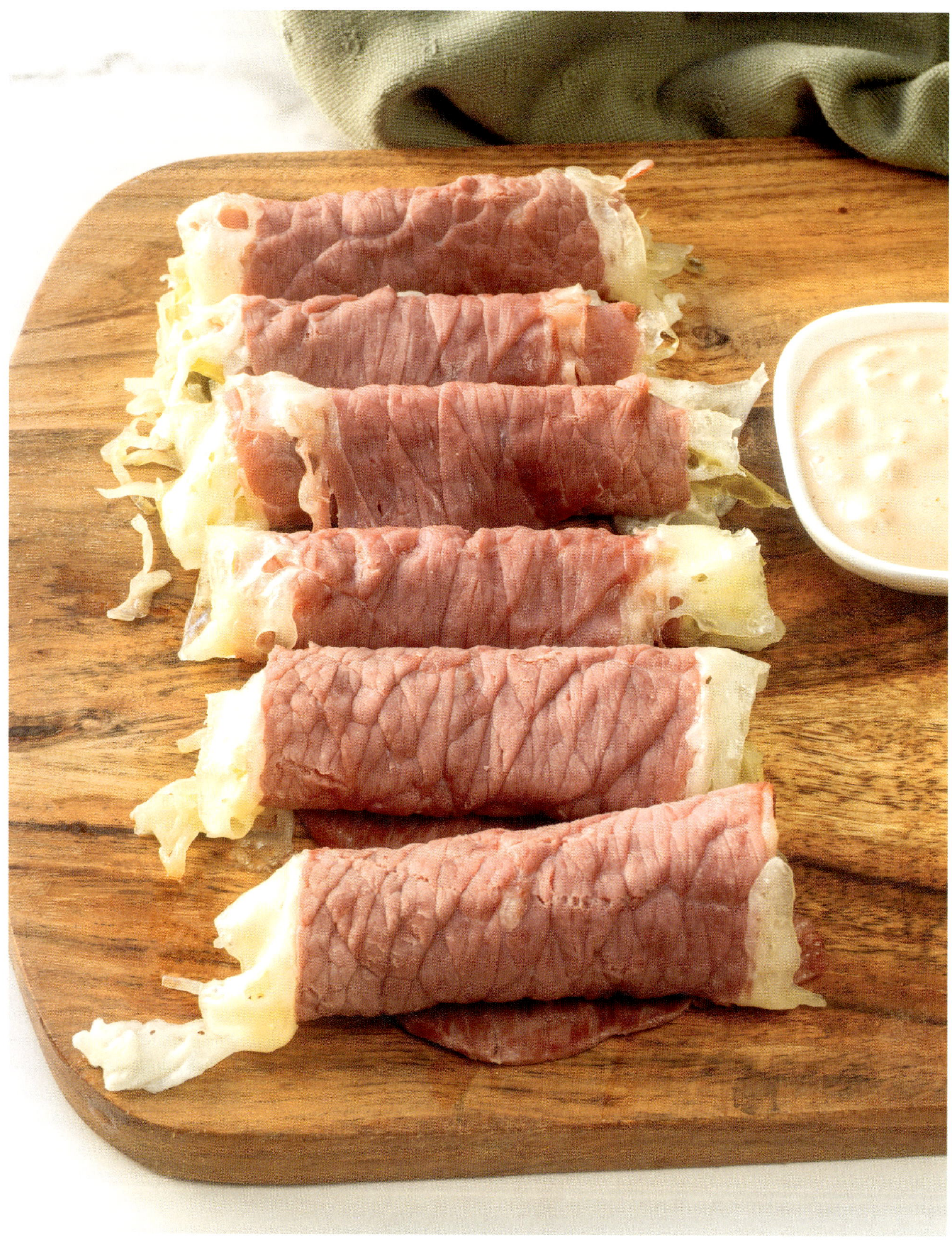

PER SERVING (with 1 tablespoon dressing)	calories: **513** | fat: **43g** | protein: **26g** | carbs: **2g** | macro split: **77/21/2**

YIELD: 1 serving

PREP TIME: 5 minutes

COOK TIME: 5 minutes

REUBEN ROLL-UPS

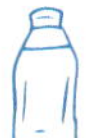
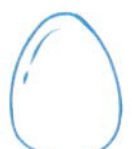

These roll-ups are everything you love about the classic sandwich—just without the bread! They're quick to prepare, incredibly satisfying, and even easier to enjoy. Pair them with a side of my keto Thousand Island dressing, and you won't miss the bread one bit. Plus, with minimal cleanup, they're as convenient as they are delicious!

FOR THE ROLL-UPS:

6 slices thin-cut corned beef lunchmeat

6 slices thin-cut Swiss cheese

¼ cup sauerkraut

FOR THE THOUSAND ISLAND DRESSING:

(Makes ¾ cup)

½ cup avocado oil mayonnaise

2 tablespoons minced dill pickles

2 tablespoons sugar-free ketchup

1 teaspoon distilled white vinegar

Pinch of salt

Pinch of ground black pepper

1. Preheat the oven to 375°F. Line a sheet pan with parchment paper or a silicone baking mat.
2. Lay the corned beef slices on the prepared pan, spacing them evenly. Top with the Swiss cheese slices and then the sauerkraut, using about 2 teaspoons per stack.
3. Bake for 5 minutes, or until the cheese is fully melted.
4. While the stacks are baking, stir together all of the ingredients for the dressing until smooth. Set aside.
5. Remove the pan from the oven and allow the stacks to cool for 2 minutes. Then roll each stack into a cigar shape.
6. Serve immediately with the dressing on the side. Leftover dressing can be stored in the refrigerator for up to 5 days.

YIELD: 4 servings

PREP TIME: 12 minutes (not including time to cook bacon)

COOK TIME: 35 minutes

GARLICKY SMOTHERED GREEN BEANS

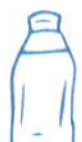

Smothered green beans are a delicious and satisfying addition to any meal, especially if you are looking for a low-toxin vegetable option. Naturally mild and easy to prepare, green beans shine when slow-cooked with rich flavors like bacon and a touch of seasoning. This dish has become a staple for us when planning our monthly keto cheat meal. The tender, savory beans pair perfectly with any main course, adding a comforting and hearty side that's both low in carbs and high in flavor.

½ cup bacon grease

1 pound green beans, trimmed

12 cloves garlic, peeled, divided

½ cup chopped green onions

1 tablespoon garlic powder

1 tablespoon onion powder

Pinch of ground white pepper

Pinch of salt

4 strips bacon, cooked and crumbled

½ cup shaved Asiago, Parmesan, and/or Romano cheese (see note, page 323)

1. Melt the bacon grease in a large frying pan, preferably ceramic or seasoned cast iron, over medium heat. Put the green beans and six of the garlic cloves in the pan, then cover with a lid or a piece of aluminum foil. Allow the beans to slowly steam and brown, stirring occasionally, until they are cooked down and softer but still crisp. This will take 20 to 30 minutes.
2. Using a garlic press, press the remaining six garlic cloves into the pan. Then add the green onions, spices, and salt. (When adding salt, keep in mind that the bacon and shaved cheese will add a salty element.) Cook for another 5 minutes, or until the beans are tender but still slightly crisp. You don't want them to be mushy.
3. Add the crumbled bacon and stir to combine, then top with the cheese. When the cheese is melty, it is ready to serve.

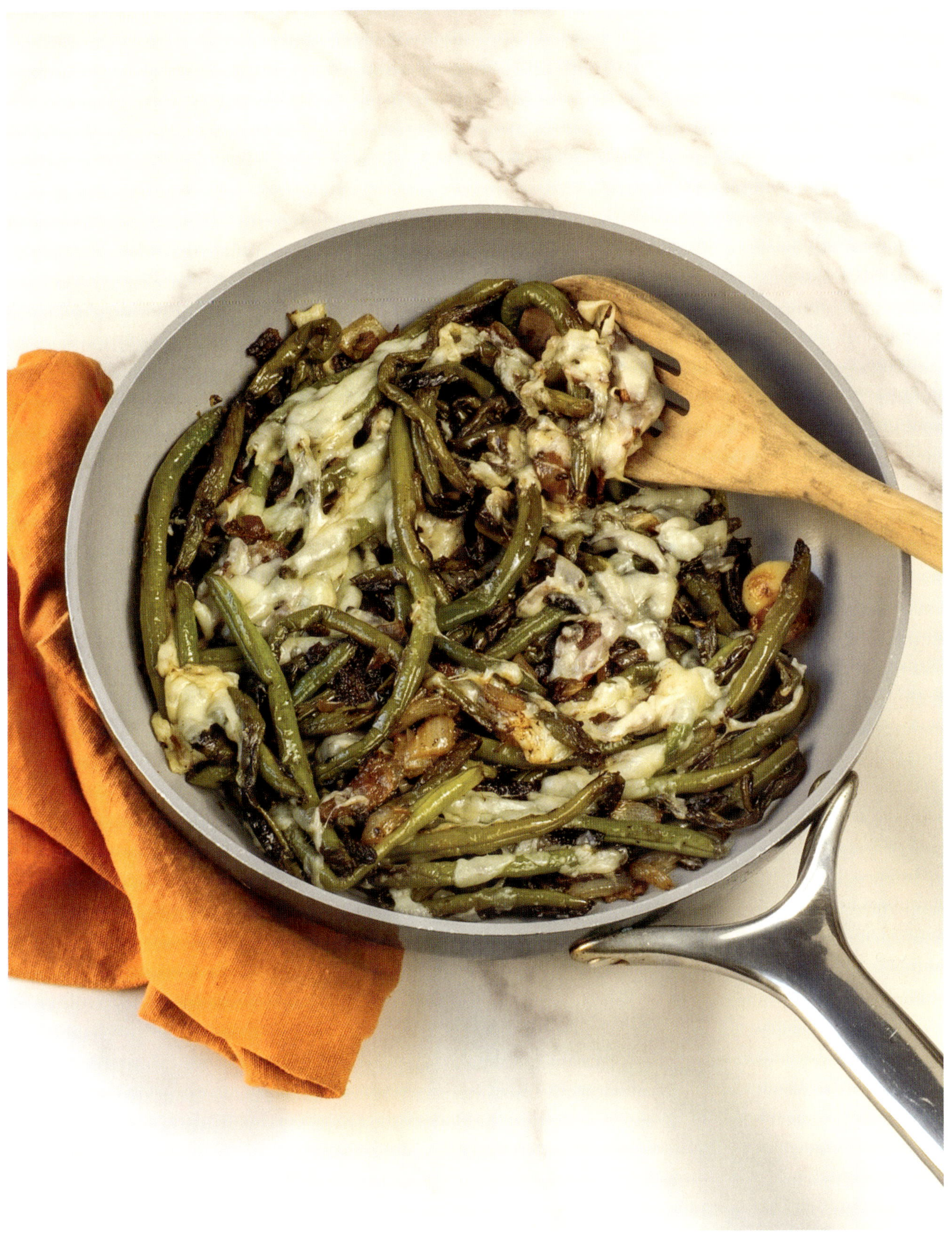

PER SERVING (½ cup)	calories: **389** | fat: **32g** | protein: **8g** | carbs: **17g** | macro split: **74/8/18**

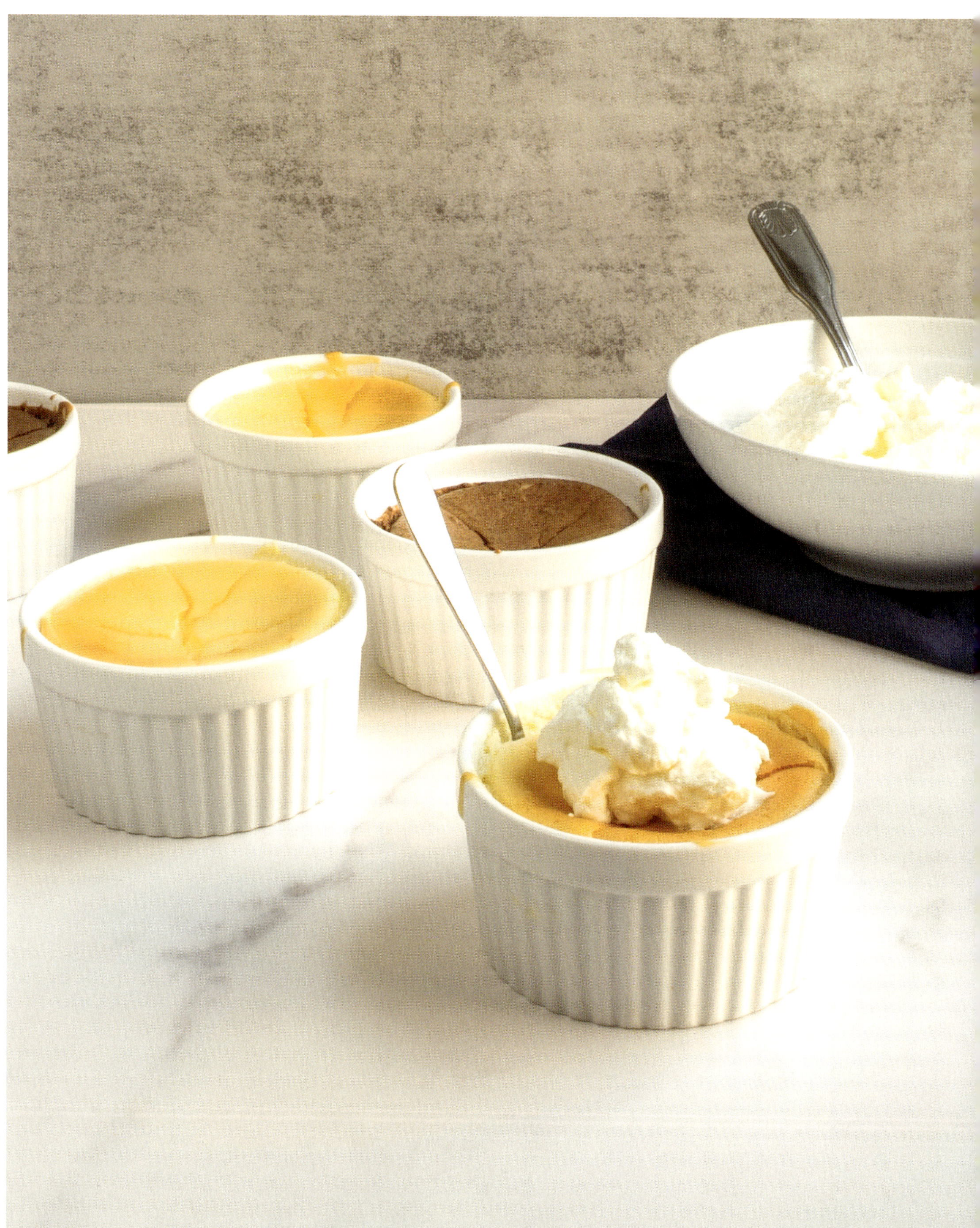

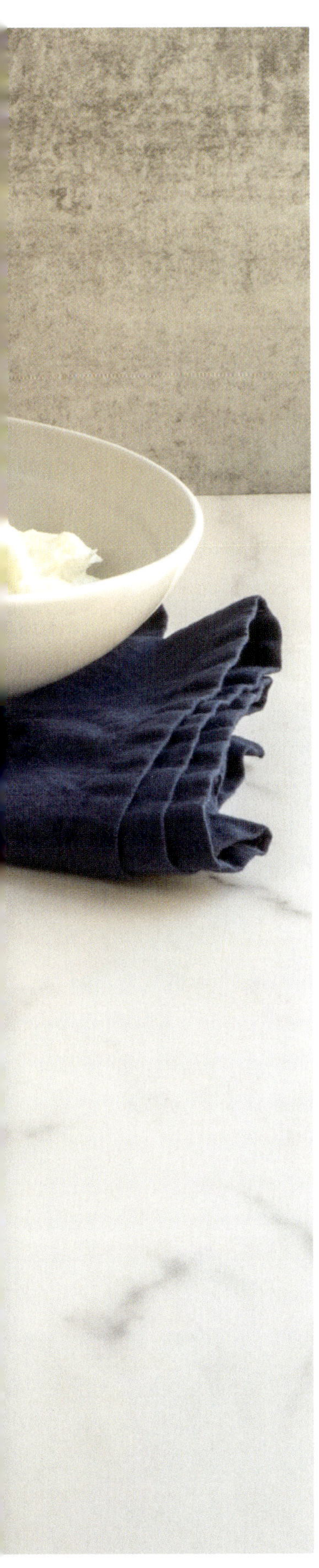

CHAPTER 16
DESSERTS

333 Butter Bites

334 Carnivore Ice Cream

337 Carnivore Ice Cream Sandwiches—Two Ways

338 Mini Cheesecakes

341 Whipped Cream & Mascarpone

342 Whipped Tallow Bites

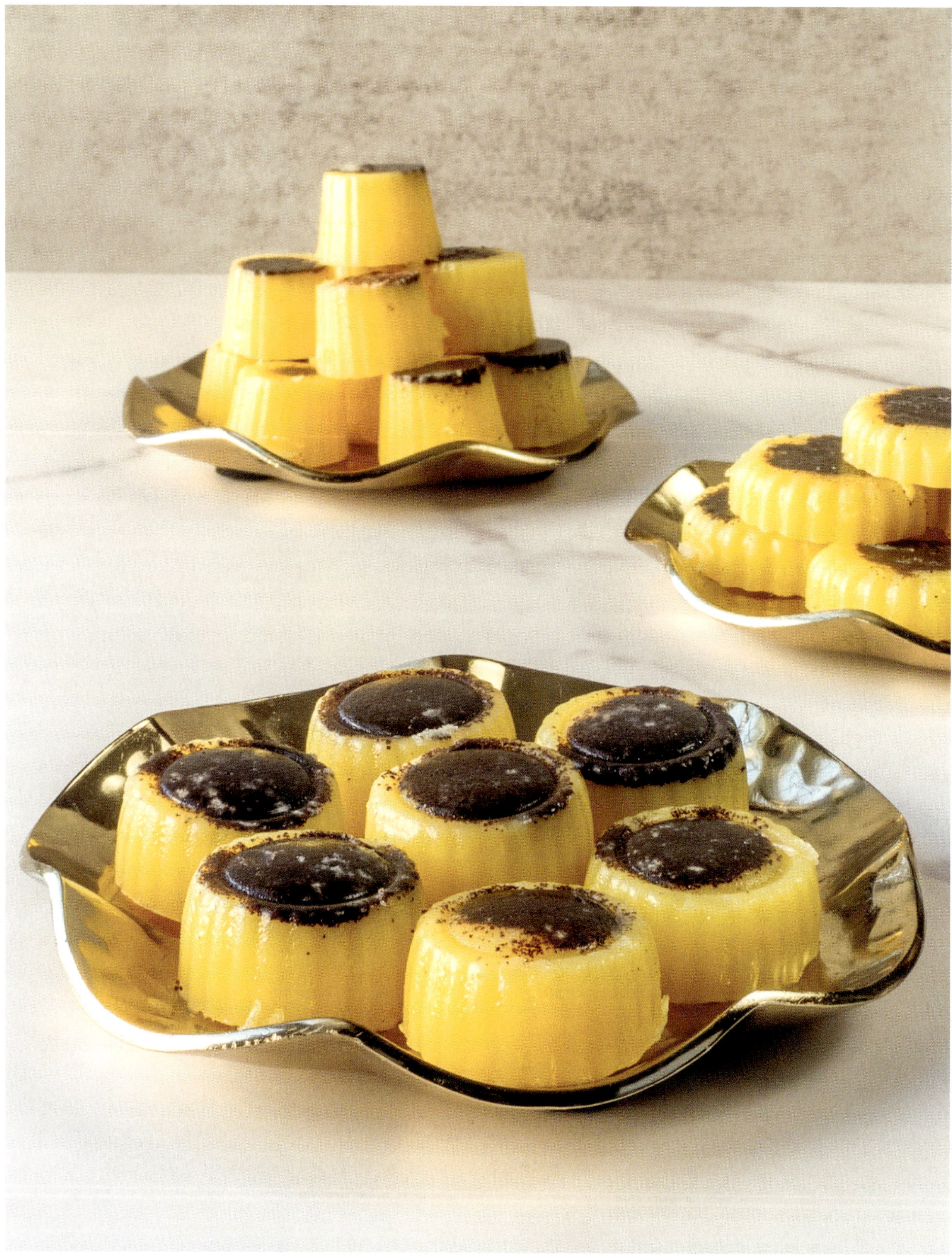

PER SERVING	calories: **200** | fat: **22g** | protein: **0g** | carbs: **0g** | macro split: **100/0/0**

YIELD: 16 bites (2 per serving)

PREP TIME: 5 minutes, plus 2 hours to chill

COOK TIME: 2 or 15 minutes, depending on whether butter is browned or just melted

BUTTER BITES

When I need a quick bite of fat, I make these bites. There are several ways to modify this recipe. You can brown the butter first to give the bites a caramelized taste, or you can simply melt the butter (which is what I prefer). I like to add chocolate-caramel electrolyte powder to make little chocolaty, salty-sweet fat bombs. If you prefer a savory protein bite, mix in about ½ cup of Dehydrated Ground Meat (page 212), either as is or ground into a fine powder.

1 cup (2 sticks) salted butter

1 (6g) packet chocolate-caramel electrolyte powder or other flavor of choice (optional)

SPECIAL EQUIPMENT:

Silicone candy mold(s) with a total of 16 (1-tablespoon) cavities (optional)

1. If using browned butter, put the butter in a medium frying pan and set over medium-low heat. Allow to slowly melt, stirring occasionally. You don't want to cook it too fast or it will burn. As the butter cooks, it will begin to foam up, which is normal. As soon as it reaches a light caramel color and you see little brown bits on the bottom of the pan, remove the pan from the heat. Pour the browned butter into a liquid measuring cup.

   If using plain melted butter, simply microwave the butter in a microwave-safe glass measuring cup until fully melted, 1 to 2 minutes. It will separate into a milky part and a clear yellow part. I have found that the clarified butter that rises to the top of the cup is best for making butter bites. The white milky part that settles to the bottom does not solidify well, so I don't use it.

2. Put the silicone candy mold(s) on a small sheet pan for easier transport to the refrigerator. Fill the cavities in the mold(s) almost to the top with the browned or plain melted butter, then sprinkle with the electrolyte powder, if using. You can also pour a thick layer in a standard-size (18 by 13-inch) sheet pan to make butter bars.

3. Place the pan in the fridge for at least 2 hours to allow the butter to cool and solidify.

4. Remove the butter bites from the molds or cut into sixteen bars. Store in an airtight container in the refrigerator for up to 3 months.

YIELD: 3 cups (½ cup per serving)

PREP TIME: 15 minutes, plus overnight to chill base and time to churn

COOK TIME: 25 minutes

CARNIVORE ICE CREAM

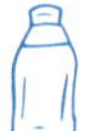
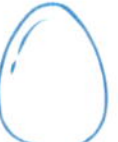

This creamy, indulgent treat is made with heavy cream, half-and-half, and allulose for a touch of sweetness with very few carbs. Each spoonful delivers a rich, velvety texture while a cinnamon stick infuses the ice cream with a subtle undertone of warmth and spice, elevating the classic vanilla flavor. Perfect for those on a carnivore diet seeking a satisfying sugar-free dessert that fits into their lifestyle!

1½ cups heavy cream

1½ cups half-and-half

1 tablespoon salted butter, melted

½ cup powdered allulose or other sweetener of choice (optional)

1 teaspoon vanilla extract

Pinch of salt

5 large egg yolks

1 cinnamon stick

SPECIAL EQUIPMENT:

Ice cream maker

1. In a medium saucepan over medium heat, bring the cream and half-and-half to a low boil. Turn down the heat to low and add the butter, allulose (if using), vanilla, and salt, stirring to combine.
2. Put the egg yolks in a small heat-safe bowl and whisk with a fork to break them up a bit. Then, while continuing to whisk, slowly add one ladle of the hot dairy mixture to the bowl to temper the yolks. Repeat with another two ladles of the dairy while whisking. Then slowly pour the tempered yolks into the saucepan with the dairy while whisking the mixture. This tempering step will ensure the yolks don't cook too fast and curdle, creating chunks of yolk in your ice cream.
3. Drop in the cinnamon stick and allow the ice cream base to gently simmer and thicken over low heat, stirring every minute. It is ready when it coats the back of a spoon. This will take about 5 minutes.
4. Remove the pan from the heat and strain the base through a fine-mesh strainer into a clean medium bowl. Return the cinnamon stick to the strained base. Cool the base in an ice bath so it's no longer piping hot, then place the base in the refrigerator overnight to cool completely.
5. Remove the cinnamon stick from the ice cream base, then pour the base into an ice cream maker and churn following the manufacturer's instructions.
6. Store the ice cream in a freezer-safe glass storage container in the freezer for up to 2 weeks.

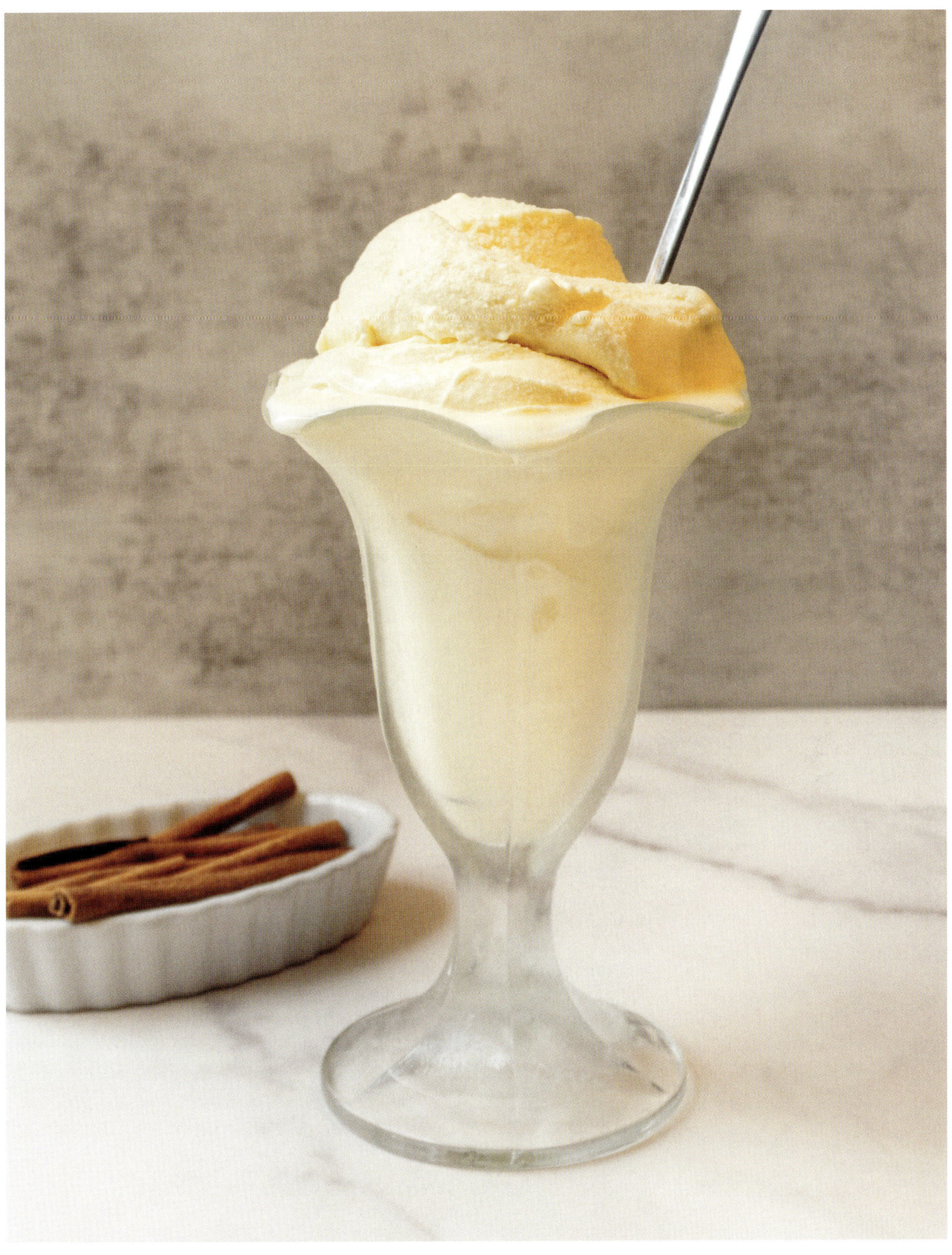

PER SERVING	calories: **343** | fat: **34g** | protein: **6g** | carbs: **5g** | macro split: **88/6/5**

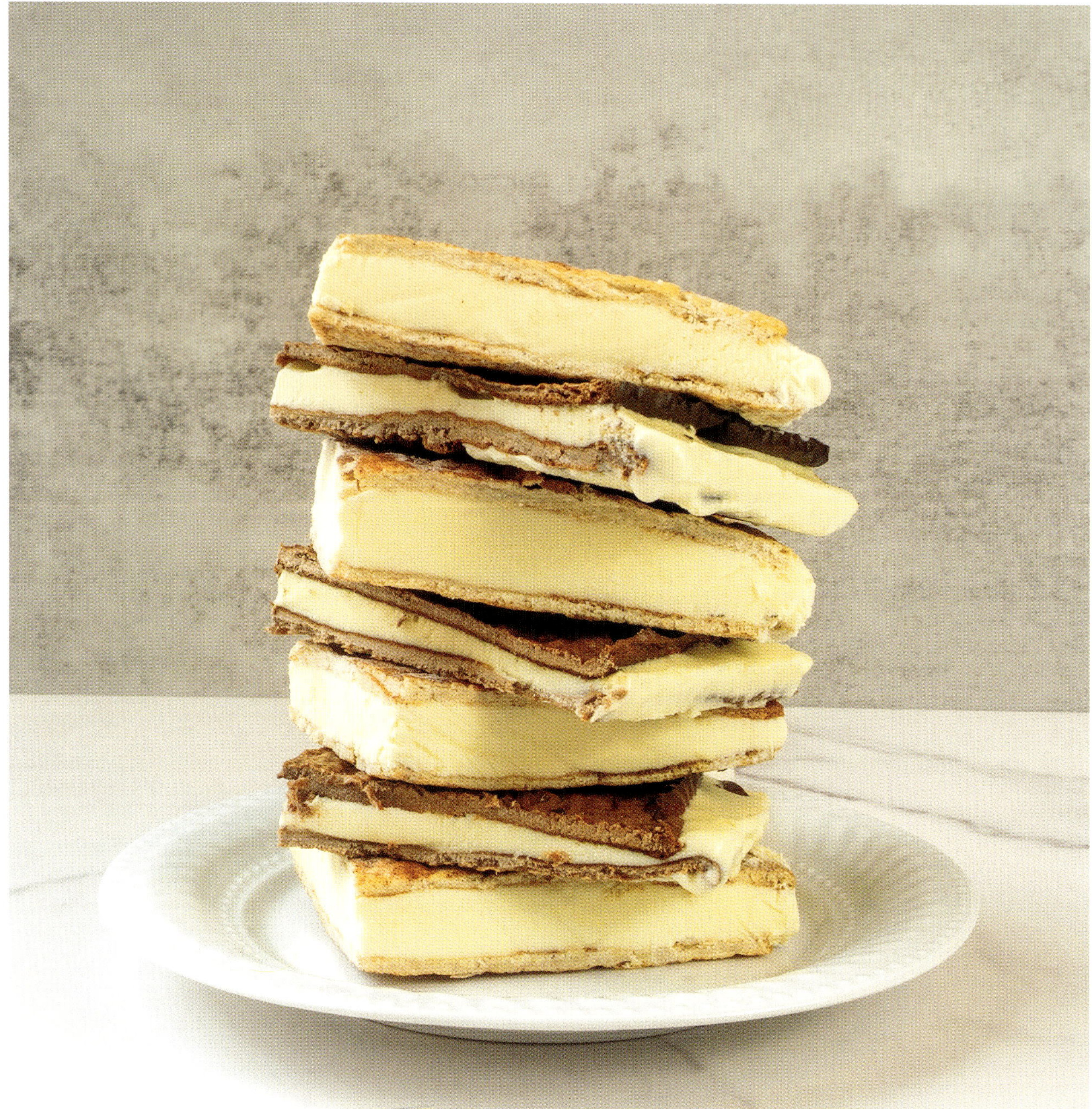

Note

I recommend using freshly churned ice cream, taken directly from the ice cream maker, because it spreads more easily, so I suggest working out the timing of the ice cream to coincide with the completion of the cookies. If you've made the ice cream ahead, allow it to soften on the counter for 15 to 20 minutes before spreading it on the baked cookie.

PER ICE CREAM SANDWICH

calories: **336** | fat: **29g** | protein: **13g** | carbs: **6g** | macro split: **77/16/7**

YIELD: 8 ice cream sandwiches

PREP TIME: 10 minutes, plus 3 hours to freeze (not including time to make ice cream)

COOK TIME: 40 minutes

CARNIVORE ICE CREAM SANDWICHES—TWO WAYS

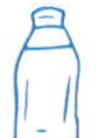 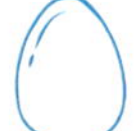

Growing up, my dad always kept ice cream sandwiches in the freezer. Unfortunately, they're off-limits on carnivore with all of the additives, gluten, and sugar. So I decided to experiment with my Cottage Cheese Flatbread (page 371), sweetening the base and adding flavorings to create two carnivore cookie options: cinnamon graham cracker and chocolate. Both turned out great—perfect for assembling your own easy carnivore-friendly ice cream sandwiches. I often make the cookies a day or two ahead. Because making individual ice cream sandwiches one by one is way too time-consuming, you bake the cookie dough in two large sheets, slather one with ice cream, and place the other cookie on top. After it's frozen solid, you simply cut the sandwiches.

FOR THE COOKIE BASE:

2 cups cottage cheese (4% milkfat)

4 large eggs

2 tablespoons Swerve brown sugar

¼ teaspoon vanilla extract

FOR THE GRAHAM CRACKER CINNAMON COOKIE:

½ teaspoon ground cinnamon

FOR THE CHOCOLATE COOKIE:

2 tablespoons cacao powder

2 tablespoons powdered allulose

1 batch Carnivore Ice Cream (page 334), freshly churned or softened (see note)

1. Preheat the oven to 360°F and line two 13 by 9-inch sheet pans (aka quarter sheet pans) with parchment paper. Grease the sides of the pans that aren't covered with parchment paper with a bit of butter.
2. In a blender or mini food processor, blend the ingredients for the cookie base, along with the cinnamon or the cacao powder and allulose, until smooth. Divide the dough into two equal portions and spread half in each of the prepared pans. Bake for 35 to 40 minutes, until the dough is cooked through in the middle and a bit crispy on the edges. Let cool in the pans for 10 minutes.
3. Once the cookie sheets are completely cool, flip one of them over onto a larger sheet pan and trim any burnt edges. Using a silicone spatula, evenly spread the entire batch of ice cream all the way to the edges of the cookie. Top with the second cookie and press any ice cream that is coming out the sides back into the cookies.
4. Put the pan in the freezer for at least 3 hours to fully harden. Then, using a chef's knife warmed under hot water, cut into eight ice cream sandwiches. Individually wrap them in plastic wrap so they are ready to eat whenever you choose.

YIELD: 6 mini cheesecakes (1 per serving)

PREP TIME: 15 minutes, plus 3 hours to cool/chill

COOK TIME: 55 minutes

MINI CHEESECAKES

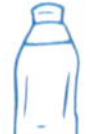
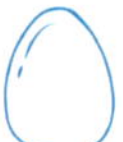

Sometimes you need a sweet treat, and cheesecake is an excellent option. I make these in 6-inch ramekins so I have individual servings instead of a whole cheesecake. I like to top them with either freshly whipped cream or Whipped Cream & Mascarpone (page 341). If you are doing a keto cheat meal, you could top them with some strawberries or mix in some cacao powder for a chocolate version.

2 (8-ounce) packages full-fat cream cheese, at room temperature

¾ cup full-fat sour cream

3 large eggs

¾ cup powdered allulose (optional)

1 teaspoon vanilla extract (optional)

2 tablespoons salted butter, melted

2 tablespoons cacao powder (optional, for keto version)

SPECIAL EQUIPMENT:

6 (6-inch) ramekins

1. Preheat the oven to 350°F. Grease six 6-inch ramekins with bacon grease or butter.
2. Put the cream cheese and sour cream in a large bowl or the bowl of a stand mixer fitted with the whisk attachment. Using a hand mixer or the stand mixer, beat until well blended. Then, with the mixer running, slowly add the other ingredients one at a time: the eggs one by one, the allulose (if using), vanilla (if using), and butter. If making chocolate cheesecakes, add the cacao powder and mix briefly to combine.
3. Ladle the mixture into the prepared ramekins, filling each one to about an inch from the top.
4. Place the ramekins in a 13 by 9-inch baking dish and set the dish in the oven. Pour hot water into the dish until it comes about halfway up the sides of the ramekins.
5. Bake for 55 minutes, or until the cheesecakes jiggle only slightly when gently shaken.
6. Turn off the oven, crack open the door, and allow the cheesecakes to cool in the oven for 30 minutes. Then pull the baking dish from the oven and let the cheesecakes cool in their water bath for another 30 minutes. Finally, put the ramekins in the refrigerator until chilled, at least 3 hours.
7. Once chilled, eat the cheesecakes straight out of the ramekins.

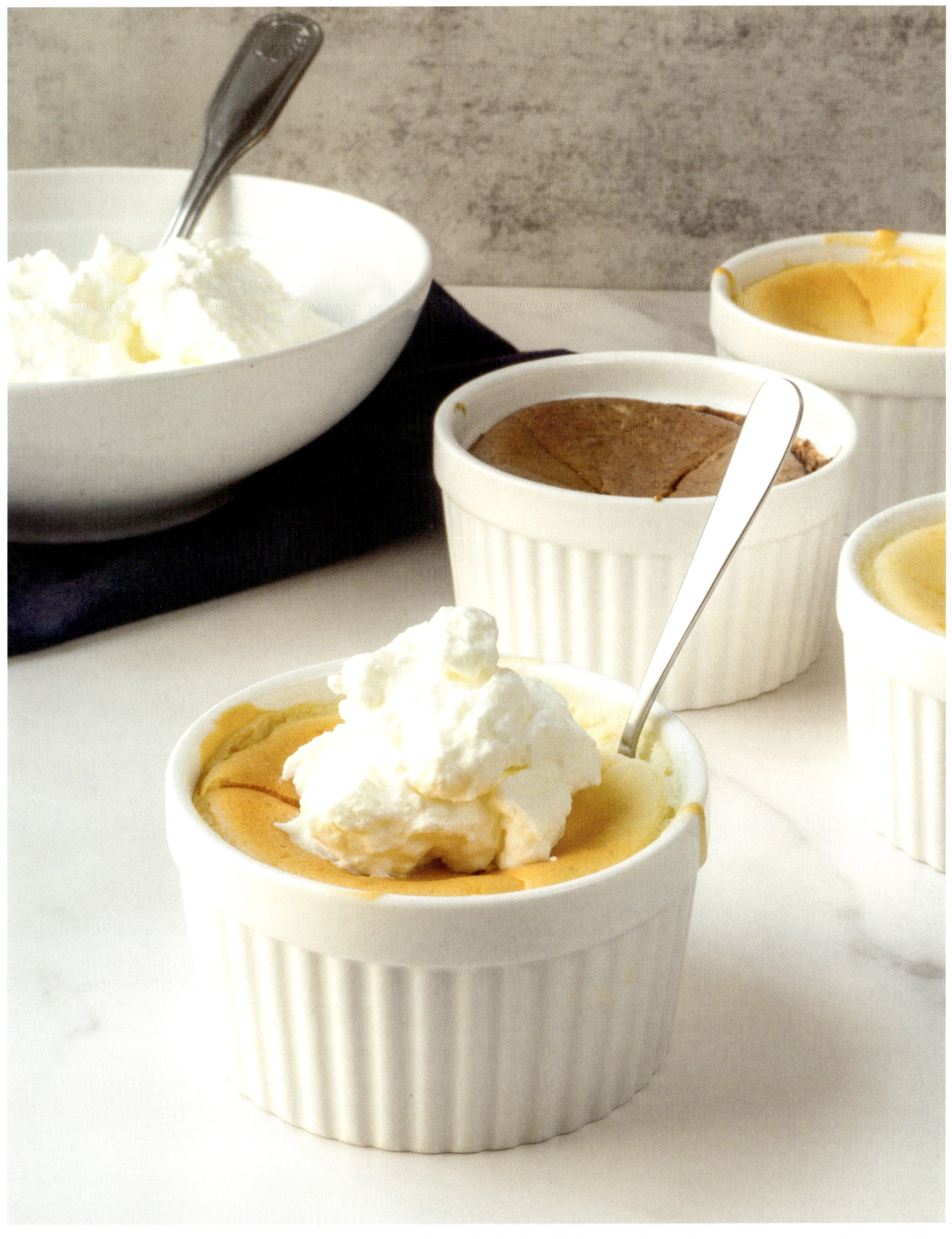

(the carbs in the allulose don't count, so net carbs are closer to 4g)

PER SERVING (without cacao powder)	calories: **398** | fat: **39g** | protein: **10g** | carbs: **28g** | macro split: **87/9/4**

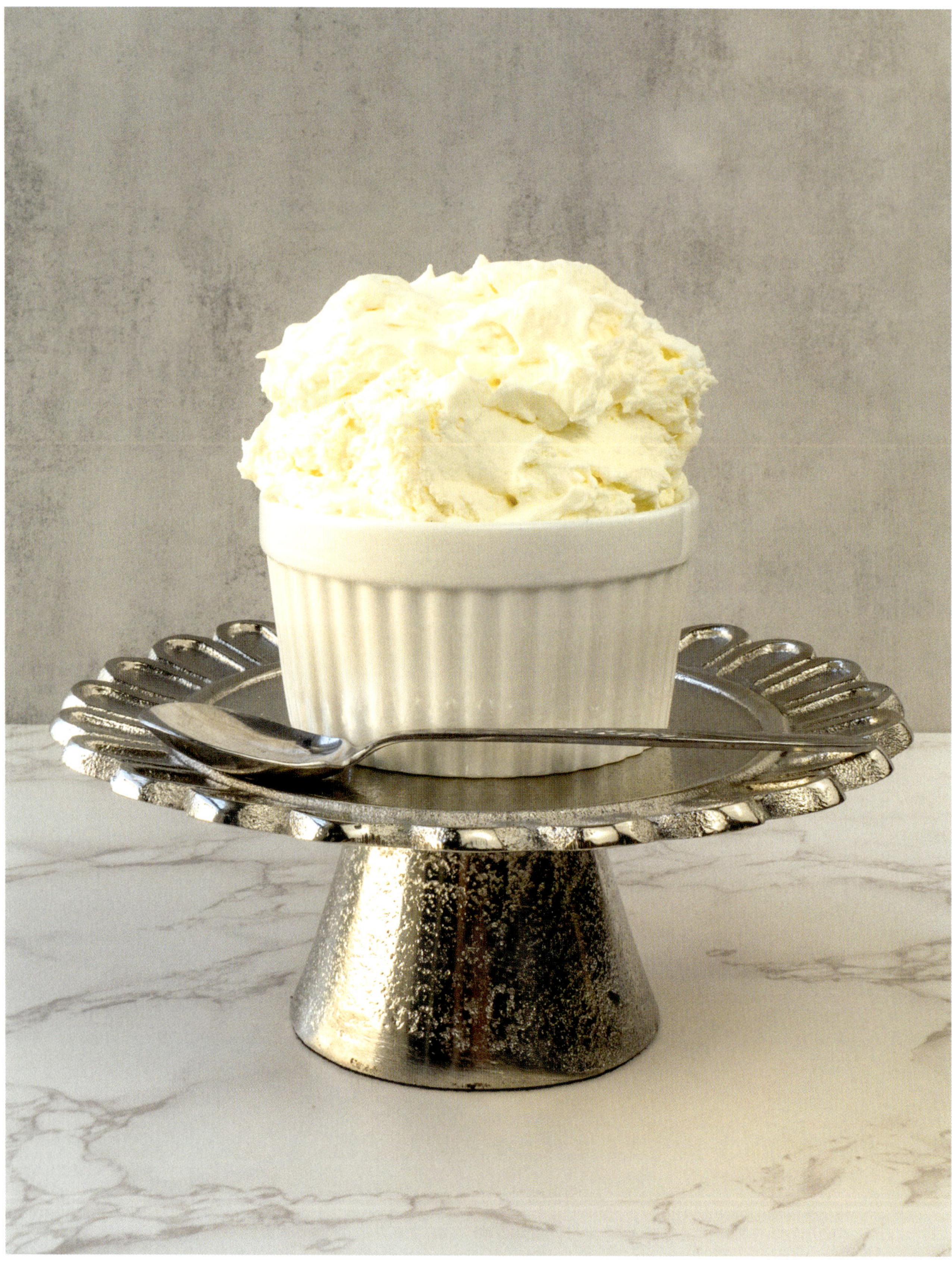

PER SERVING | calories: **222** | fat: **25g** | protein: **3g** | carbs: **1g** | macro split: **94/4/1**

YIELD: 2 cups
(2 tablespoons per serving)

PREP TIME: 10 minutes

WHIPPED CREAM & MASCARPONE

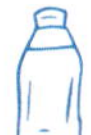

This simple and delicious topping can be eaten as a dessert on its own. I like to use it to top my Egg Pudding (page 215), Pumpkin Spice Cheesecake (page 314), Mini Cheesecakes (page 338), and Carnivore Ice Cream (page 334). If you are having a keto cheat meal, adding some of this whipped topping to fresh berries would be amazing.

1 (8-ounce) container mascarpone cheese

1 cup heavy cream

1 teaspoon vanilla extract (optional)

½ cup powdered allulose, or ¼ teaspoon liquid stevia (optional)

1. Put the mascarpone, cream, and vanilla (if using) in a large mixing bowl or the bowl of a stand mixer fitted with the whisk attachment. Whip on medium speed using a hand mixer or the stand mixer until soft peaks form.
2. If using allulose, slowly add it to the mascarpone mixture with the mixer running to prevent clumping. If using liquid stevia, just add it to the mixture and fold in by hand.
3. Transfer the finished whipped topping to a storage container. You can serve it right away, or it will keep in the refrigerator for up to 1 week.

YIELD: 16 bites (2 per serving)

PREP TIME: 15 minutes, plus 2 hours to freeze (not including time to make dehydrated beef)

WHIPPED TALLOW BITES

These whipped tallow bites hit the spot and help keep your fat intake high. They hold their shape best when cold, so be sure to eat them quickly once you take them out of the fridge or freezer.

- 2 cups beef tallow, at room temperature (see note)
- ½ cup dehydrated ground beef (page 212), ground into a powder
- ½ teaspoon salt
- 1½ tablespoons raw honey (optional)

SPECIAL EQUIPMENT: Silicone candy mold(s) with a total of 16 (1-tablespoon) cavities (optional)

1. Put the softened tallow in the bowl of a stand mixer or in a large mixing bowl and whip with the stand mixer or a hand mixer on high speed until creamy and fluffy.
2. Turn the mixer to low and slowly add the powdered ground beef, salt, and honey, if using.
3. Once all of the ingredients are fully incorporated, turn off the mixer and use a small spoon to fill sixteen cavities in the candy mold(s) all the way to the top with the mixture. Use the back of the spoon to press the whipped mixture into the cavities, adding more to top them off if needed. You can also spread a thick layer in a standard-size (18 by 13-inch) sheet pan to make whipped tallow bars.
4. Place the candy mold(s) or sheet pan in the freezer for at least 2 hours. Once the bites are fully set, pop them out of the molds; if you used a sheet pan, cut into sixteen bars. Store in an airtight container in the freezer for up to 6 months.

Note

The tallow will not whip if it is liquefied. It should be softened but still solid, like the texture of butter kept at room temperature.

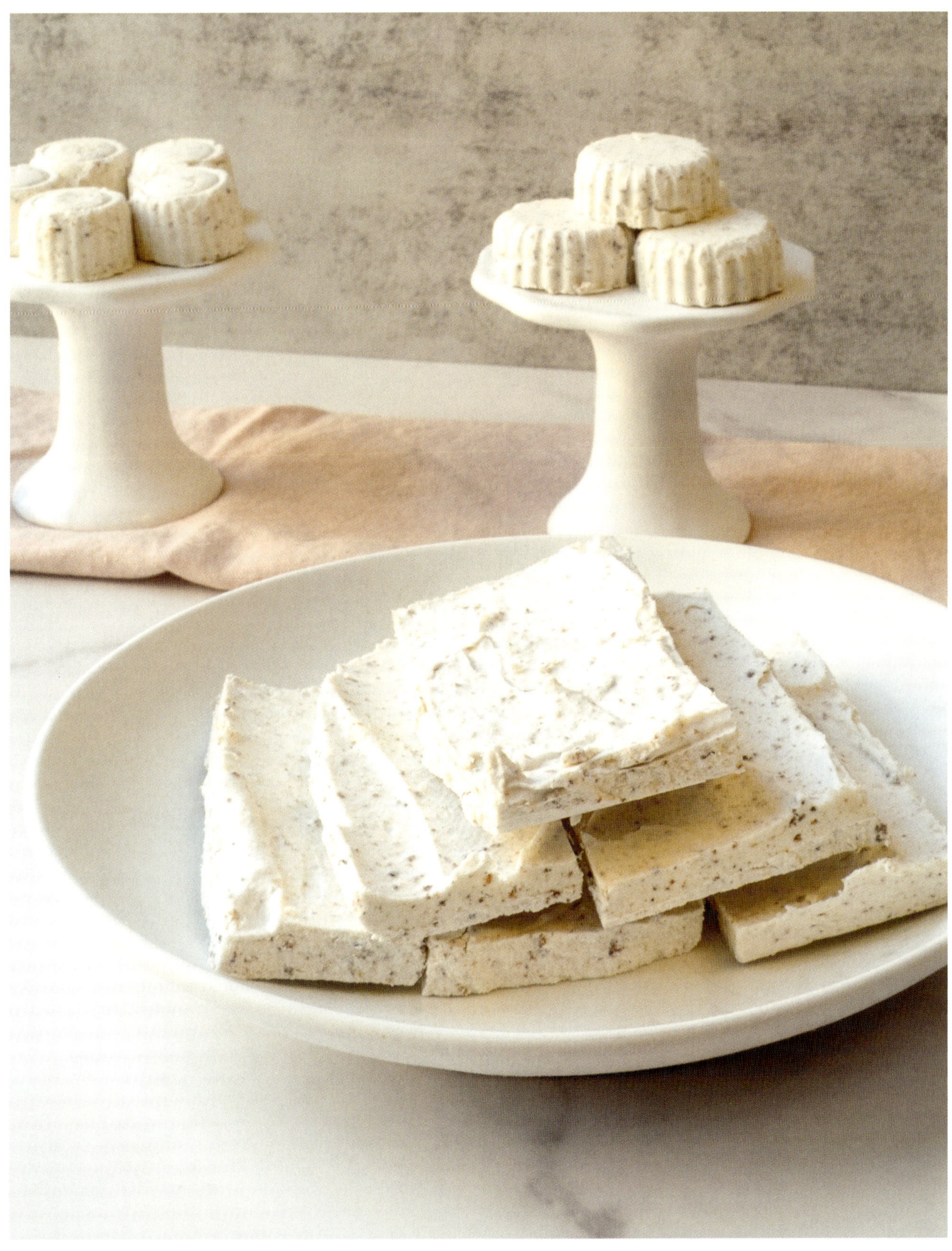

PER SERVING	calories: **274** | fat: **29g** | protein: **3g** | carbs: **2g** | macro split: **94/4/2**

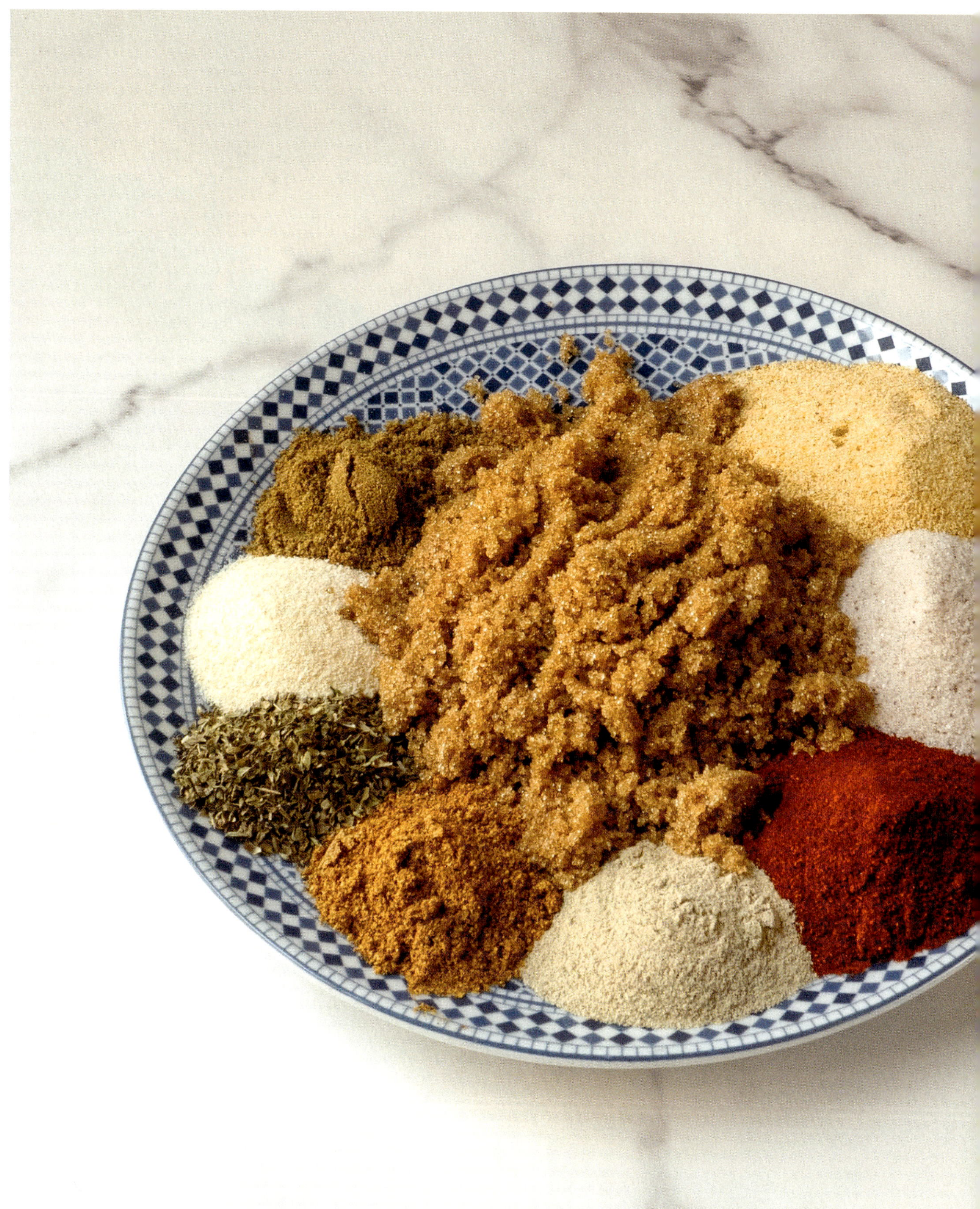

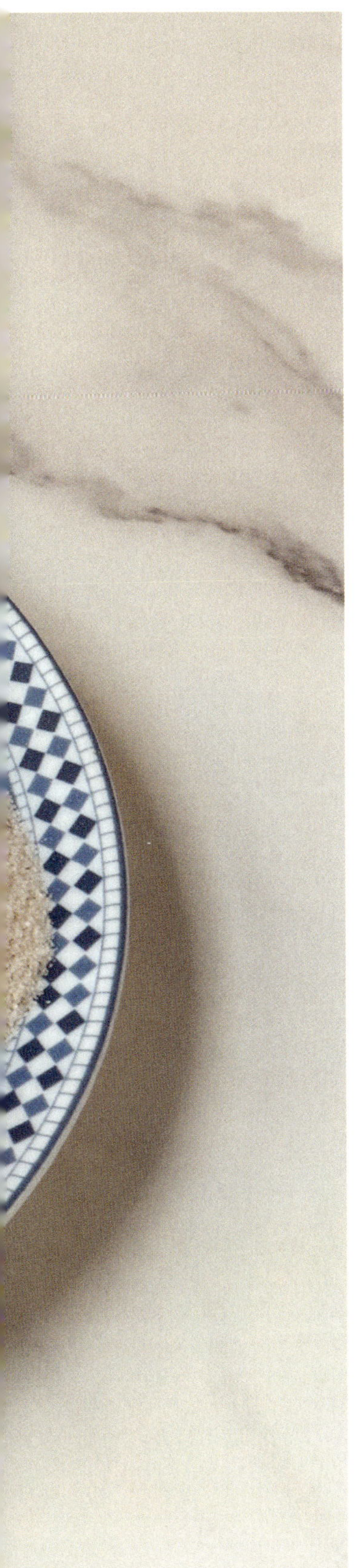

CHAPTER 17

SPICE MIXES, SAUCES, AND DRESSINGS

346 Cajun Seasoning

347 BBQ Spice Rub

348 Chicken & Pork Seasoning

349 Chili Spice Seasoning

350 Taco Seasoning

351 Alfredo Sauce

352 Bacon Mayonnaise

355 Marrownaise

356 Spicy Mayonnaise

357 American Kajmak

359 Bone Marrow Butter

361 Buttermilk Ranch Dressing

YIELD: ½ cup plus 2 teaspoons

PREP TIME: 5 minutes

CAJUN SEASONING

Incorporating seasonings into your version of the carnivore diet can really enhance your meals and add a whole new layer of flavor. I incorporate them often. This spice mix is one of my favorites—it's my special blend, featured in my Crab Cakes with Rémoulade (page 293) and my Spiced Pumpkin-Shaped Cheese Ball (page 305). It's perfect whenever you want to add a bold, zesty kick to dishes. Whether you're using it to season seafood, meats, or even eggs, this seasoning mix brings a delightful balance of heat and smokiness and depth of flavor.

- 2 tablespoons garlic powder
- 2 tablespoons Italian seasoning
- 2 tablespoons smoked paprika
- 1 tablespoon ground white pepper
- 1½ teaspoons salt
- 1½ teaspoons onion powder
- 1 teaspoon cayenne pepper (optional)
- 1 teaspoon red pepper flakes (optional)

Put all of the ingredients in a small bowl and mix thoroughly. Store in an airtight jar or container for up to 3 months.

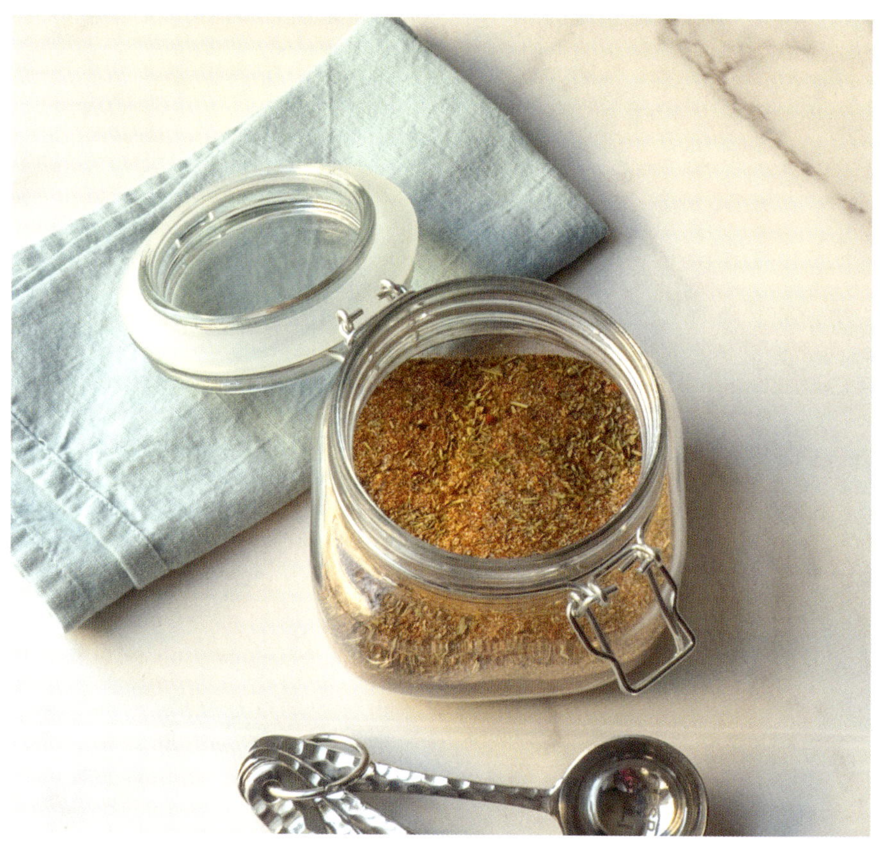

YIELD: 1 scant cup

PREP TIME: 5 minutes

BBQ SPICE RUB

Use this BBQ spice rub for ribs, brisket (page 206), or anything you want to throw on the grill. It's the perfect way to bring rich, smoky flavor to your favorite cuts of meat. For best results, I generally use 1 tablespoon of this spice rub per pound of meat, ensuring every bite is packed with flavor. Whether you're smoking, grilling, or slow-cooking, this spice blend helps create that mouthwatering caramelized crust on the outside while enhancing the natural flavors of the meat. It's an essential seasoning for taking your BBQ game to the next level!

- 1/3 cup Swerve brown sugar
- 2 tablespoons garlic powder
- 2 tablespoons smoked paprika
- 2 tablespoons salt
- 2 teaspoons ground white pepper
- 2 teaspoons cayenne pepper
- 2 teaspoons chili powder
- 2 teaspoons ground cumin
- 2 teaspoons onion powder
- 2 teaspoons dried oregano leaves

Put all of the ingredients in a small bowl and mix thoroughly. Store in an airtight jar or container for up to a month.

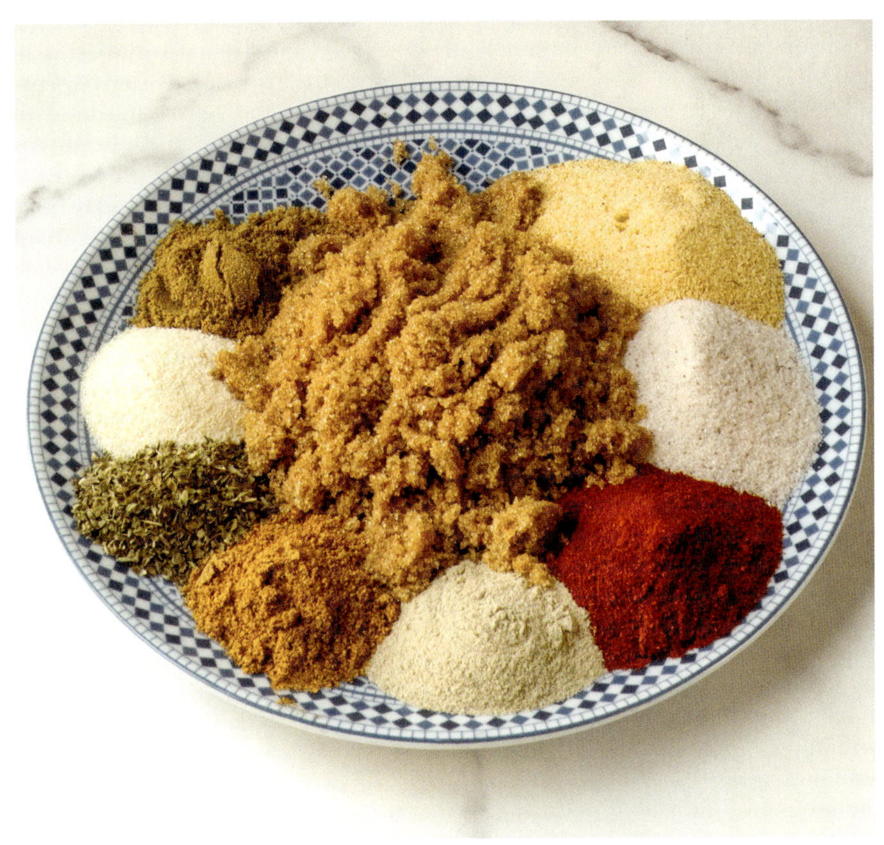

YIELD: ½ cup

PREP TIME: 5 minutes

CHICKEN & PORK SEASONING

This versatile seasoning is a go-to for adding bold flavor to a variety of meats on the carnivore diet. It's perfect for wings, drumsticks, chicken thighs, or pork chops, effortlessly enhancing their taste with a smoky, savory kick. Whether you're grilling, roasting, or pan-frying, this spice mix makes it easy to elevate your favorite cuts of chicken or pork.

- 2 tablespoons garlic powder
- 2 tablespoons onion powder
- 2 tablespoons salt
- 1 tablespoon smoked paprika
- 1 tablespoon ground white pepper

Put all of the ingredients in a small bowl and mix thoroughly. Store in an airtight jar or container for up to 3 months.

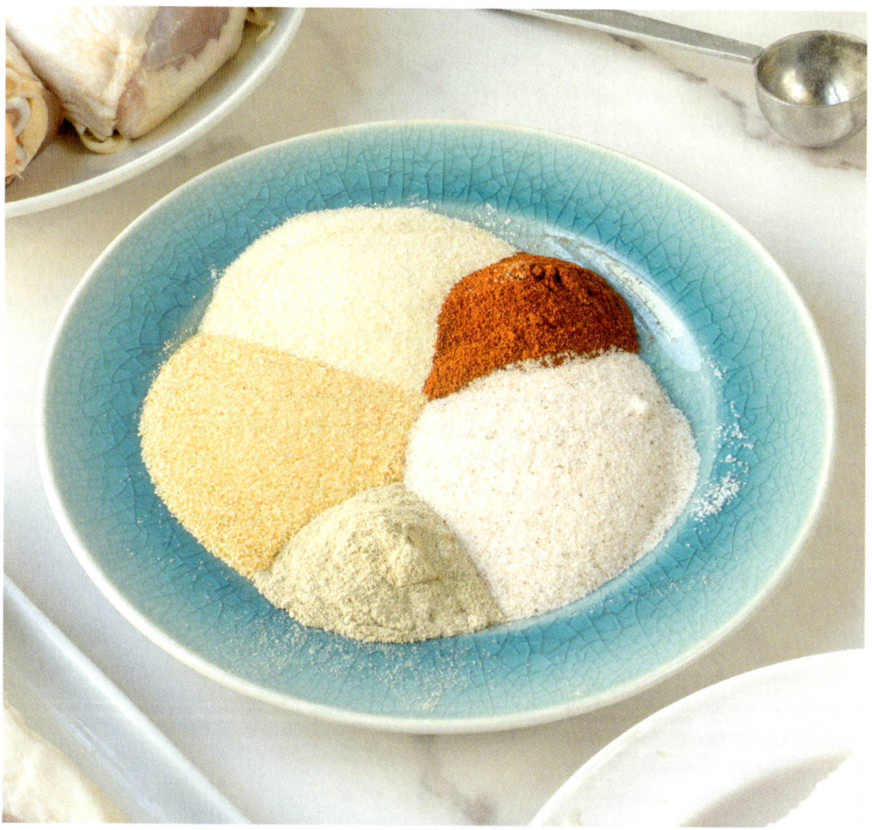

YIELD: ½ cup

PREP TIME: 5 minutes

CHILI SPICE SEASONING

To make this spice mixture, I take chili powder and ramp it up with extra cumin and garlic powder, along with onion powder and smoked paprika. I use this blend in my Chili Cheese Dog Meatballs (page 290), which is a favorite recipe of mine on the carnivore diet. The spice mix adds a savory depth and a bit of heat, perfectly complementing the rich flavors of the beef and cheese. It's the perfect way to season the meat and give any dish that extra punch of flavor without any carbs. Since the mix is so easy to prepare and store in bulk, I always have it on hand whenever I need a quick seasoning boost. It's one of those simple yet essential ingredients that makes meals so much more satisfying!

- 2½ tablespoons chili powder
- 1 tablespoon ground cumin
- 1 tablespoon garlic powder
- 1 tablespoon onion powder
- 1 tablespoon ground white pepper
- 1 tablespoon smoked paprika
- 1½ teaspoons salt
- ½ teaspoon cayenne pepper (optional)

Put all of the ingredients in a small bowl and mix thoroughly. Store in an airtight jar or container for up to 3 months.

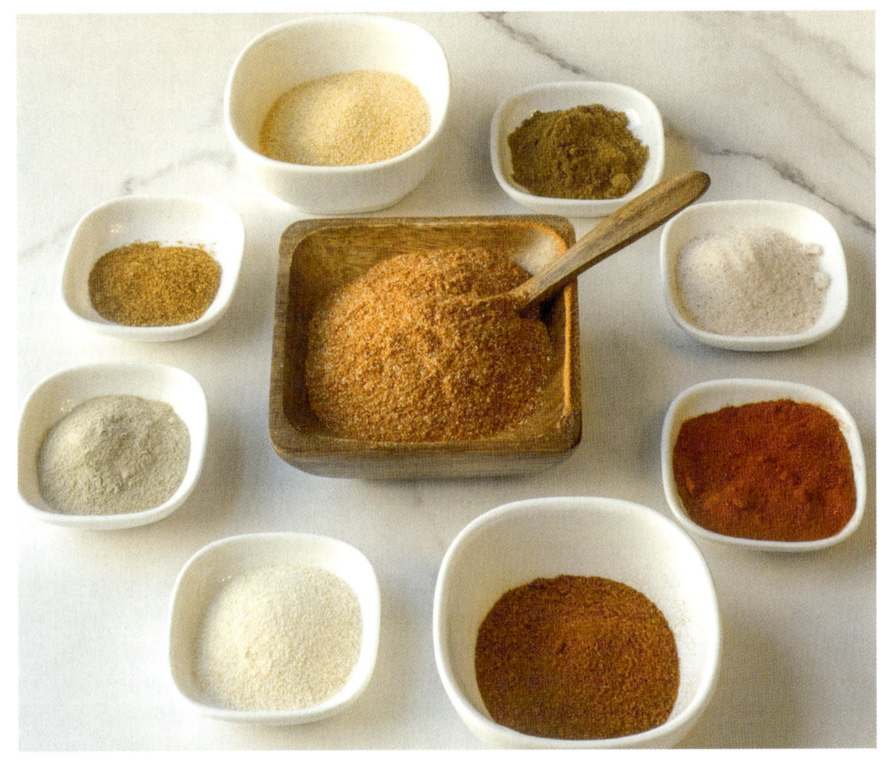

YIELD: 1/3 heaping cup

PREP TIME: 5 minutes

TACO SEASONING

Of all the spice mixes in this chapter, this is the one I use by far the most frequently. I love that I have full control over the quality of every ingredient that goes into it, ensuring it's made with only the best spices. Plus, it's incredibly convenient—I can prepare a big batch in advance and store it so it's ready to go whenever I need a quick seasoning boost. Whether I'm making tacos (see page 289) or seasoning meat, this mix is my go-to. It's a versatile, time-saving staple that never disappoints!

- 1½ tablespoons ground cumin
- 1 tablespoon chili powder
- 1 tablespoon garlic powder
- 1 tablespoon onion powder
- 1 tablespoon red pepper flakes
- 1 teaspoon salt
- 1 teaspoon ground white pepper
- ¼ teaspoon cayenne pepper (optional)

Put all of the ingredients in a small bowl and mix thoroughly. Store in an airtight jar or container for up to 3 months.

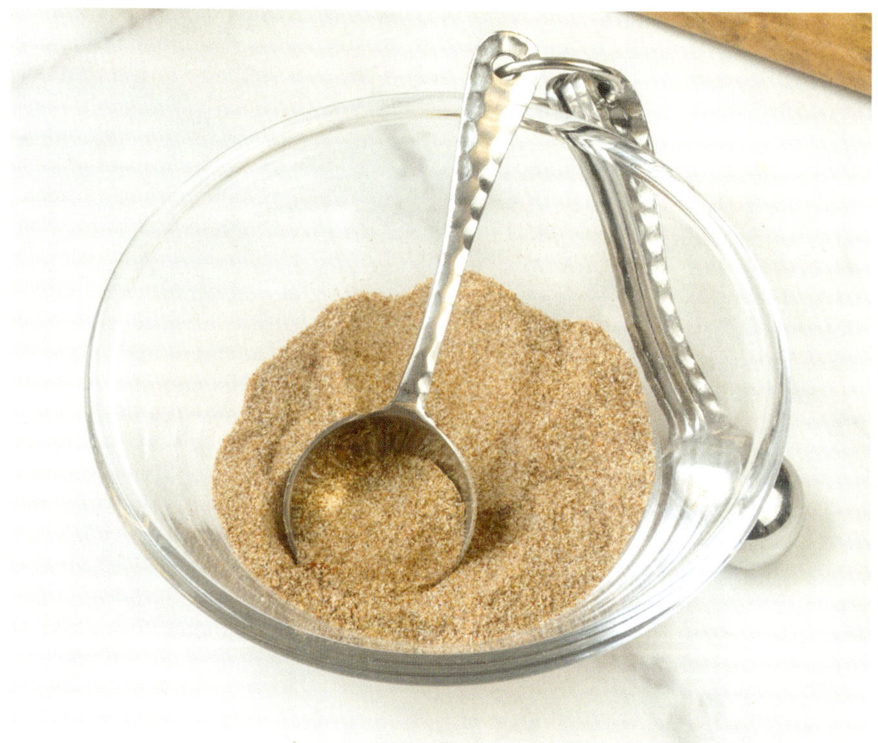

YIELD: 1 cup
(½ cup per serving)

PREP TIME: 5 minutes

COOK TIME: 5 minutes

ALFREDO SAUCE

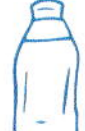

Alfredo sauce is simple and versatile. I use it in my Turkey Alfredo (page 310) and on Carnivore White Pizza (page 283). You could also top Carnivore Noodles (page 364) with some leftover meat and this delicious sauce for an amazing meal. The sauce can be made ahead and stored in the refrigerator for up to a week. When you are ready to use it, simply reheat it in a saucepan.

- ¼ cup (½ stick) salted butter
- ¾ cup heavy cream
- 1¼ cups grated Parmesan cheese
- 1 teaspoon garlic powder (optional)

1. Put the butter and cream in a medium saucepan and whisk over low heat until the butter is melted and combined with the cream.
2. Add the Parmesan cheese and garlic powder, if using, and continue whisking until the cheese is melted. The sauce is ready when it is smooth. Serve immediately.

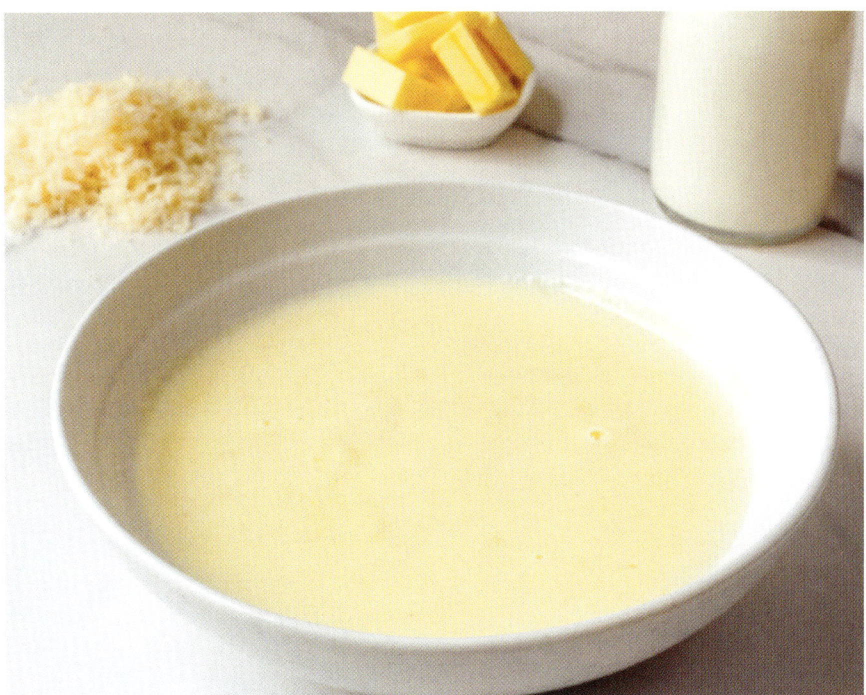

PER SERVING

calories: **772** | fat: **73g** | protein: **21g** | carbs: **10g** | macro split: **84/11/5**

YIELD: 1 cup
(1 tablespoon per serving)

PREP TIME: 10 minutes, plus 2 hours to chill if desired (not including time to cook bacon)

BACON MAYONNAISE

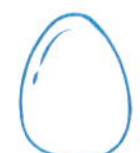

I cook bacon several times a week, which means I always have extra bacon grease on hand. One of my favorite ways to use it is in this incredible mayonnaise recipe, which is always a hit. Bacon grease gives mayo a savory depth that regular oils just can't match, turning it into a luxurious, flavor-packed spread. You can use an immersion blender, a countertop blender, or a mini food processor, depending on what you have in your kitchen.

3 large egg yolks

2 teaspoons prepared yellow mustard

1 cup bacon grease, slightly warmed so it is liquid

1 tablespoon freshly squeezed lemon juice

2 teaspoons white wine vinegar

½ teaspoon salt

Pinch of ground white pepper

2 strips bacon, cooked and crumbled

IMMERSION BLENDER INSTRUCTIONS:

1. Put the egg yolks and mustard in a wide-mouth 16-ounce mason jar. Insert an immersion blender and blend briefly.
2. Gradually drizzle in the bacon grease while blending continuously until the ingredients are fully incorporated and the consistency is thick but spreadable. Once emulsified, remove the blender from the jar and add the lemon juice, vinegar, salt, and pepper. Blend again briefly to combine.
3. Add the crumbled bacon to the mayo and stir with a spoon. For best results, chill the mayo for 2 hours before serving. Store in the refrigerator for up to 2 weeks.

COUNTERTOP BLENDER/FOOD PROCESSOR INSTRUCTIONS:

1. Put the egg yolks and mustard in a blender or mini food processor and blend until combined.
2. With the machine running, very slowly drizzle in the bacon grease, starting with just a little to begin emulsifying it with the yolks. This step is critical, as it determines the success of the mayonnaise. Once all of the grease has been incorporated, stop the machine. The consistency should be thick but spreadable, not runny.
3. Add the lemon juice, vinegar, salt, and pepper. Pulse a few times to mix everything together.
4. Transfer the mayo to a 16-ounce mason jar, then add the crumbled bacon and stir with a spoon. For best results, chill the mayo for 2 hours before serving. Store in the refrigerator for up to 2 weeks.

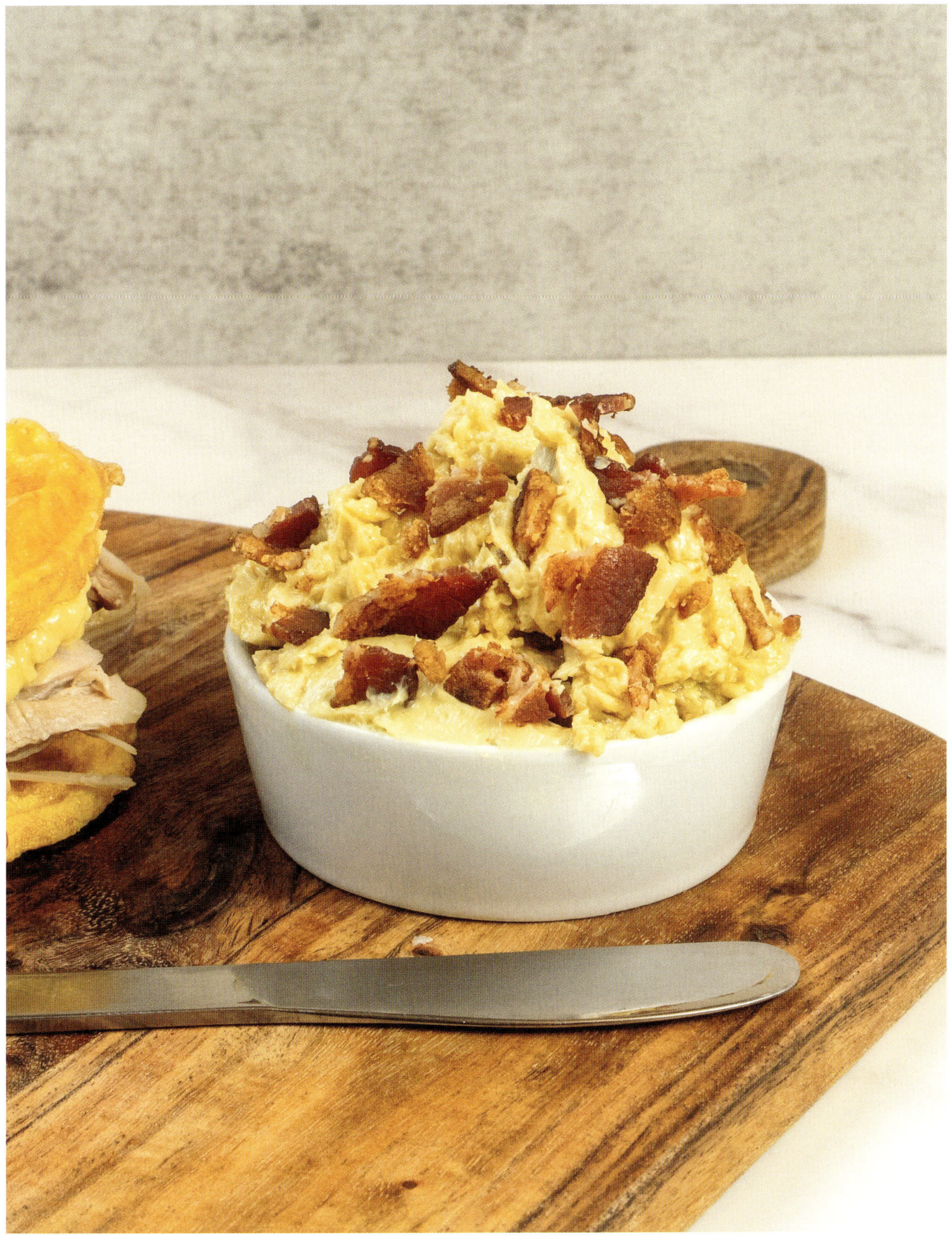

PER SERVING	calories: **99** | fat: **10g** | protein: **0g** | carbs: **0g** | macro split: **100/0/0**

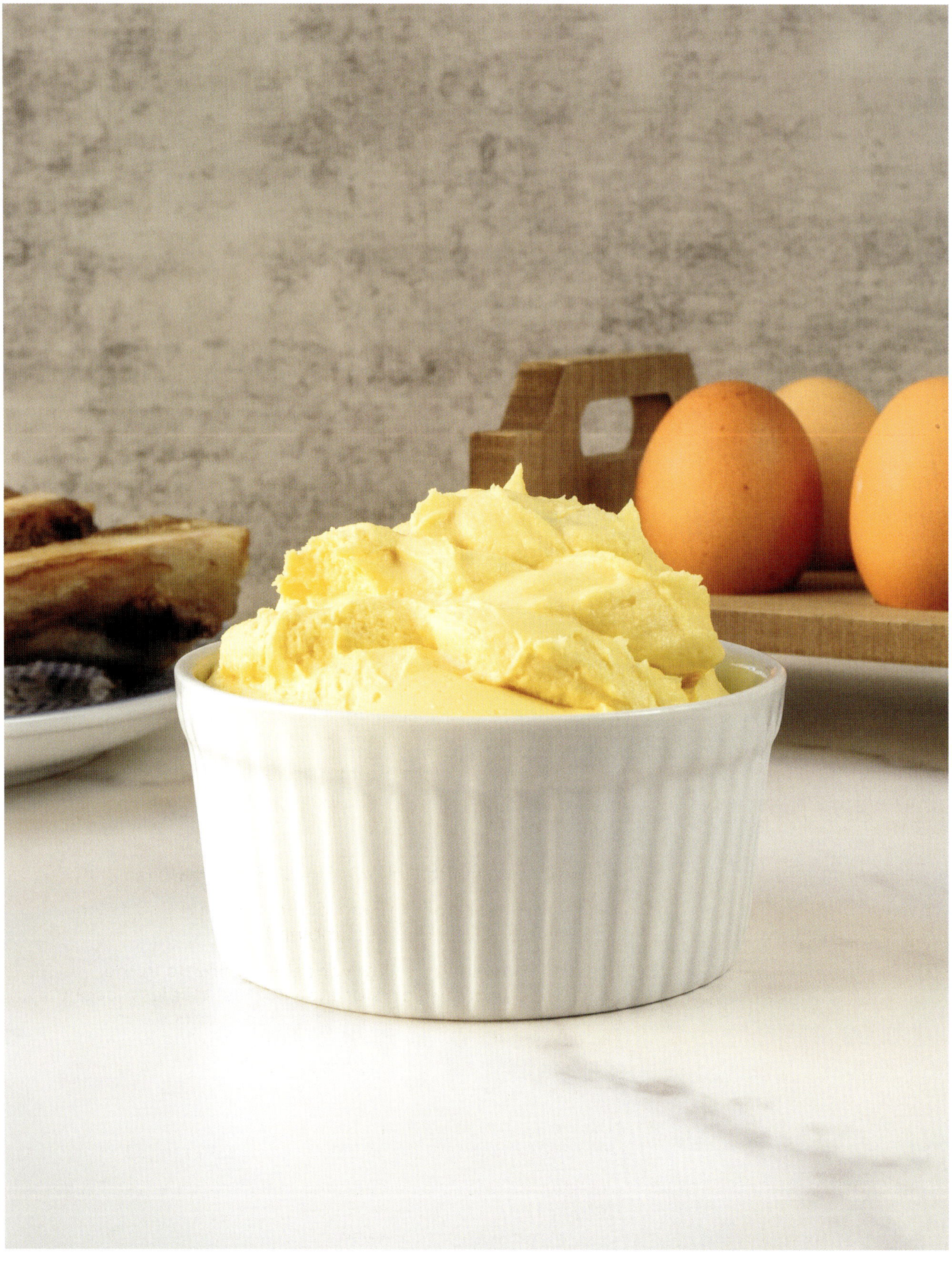

PER SERVING

calories: **116** | fat: **12g** | protein: **1g** | carbs: **0g** | macro split: **95/5/0**

YIELD: 1 cup
(1 tablespoon per serving)

PREP TIME: 10 minutes, plus 2 hours to chill if desired (not including time to roast marrow bones)

MARROWNAISE

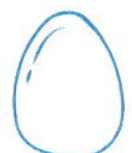

Marrownaise, a bone marrow mayonnaise, offers an unparalleled depth of flavor. Whenever I cook bone marrow, I save the liquid fat to create this rich and delicious condiment. It's perfect for elevating any dish that calls for mayonnaise! You can use an immersion blender, countertop blender, or mini food processor, depending on what you have in your kitchen.

- 3 large egg yolks
- 3 teaspoons prepared yellow mustard
- 1 cup bone marrow fat (saved from roasting marrow bones; see page 205), slightly warmed so it is liquid-y
- 1 tablespoon freshly squeezed lemon juice (optional, but strongly recommended)
- 2 teaspoons white wine vinegar
- 1 large egg white
- ½ teaspoon salt
- Pinch of ground white pepper

IMMERSION BLENDER INSTRUCTIONS:

1. Put the egg yolks and mustard in a wide-mouth 16-ounce mason jar. Insert an immersion blender and blend briefly.
2. Gradually drizzle in the liquid bone marrow fat while blending continuously until the ingredients are fully incorporated and the consistency is thick but spreadable. Once emulsified, remove the blender from the jar and add the lemon juice (if using), vinegar, egg white, salt, and pepper. Blend again briefly to combine.
3. For best results, chill the mayo for 2 hours before serving. Store in the refrigerator for up to 2 weeks.

COUNTERTOP BLENDER/FOOD PROCESSOR INSTRUCTIONS:

4. Put the egg yolks and mustard in a blender or mini food processor and blend until combined.
5. With the machine running, very slowly drizzle in the liquid bone marrow fat, starting with just a little to begin emulsifying it with the yolks. This step is critical, as it determines the success of your mayonnaise. Once all of the oil has been incorporated, stop the machine. The consistency should be thick but still spreadable.
6. Add the lemon juice (if using), vinegar, egg white, salt, and pepper. Pulse a few times to mix everything together.
7. Transfer the mayo to a 16-ounce mason jar. For best results, chill the mayo for 2 hours before serving. Store in the refrigerator for up to 2 weeks.

YIELD: 1 heaping cup (1 tablespoon per serving)

PREP TIME: 5 minutes, plus 2 hours to chill if desired

SPICY MAYONNAISE

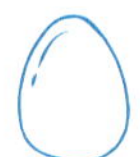

In my opinion, spicy mayonnaise is a must-have. It's easy to make using your favorite hot sauce, but combining Sriracha and hot sauce takes it to the next level. This blend adds a rich depth of flavor to any dish.

1 cup avocado oil mayonnaise

1 to 2 tablespoons Sriracha, according to taste

1 to 2 tablespoons medium-hot hot sauce, such as Cholula, according to taste

Pinch of salt

1. Put the mayonnaise in a small bowl and add the Sriracha and hot sauce. Stir until fully blended, then season with the salt. Taste and add more Sriracha, hot sauce, and/or salt, if needed.
2. Pour the spicy mayo into a mason jar. For best results, chill the mayo for 2 hours before serving. Store in the refrigerator for up to 2 weeks.

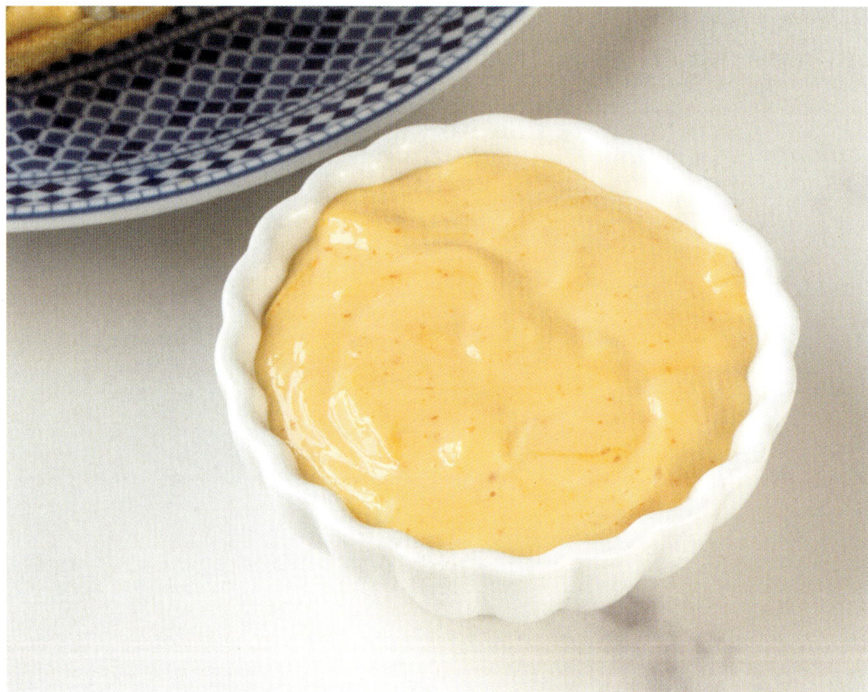

PER SERVING

calories: **100** | fat: **12g** | protein: **0g** | carbs: **0g** | macro split: **100/0/0**

YIELD: 2¼ cups
(2 tablespoons per serving)

PREP TIME: 10 minutes

AMERICAN KAJMAK

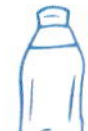

Kajmak is a Serbian spread for bread, but it is mostly served with Serbian burgers (see page 222). The American version is much less labor-intensive than the traditional clotted cream version that can take days to make. I eat it with Serbian sausages (see page 225) or as a dip for any kind of grilled meat. Simply delicious!

2½ (8-ounce) packages full-fat cream cheese, at room temperature

1 pound (4 sticks) salted butter, at room temperature

1. Put the cream cheese and butter in a medium bowl or the bowl of a stand mixer. Mix with a hand mixer or the stand mixer on medium speed until fully combined and creamy.
2. Transfer to a small storage container and store in the refrigerator for up to 2 weeks. When you are ready to use it, pull the portion you need from the refrigerator and allow it to come to room temperature for about 30 minutes before serving so that it will be soft enough to spread.

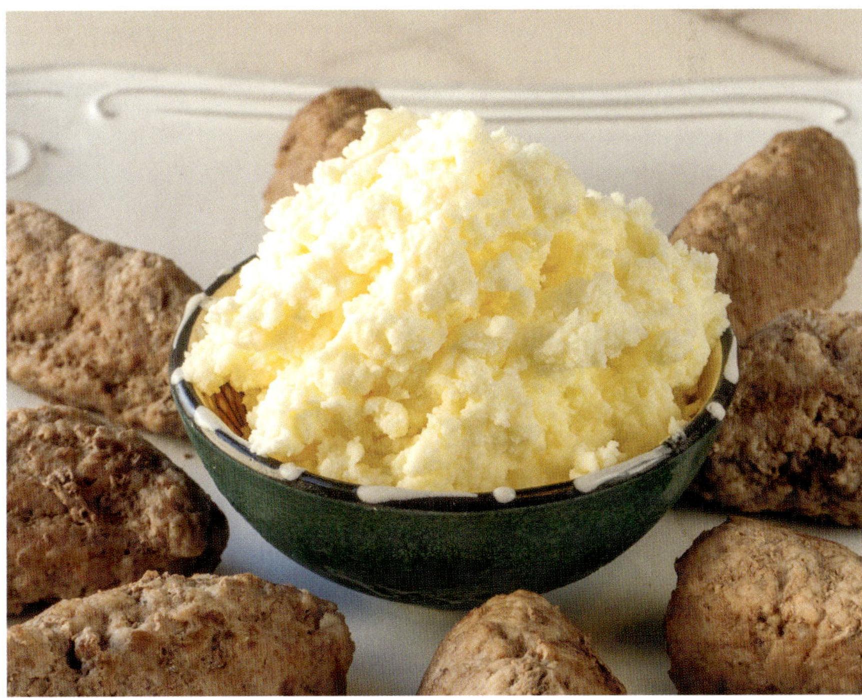

PER SERVING	calories: **258** | fat: **28g** | protein: **1g** | carbs: **1g** | macro split: **96/2/2**

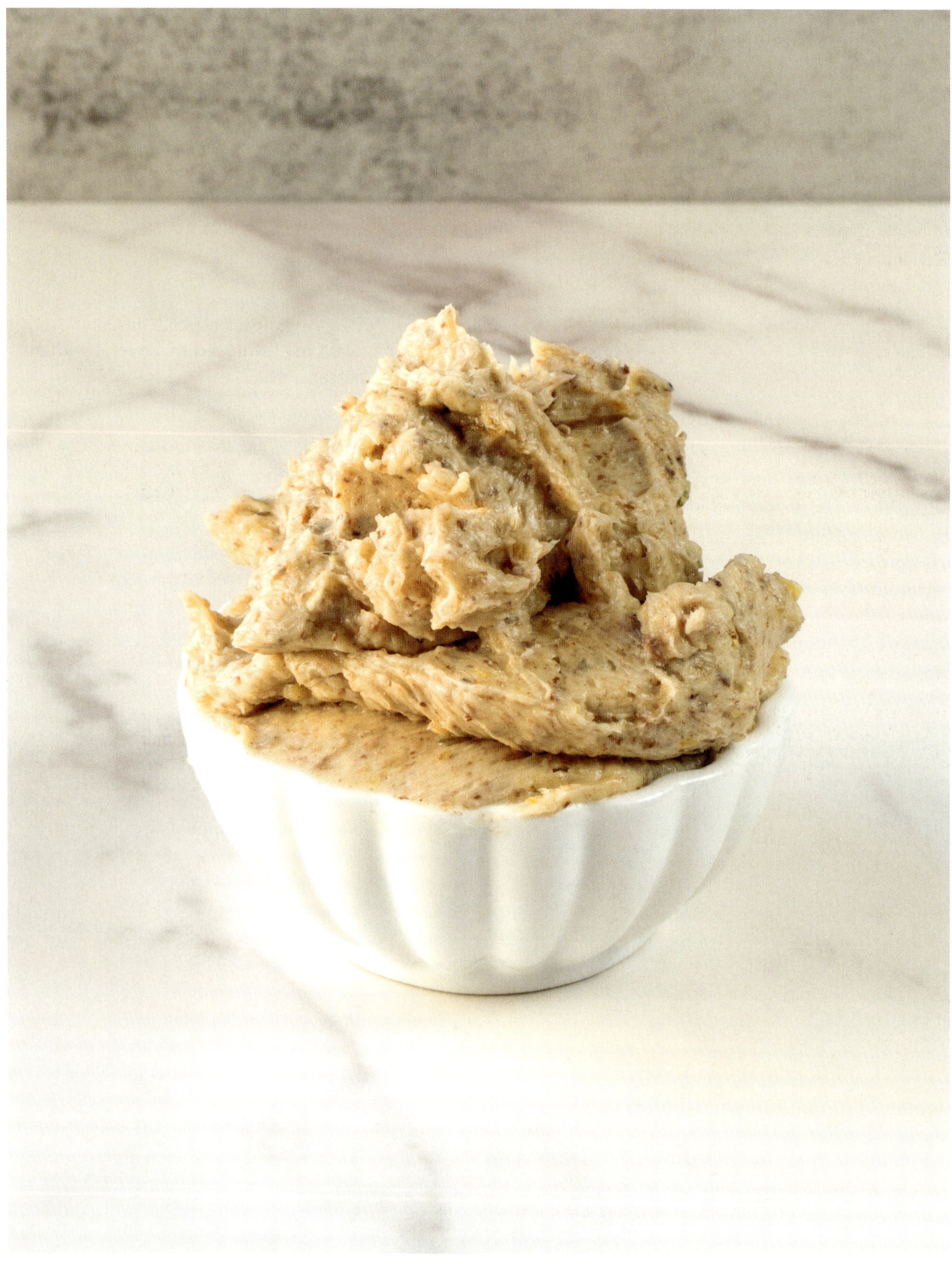

PER SERVING	calories: **107** | fat: **11g** | protein: **1g** | carbs: **1g** | macro split: **94/2/4**

YIELD: ½ cup
(1 tablespoon per serving)

PREP TIME: 10 minutes
(not including time to roast marrow bones)

BONE MARROW BUTTER

I love bone marrow, and I love butter. Combine the two in equal parts and I am *obsessed.* Any time you want to elevate a dish, cover it with a few tablespoons of this flavorful butter.

¼ cup Roasted Bone Marrow (page 205), at room temperature (see note)

¼ cup (½ stick) salted butter, at room temperature

8 cloves garlic, peeled

⅛ teaspoon dried rosemary needles

⅛ teaspoon dried ground thyme

Salt

SPECIAL EQUIPMENT:
Immersion blender

1. Put the marrow and butter in a large mason jar or small bowl and use an immersion blender to fully blend the two together. Then, using a garlic press, press the garlic cloves into the marrow butter. Add the dried herbs and blend again. Season with salt to taste and blend one final time.
2. Store in an airtight container in the refrigerator for up to a week.

Note

Once you've completed the Roasted Bone Marrow recipe and have scraped the cooked marrow from each bone, you should end up with about ¼ cup of marrow. If you end up with a little less or a little more, simply adjust the amount of butter to match. This recipe is a simple ratio of equal parts marrow to butter.

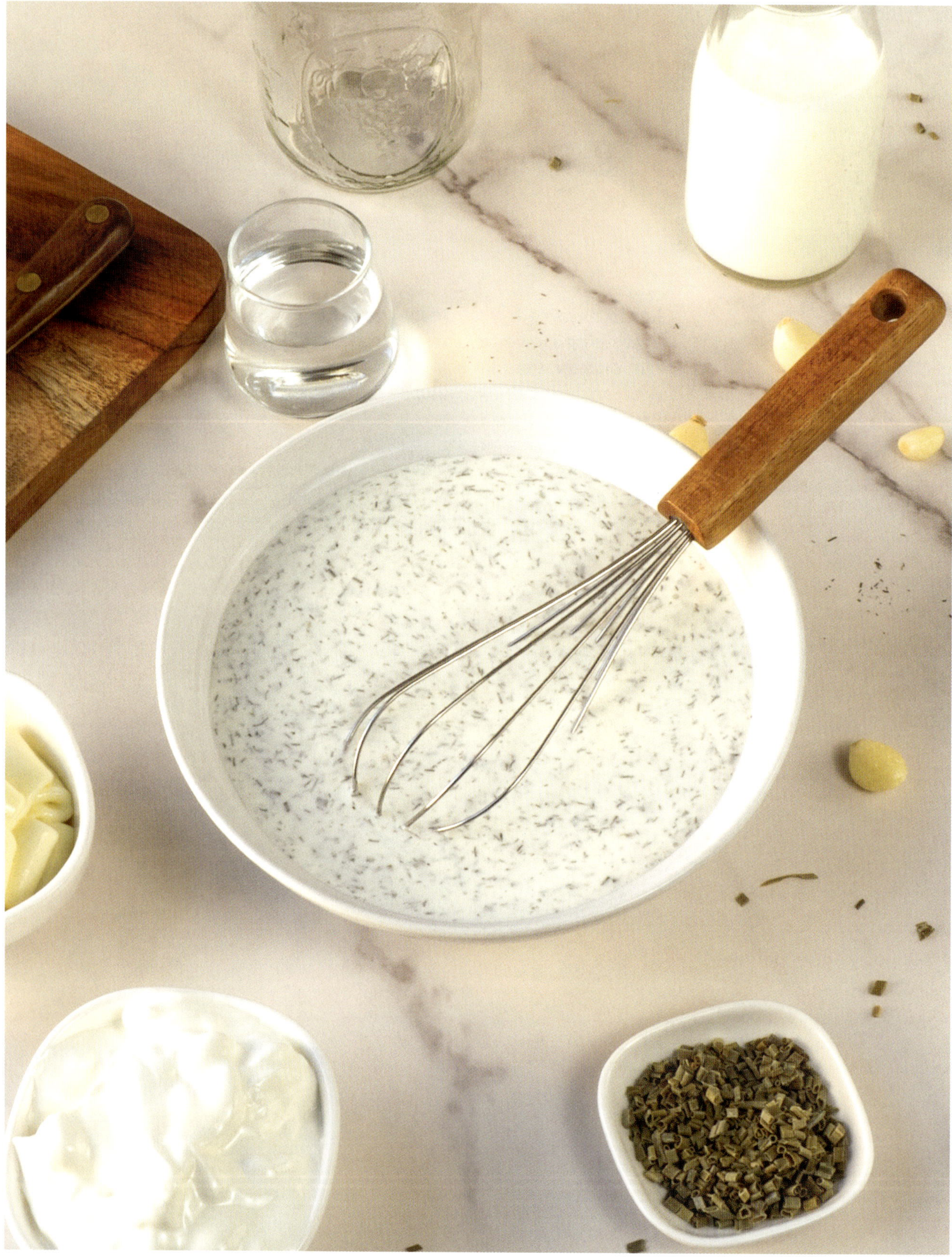

PER SERVING

calories: **70** | fat: **7g** | protein: **1g** | carbs: **1g** | macro split: **90/3/7**

YIELD: 2 cups
(2 tablespoons per serving)

PREP TIME: 10 minutes, plus 2 hours to chill

BUTTERMILK RANCH DRESSING

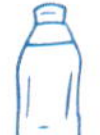
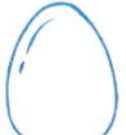

Ranch dressing is a classic that pairs perfectly with just about everything. However, many store-bought versions are loaded with seed oils, preservatives, and other additives that you want to avoid. That's why making your own ranch at home is a game changer. Not only is it free from unwanted ingredients, but it also tastes fresher and is more flavorful! If you're a fan of blue cheese, this recipe also works as the perfect base for a blue cheese dressing—just mix in some crumbled blue cheese and you're good to go. Once you've tried this homemade version, you'll never want to go back to store-bought!

½ cup avocado oil mayonnaise

½ cup full-fat sour cream

½ cup buttermilk

2 tablespoons white wine vinegar

1 tablespoon freshly squeezed lemon juice (optional)

1 tablespoon dried dill weed

1 tablespoon dried parsley

2 teaspoons dried chives

1 teaspoon onion powder

1 teaspoon salt

2 to 6 cloves garlic, pressed with a garlic press (optional)

1. Put all of the ingredients in a small mixing bowl and whisk together. If you are adding garlic, start with two cloves and taste. I prefer a lot of garlic, so I add up to six cloves.
2. Pour the dressing into a 16-ounce mason jar. Chill the dressing for 2 hours before serving. Store in the refrigerator for up to a week.

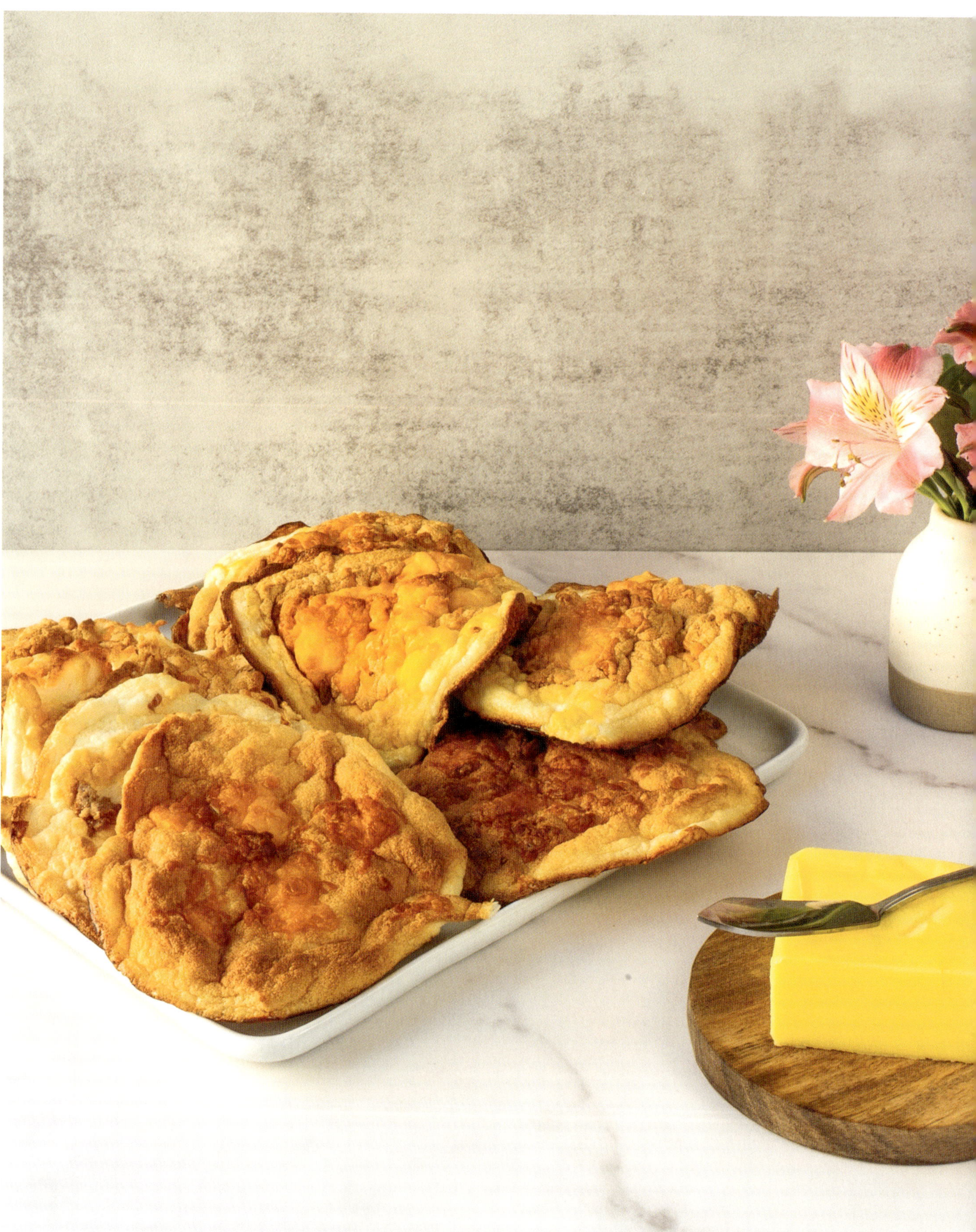

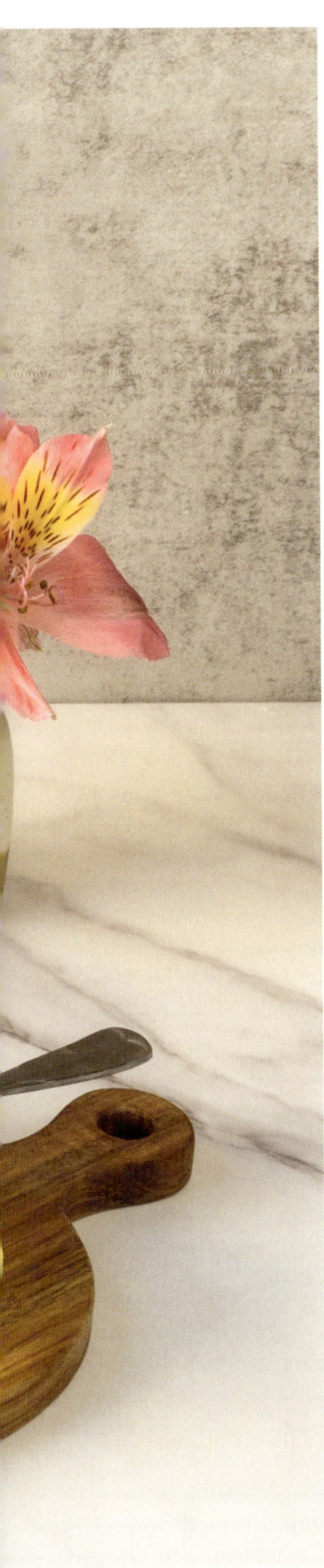

CHAPTER 18
BREADS

364 Carnivore Crepes/Noodles

367 Carnivore Flatbread

368 Chaffles

371 Cottage Cheese Flatbread

372 Cloud Bread Loaf or Buns

YIELD: 3 crepes or 2 cups noodles (1 crepe or ⅔ cup noodles per serving)

PREP TIME: 5 minutes

COOK TIME: 12 minutes

CARNIVORE CREPES/NOODLES

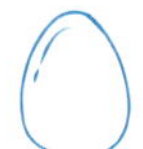

I originally found this recipe on Indigo Nili's YouTube channel (you should definitely check her out; she has a ton of great recipes). It requires only a few ingredients, so it's simple to make. Plus, you can use these versatile crepes in a lot of different ways. I like to cut them into noodles for Beef Stroganoff (page 276) or use them as is to make Sweet Cream Cheese–Filled Crepes (page 239). These crepes are much easier to cook and flip using a crepe pan and a crepe flipper, but they can be cooked with an ordinary frying pan and a spatula.

4 large egg whites

1 whole large egg

2 tablespoons unflavored beef gelatin powder

1½ tablespoons salted butter or other animal fat of choice, for the pan

SPECIAL EQUIPMENT: Immersion blender (optional), 10-inch nonstick crepe pan, crepe flipping tool (optional)

1. Put the egg whites and whole egg in a 2-cup liquid measuring cup. Add the gelatin and blend thoroughly with an immersion blender for at least 1 minute, until the gelatin is dissolved and the mixture is smooth with no clumps remaining. (You could also use a whisk and some elbow grease.)
2. Set a 10-inch crepe pan or nonstick frying pan over medium heat. Heat one-third of the butter in the pan until it bubbles. Pour one-third of the crepe batter into the center of the pan and then immediately pick up the pan and tilt it to evenly distribute the batter across the bottom, all the way to the edges. It's imperative that you move quickly to avoid thick crepes.
3. These crepes cook fast! As soon as the edges start to brown and curl up a bit, about 2 minutes, it's time to flip the crepe. Using a crepe flipper or spatula, flip the crepe to cook the other side for 2 minutes, then transfer to a plate. The flipping takes some practice; the first couple of times I made these, they looked terrible! But just keep practicing, and you will master this skill.
4. Repeat the process twice more with the remaining butter and crepe batter to make a total of three crepes.
5. Fill or cover the crepes with your choice of sweet or savory ingredients. To use the crepes as noodles, roll them up like a cigar and cut across the roll, then unfurl the noodles. You can make the crepes ahead of time and store them in the refrigerator for a few days before using.

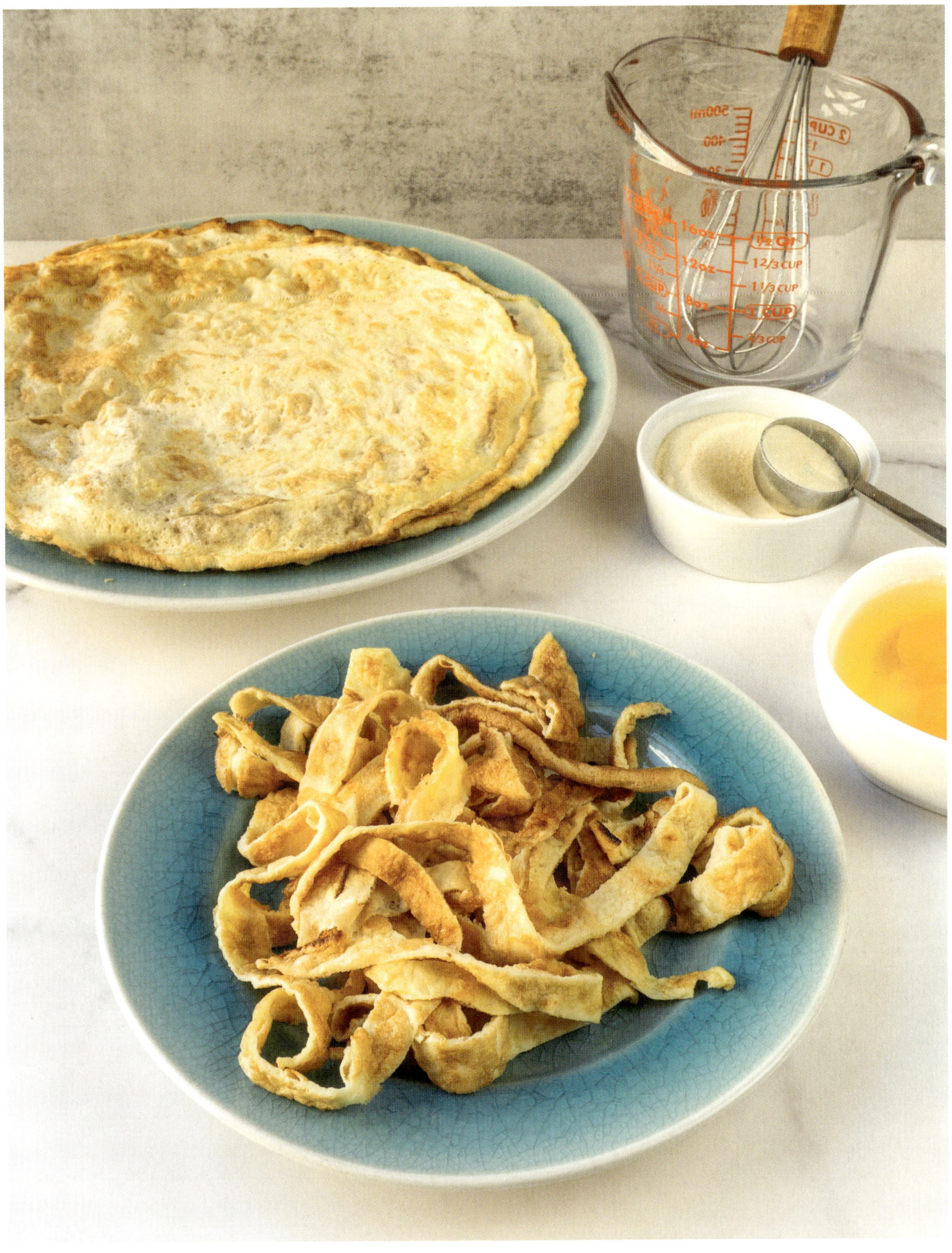

PER SERVING | calories: **360** | fat: **21g** | protein: **38g** | carbs: **4g** | macro split: **53/43/4**

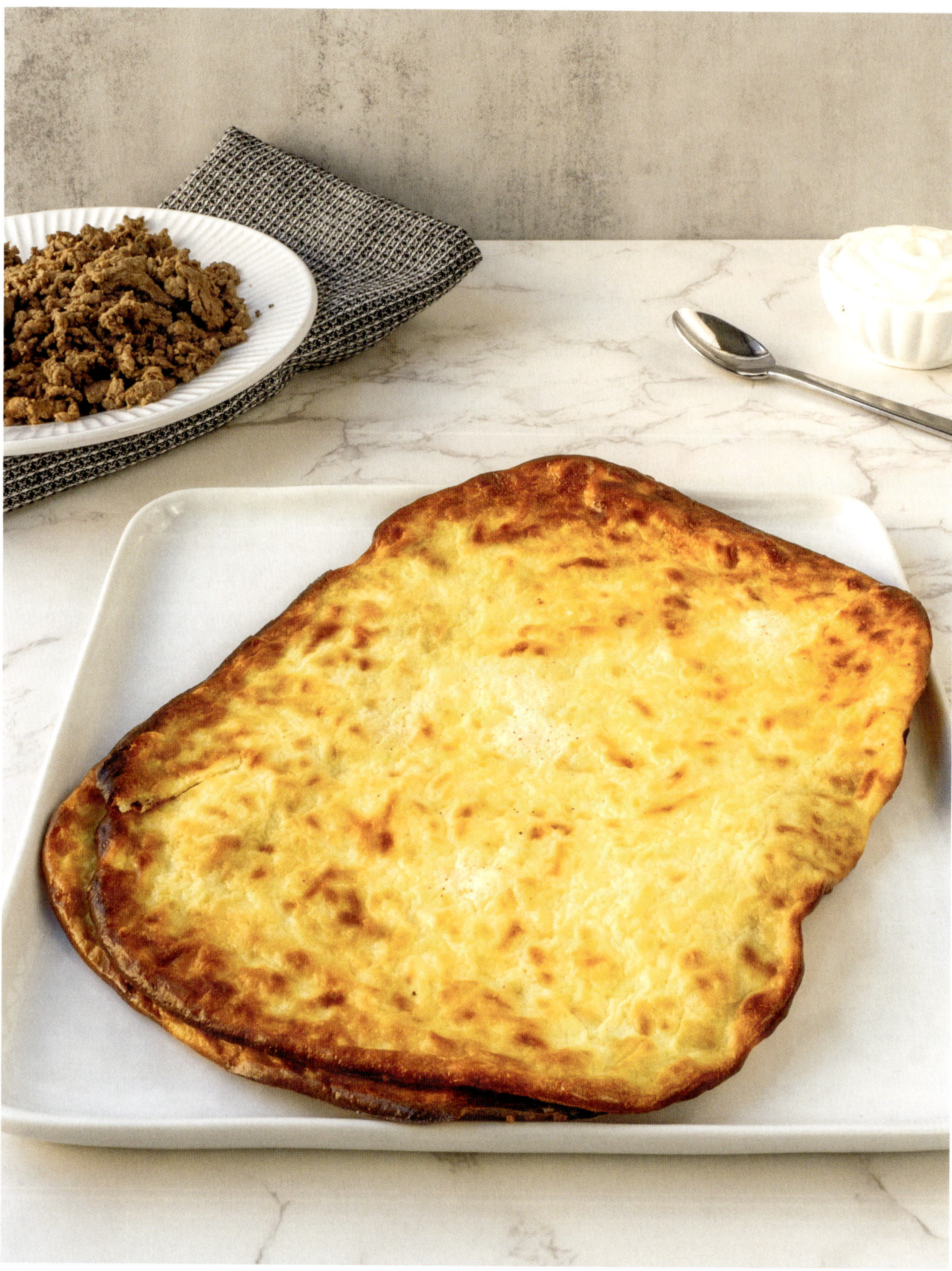

PER FLATBREAD	calories: **1148** | fat: **82g** | protein: **87g** | carbs: **16g** | macro split: **64/31/5**

YIELD: 1 large flatbread

PREP TIME: 5 minutes

COOK TIME: 20 minutes

CARNIVORE FLATBREAD

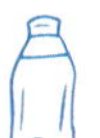
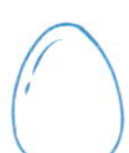

I found this recipe on *LowCarb Abode* on YouTube and made some slight modifications. This flatbread is strong enough to use for a quesadilla (see page 297) or as a sandwich wrap. You can also cut it into slices and enjoy it as a snack, either on its own or dipped in a dressing. If you want, make two smaller flatbreads by pouring the batter into two smaller circles or rectangles instead of one large one.

3 large eggs

1 cup shredded whole-milk mozzarella cheese

1 cup full-fat plain Greek yogurt

Pinch of salt

Pinch of ground white pepper

1. Preheat the oven to 425°F. Line a sheet pan with parchment paper or a silicone baking mat.
2. Mix the eggs, cheese, yogurt, salt, and pepper in a large mixing bowl until combined.
3. Pour the batter onto the prepared pan into an oval or rectangular shape that is about ¼ to ½ inch thick.
4. Bake for 20 minutes, or until golden brown and the center is no longer liquid-y.
5. Allow to cool for 10 minutes before eating. You can make this flatbread ahead of time; it will keep in the refrigerator for a few days. Reheat in the microwave or oven to make the flatbread pliable again.

YIELD: 6 chaffles (2 per serving)

PREP TIME: 5 minutes

COOK TIME: 15 minutes

CHAFFLES

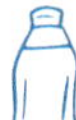
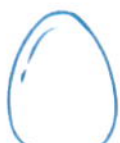

Chaffles are one of the simplest low-carb breads to whip up! I love making a few batches to keep in the fridge, ready for quick and tasty sandwiches anytime. You can also get creative by trying different cheeses or adding different spice blends to make each batch uniquely delicious!

4 large eggs

1 cup shredded cheddar or other semi-hard cheese of choice

Pinch of salt

SPECIAL EQUIPMENT:

Mini waffle maker

1 Preheat a mini waffle maker for 10 minutes.

2 Put all of the ingredients in a small bowl and mix with a fork until the eggs and cheese are fully combined.

3 Pour one-sixth of the batter onto the waffle iron. (No need to grease the iron; the oils from the cheese will be enough to lubricate the surface.) Close the lid and cook for 5 minutes, or until the chaffle is crispy and golden.

4 Remove the chaffle from the waffle iron and set on a plate. Repeat this process five more times to make a total of six chaffles.

5 Store leftovers in the refrigerator for up to a week.

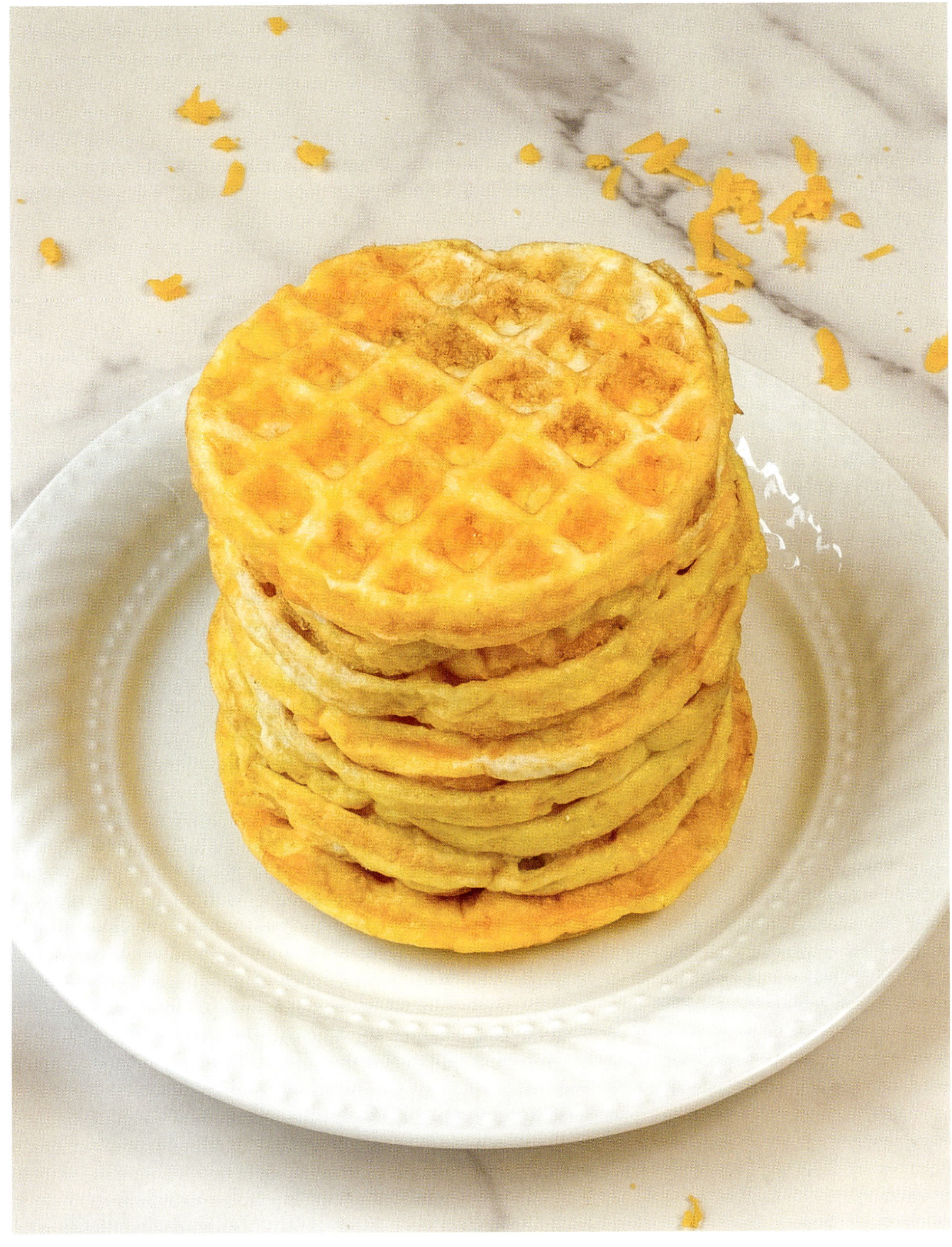

PER SERVING	calories: **121** | fat: **9g** | protein: **9g** | carbs: **1g** | macro split: **68/29/3**

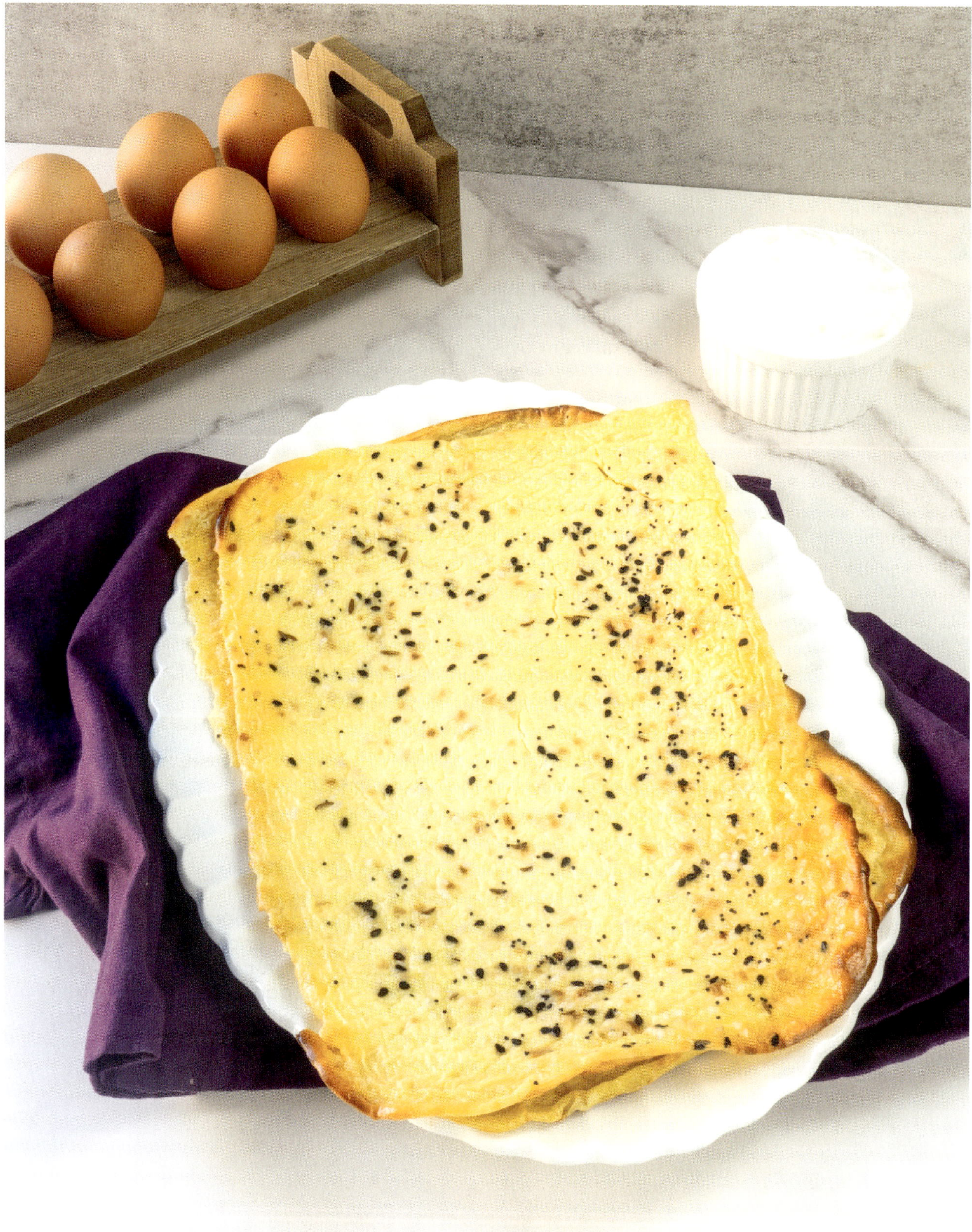

PER FLATBREAD

calories: **315** | fat: **15g** | protein: **36g** | carbs: **10g** | macro split: **42/45/13**

YIELD: one 13 by 9-inch flatbread

PREP TIME: 5 minutes

COOK TIME: 30 minutes

COTTAGE CHEESE FLATBREAD

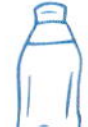
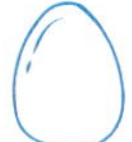

Cottage cheese recipes took the spotlight in 2024. I experimented with a few different cottage cheese flatbread recipes, and this one became a go-to for its perfect texture and delicious flavor every time. This recipe makes one medium-sized flatbread; it's great for wraps or can be sliced into pieces for a satisfying snack. You can use this same recipe to make twelve individual-sized flatbread rounds for sliders (see page 250) and other sandwiches; see the variation below.

1 cup cottage cheese (4% milkfat)

2 large eggs

½ teaspoon salt

1 teaspoon everything bagel seasoning (optional)

1. Preheat the oven to 350°F. Line a 13 by 9-inch sheet pan (aka quarter sheet pan) with parchment paper.
2. Blend the cottage cheese, eggs, and salt in a blender or food processor until smooth. Pour into the prepared pan. Sprinkle with the everything bagel seasoning, if using.
3. Bake for 30 minutes, or until golden brown and bubbly.
4. Allow to cool in the pan for 10 minutes before serving. These can be made ahead of time and stored in the refrigerator for a few days. Reheat in the microwave or oven to make it pliable again.

VARIATION:

Individual Cottage Cheese Flatbread Rounds. Instead of pouring the entire batch onto a quarter sheet pan, use a ladle to take one-twelfth of the batter and pour it onto a standard-size sheet pan lined with parchment paper. Repeat eleven times, leaving a couple of inches between rounds. (You may need to use two sheet pans.) Bake at 360°F for 15 to 20 minutes, until the breads are golden brown and bubbly.

YIELD: 1 large loaf (12 slices) or 12 buns (1 slice or bun per serving)

PREP TIME: 15 minutes

COOK TIME: 20 minutes for buns or 30 minutes for loaf

CLOUD BREAD LOAF OR BUNS

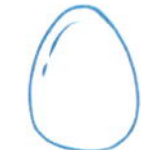

This recipe began with Maria Emmerich's Protein Sparing Wonder Bread, an incredibly creative approach to protein-based baking. While the original version is excellent, I found it a touch dry, so I modified it by adding extra fat in the form of egg yolks for more moisture and flavor.

2 cups egg whites (prepackaged or fresh from about 16 large eggs)

¼ cup powdered allulose

1 teaspoon salt

1 cup egg white protein powder

3 large egg yolks, whisked

1. Preheat the oven to 325°F. If making a loaf of bread, grease a 9 by 5-inch loaf pan with butter or avocado oil spray or line it with parchment paper; if making buns, line two sheet pans with parchment paper or silicone baking mats.
2. Put the egg whites, allulose, and salt in a stand mixer fitted with the whisk attachment and whip on high speed until stiff peaks form. (You can also use a large metal bowl and a hand mixer for this step.)
3. Turn the mixer to low and slowly add the protein powder until fully combined.
4. Turn off the mixer. Using a silicone spatula, slowly fold in the egg yolks. Do this carefully to prevent the egg whites from deflating.
5. To make a loaf, scoop the mixture into the prepared loaf pan, then smooth the top with the spatula and form it into a bread shape, making it slightly higher in the middle. It should be a couple of inches taller than the sides of the pan, then rounded and smoothed. If making buns, scoop up about ½ cup of the mixture and mound it high on one of the prepared sheet pans. Use the spatula to form it into a round bun shape that is about 4 inches in diameter. Repeat with the rest of the mixture to make 12 bunlike shapes on the prepared sheet pans, six per pan, leaving an inch or so between the buns. These will deflate a bit after baking.
6. Bake until the top of the loaf or buns is golden brown and lightly crackled. This will take about 30 minutes for the loaf or 20 minutes for the buns.

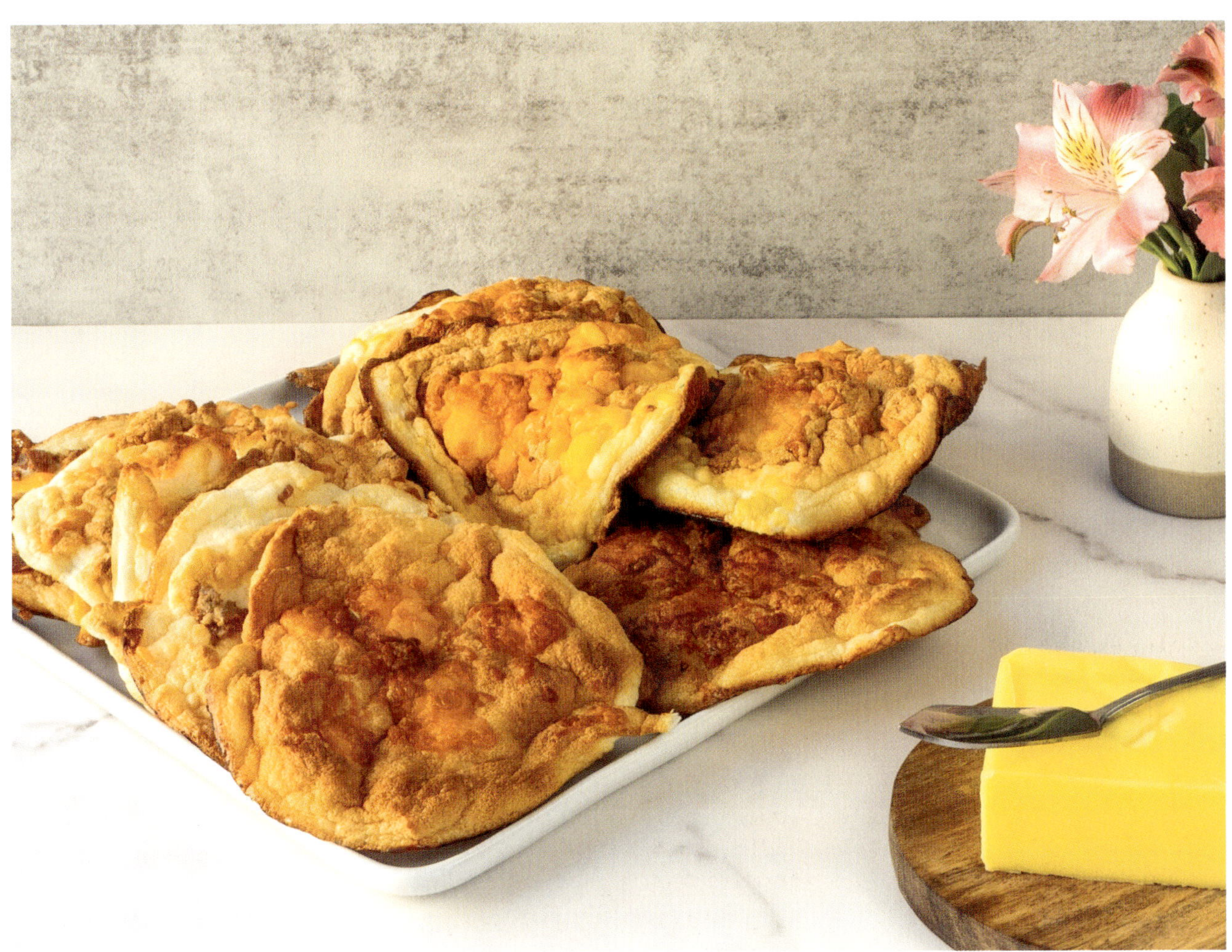

7 Let cool for 15 minutes before cutting and serving. Store in the refrigerator for up to 1 week. You can toast the bread, but watch very carefully, as the edges will toast much faster than the inside.

VARIATIONS:

Cheddar Cheese Cloud Bread Loaf/Buns. After completing Step 4, gently fold in ½ cup of finely shredded cheddar cheese. Once you've completed Step 5, forming the mixture into a loaf or buns, sprinkle the loaf or buns with another ½ cup of cheese, then bake as directed.

Bacon & Cheese Cloud Bread Loaf/Buns. After completing Step 4, gently fold in ½ cup of finely shredded cheddar cheese and ½ cup of cooked and crumbled bacon. Once you've completed Step 5, forming the mixture into a loaf or buns, sprinkle the loaf or buns with another ½ cup of cheese and ½ cup of bacon, then bake as directed.

PER SERVING | calories: **41** | fat: **1g** | protein: **6g** | carbs: **0g** | macro split: **30/70/0**

APPENDIX A: HOW TO QUICKLY EVALUATE THE QUALITY OF A SCIENTIFIC PAPER

Being able to quickly determine whether a scientific paper is worth worrying about is a vital skill—especially today, when Big Food and Big Pharma are funding more "research" than ever. It is estimated that at least half of all scientific papers are misleading and/or have such strong conflicts of interest that they cannot be taken seriously. But the media continues to use weak studies and sensational headlines to garner attention.

Attempting to read scientific papers can be intimidating, especially if you haven't had prior exposure to them. But there are specific things you can look for, and with a bit of practice, you will be able to skim a paper and know within thirty seconds whether it is worth your time to read further. Given the subject of this book, I will assume that most of the papers you will be skimming will be about nutrition and diet, so I will focus on what to look for in these types of papers.

First, though, you need to have a basic understanding of the different ways studies can be conducted. There is a hierarchy, and some studies are of higher quality than others.

The highest-quality scientific evidence results from meta-analyses and systematic reviews, followed closely by randomized controlled studies, and the best meta-analyses and systematic reviews are based on the review of randomized controlled studies. (The quality of a review is based on the quality of the studies it is reviewing, so keep that in mind.) Next best are observational studies, followed by animal trials and case reports.

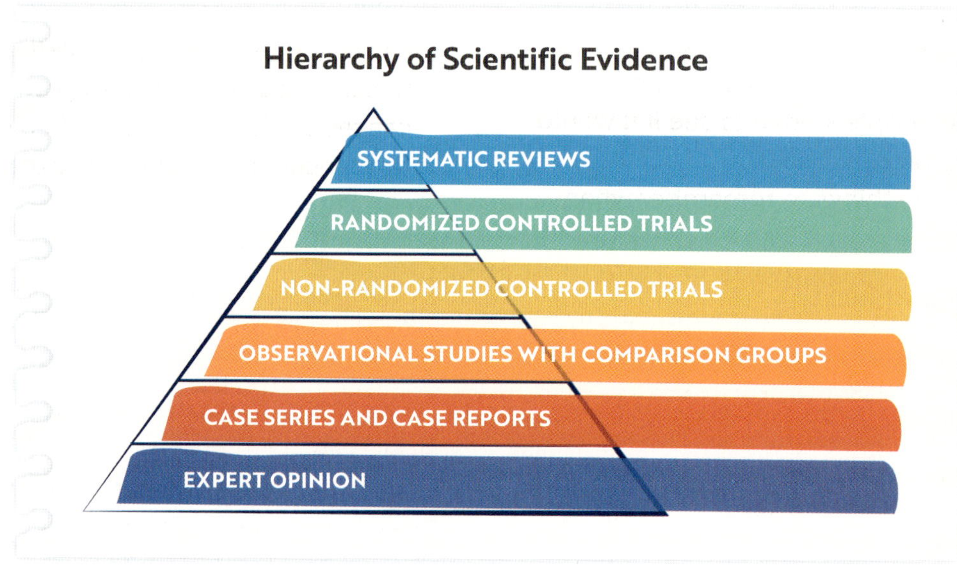

Many studies in nutrition are epidemiological, sometimes called observational, population, or cohort studies. The goal of an observational study is to look for possible relationships between some characteristic and a disease. There are two main types of observational studies: cohort and case control.

In a cohort study, the researchers are looking either forward (prospective) or backward (retrospective). Prospective studies are typically very expensive because they involve recruiting large groups of people, having the participants take some baseline tests and measurements, and then following them for years afterward to see what happens. Almost all observational studies published nowadays are retrospective studies that look back at cohort data from previous prospective studies and comb that historical data for patterns.

A case-control observational study differs from a cohort study only in that it has a control group. The control group doesn't get the treatment being tested, while the experimental group does. By looking at the differences between the two groups, scientists can see what effect the treatment has and better understand the results.

It was a case-control study that helped determine the link between smoking and lung cancer, for example. It simply would have been unethical to build a randomized controlled trial that made people smoke to see if it would give them lung cancer.

There are three things to remember when looking at epidemiological studies:

1. They can find associations, but not causation. For an observed association to be causal, the risk ratio needs to be at least 2, which is almost never the case. (A risk ratio of 1 means equal risk, a ratio above 1 means higher risk, and a ratio below 1 means lower risk.)
2. They often present relative risk instead of absolute risk. Absolute risk is the actual chance of something happening. Relative risk compares that chance between two groups. For example:
   - If 2 out of 100 people get sick without a treatment, the absolute risk is 2 percent.
   - If 1 out of 100 people get sick with the treatment, the absolute risk is 1 percent.
   - The relative risk is 1 percent divided by 2 percent, or 0.5—meaning the treatment cuts the risk in half.

So, absolute risk tells you how likely something is, while relative risk tells you how much more or less likely it is compared to another group. Statin papers often use absolute and relative risk to amplify a drug's benefits. The real benefit of a statin might be just a 1 percent drop in absolute risk. However, ads often say they reduce heart attack risk by 50 percent, which is only true when comparing relative risk. This makes the drug seem more effective than it is, because a 50 percent drop sounds bigger than a 1 percent difference.

3. They always suffer from confounders, variables that are linked to both the possible cause and the outcome. For example, if a study shows that people who carry lighters get more lung cancer, smoking is a confounder—because smoking is related to carrying a lighter and to getting lung cancer, but it isn't the identified cause of the cancer in the study; the lighter is.

Now that you have a better understanding of how most nutritional studies work, let's dive into how you can quickly skim a paper to see if it is worth your time.

I start with the abstract. It is typically the first main paragraph of the paper, under the title and author name(s). It is basically a summary of the paper and its findings. The first things I look for are the words *observational, epidemiological, population, or cohort study.*

The next words I look for in the abstract are *food questionnaire, food survey,* or something to that effect. I look for these words because food questionnaires or surveys are notoriously unreliable. Many people can't remember what they ate yesterday, let alone a week ago. Many respondents lie. Also, the survey questions can be written in ways that are confusing to the people taking the survey. Bottom line: If the data used to make a claim is coming from a food survey, that is a clear indicator to me that this study is dead in the water.

For example, let's say you are skimming a study entitled "Red Meat Causes Cancer." But when you skim the abstract, you see that this is an *observational study* using *24-hour food survey* data from the UK Biobank that is fifteen years old. From such weak data, the researchers cannot make a reliable claim that eating red meat *causes* cancer. Were the subjects actually eating what they said they were eating? Were they excluding or including certain foods? How can we know if one twenty-four-hour period was representative of how each participant ate every day for the next however many years? These questions alone make me discount any associations the researchers find.

But let's say their food survey data wasn't fatally flawed. Even then, the researchers can only come up with associations from this data and then form hypotheses from these associations. One hypothesis could be, "We think that eating any amount of red meat causes cancer," which could then be tested with a higher-quality, more rigorous study, such as a randomized controlled trial (RCT). Only after conducting an RCT could they begin to confirm or invalidate their hypothesis. And even then, the RCT would need to be repeated by other researchers to confirm that it wasn't an anomaly.

If the abstract reveals an epidemiological study and/or food survey data, I start to doubt the quality of the study. But I like to dig a bit deeper. Next, I try to figure out who funded the research. This information is typically found toward the end of the paper, before the references. Sometimes the funding source is very clear, and sometimes it is hidden. But if, for example, a study funded by a sugar manufacturer claims that sugar consumption is good for you, I throw that study in the trashcan. Unfortunately, you will find many "studies" like this.

It's also worth looking at the authors and their conflicts of interest. Authors are required to disclose any industry affiliations they have, typically in a short paragraph at the beginning or end of the paper. This can be a great place to root out glaring conflicts of interest or bias.

The final thing I check is the study design or methodology. Are the researchers measuring things correctly? Are their definitions accurate? For example, I once came across a study that claimed a keto diet doubled the risk of heart attack and stroke. But when I looked at how they were defining a "keto" diet, I discovered that the researchers allowed for up to 45 percent of a person's daily calorie intake to come from carbohydrates. That is not a keto diet. A keto diet is typically very low in carbs. Because of this inaccuracy, the researchers' claims were not valid, because they weren't studying a keto diet. You will see these types of issues in many of the papers you skim.

Let's review quickly:

- Look for words like *observational, epidemiological, food survey,* and *food questionnaire.*
- Who funded the research?
- Check out the authors' conflicts of interest and industry affiliations.
- Does the study design seem accurate or inaccurate?

You may wonder why such weak research is published in highly reputable journals. A lot of it has to do with who's pulling the strings behind the scenes. Big Food and Big Pharma have their tentacles in everything, including higher education and scientific journals. Major reform and legislation are needed to require researchers to be more honest and rigorous. But until then, become an expert study skimmer and learn to separate the wheat from the chaff.

Another great way to hone this skill is to subscribe to Zoe Harcombe's weekly newsletter. Zoe is a researcher, author, blogger, and public speaker. Her areas of expertise include public health dietary guidelines (especially dietary fat), nutrition, and obesity. Every week, she presents a study and then proceeds to tear it apart. I have learned so much from her about what to look for when evaluating the quality of a study and highly recommend her newsletter. There is a small quarterly or annual fee, but I happily pay it. Head to www.zoeharcombe.com to check out subscription options.

Pages 1–2

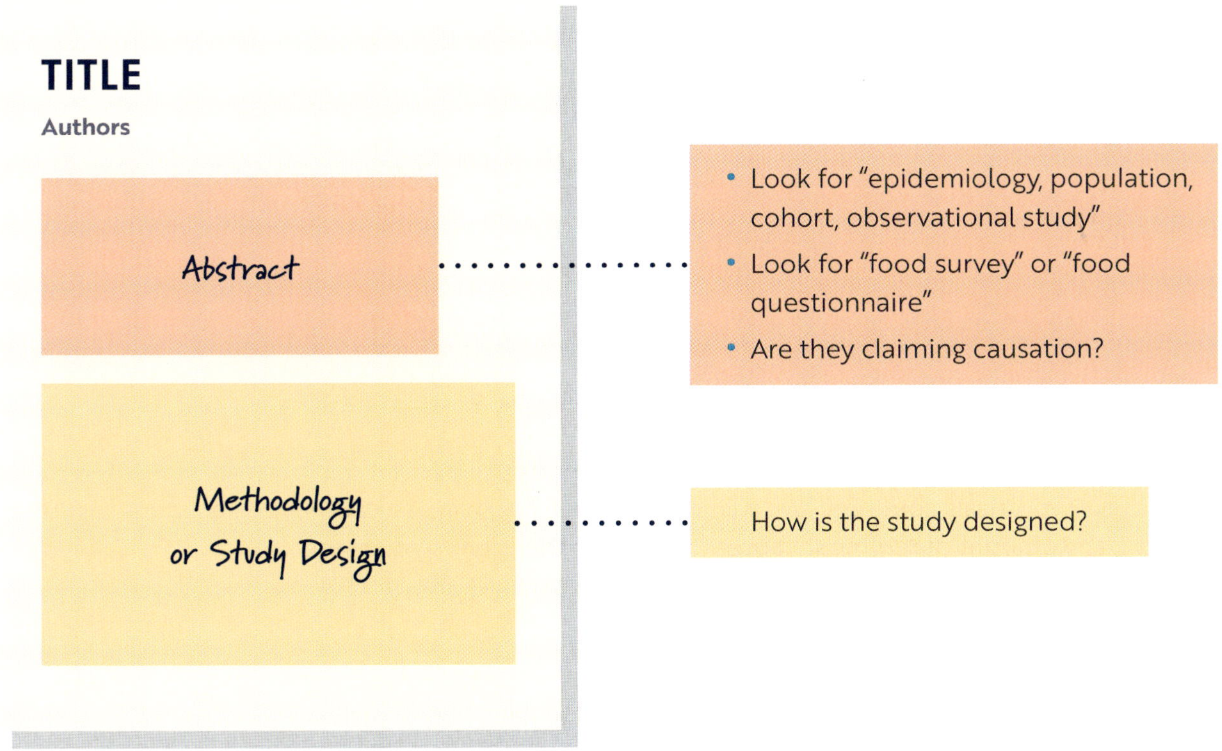

End of paper, before references

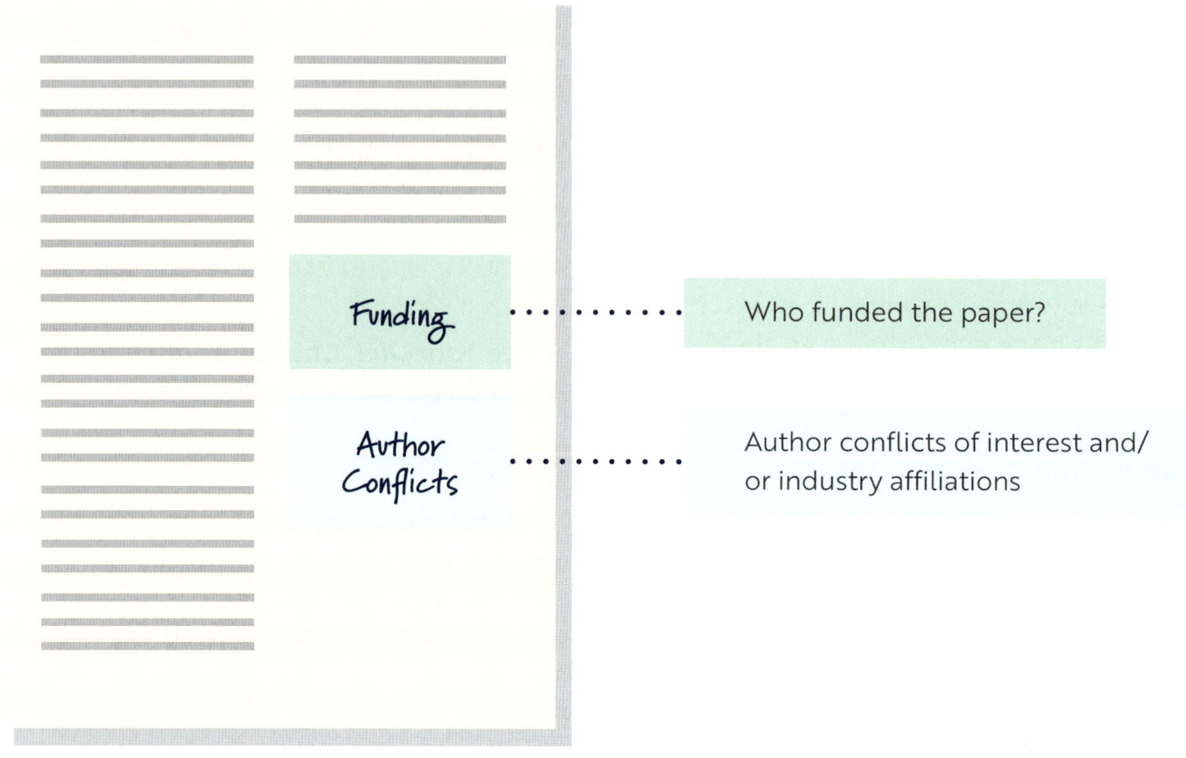

APPENDIX B: RECOMMENDED READING

There are many excellent books in this niche, and these are the ones that I have earmarked and annotated. Many of these books are paradigm shifting and may change the way you look at the world. Enjoy!

For even more of my recommended reads, head over to JennyMitich.com.

START HERE

The Big Fat Surprise by Nina Teicholz

This was the first book I read when I began my carnivore journey, and I compare it to waking up from the Matrix. It dives into why fat has been demonized and the faulty science being used to back that claim. Once you read this book, you will see the world in a different light. Teicholz spent years doing interviews and research for this book, and it shows. An absolute must-read.

The Great Plant-Based Con by Jayne Buxton

Another game-changing book that dispels vegetarian myths. This well-researched book (drawing from over 1,000 high-quality sources!) is split into three main sections covering health, the environment, and monetary interests behind the plant-based movement.

Why We Get Sick by Benjamin Bikman, PhD

Professor Bikman is one of the best sources of information on insulin resistance and its effects on the human body. This book is required reading for anyone dealing with insulin resistance because it will help you understand it better and gives you science-based solutions.

Change Your Diet, Change Your Mind by Georgia Ede, MD

Dr. Ede is a Harvard-trained psychiatrist, and her book is a must-read for anyone suffering from mental health conditions. She discusses how nutrition plays an integral role in brain function and lays out a plan for changing your diet to improve your mental health.

GREAT BOOKS ON THE CARNIVORE DIET

The Carnivore Diet by Shawn Baker, MD

The original tome on the carnivore diet, this book is a great addition to your carnivore library. Dr. Baker is measured and nuanced, never extreme, and gives excellent advice on how and why to start eating this way.

The Carnivore Code by Judy Cho, NTP

Cho is a board-certified nutritionist and the host of the Nutrition with Judy podcast. She has a clinical practice where she uses her Carnivore Cure to help people suffering from a multitude of issues, including autoimmune conditions, CIRS, and metabolic syndrome. She has taken her years of experience and turned them into an excellent carnivore resource that's backed by plenty of science and data.

Carnivore in the Kitchen by Courtney Luna

This cookbook contains eighty delicious recipes to inject some variety into your carnivore diet. Every carnivore needs a copy!

Good Fat Is Good for Women: Menopause and Eating Good Fat Is Good for Girls: Puberty and Adolescence by Dr. Elizabeth Bright

Dr. Bright believes that eating good fat is good for a woman's health at every stage of life, and I couldn't agree more. If you are approaching or in menopause, this book will give you vital information for living your best life during this time. If you have a daughter in or approaching puberty, good dietary fats are essential, and Dr. Bright's book on this topic lays out why.

Not by Bread Alone by Vilhjalmur Stefansson

The original carnivore researcher, Stefansson was an Arctic explorer and anthropologist who spent years with the Indigenous Inuit people. He lived how they lived and recorded their mostly meat-based dietary habits and good health outcomes. He estimated that over 80 percent of their diet was meat and animal products. In 1928, Stefansson did an experiment where he and a colleague consumed only meat for a year. They stayed healthy, which led Stefansson to the belief that we need to reevaluate our thoughts on what constitutes a healthy diet.

FOOD SCIENCE MUST-READS

Dark Calories: How Vegetable Oils Destroy Our Health and *How We Can Get It Back* by Catherine Shanahan, MD

Dr. Shanahan is a Cornell-trained biochemist turned family physician. This book discusses her research on the topic of oxidation-related diseases and how they connect to vegetable oils and helps us understand why it is so important to avoid consuming these oils.

Gut and Physiology Syndrome (GAPS) by Natasha Campbell-McBride, MD

This book explains how a compromised gut can drive chronic inflammation, autoimmune disease, allergies, asthma, skin issues, and many other physical disorders. Through the GAPS Nutritional Protocol, it provides a roadmap to healing the gut lining and restoring overall health. A must read for anyone suffering from an autoimmune condition.

Salt Your Way to Health; Iodine: Why You Need It, Why You Can't Live Without It; The Miracle of Natural Hormones; and *Overcoming Thyroid Disorders* by David Brownstein, MD

Brownstein is a Michigan-based doctor with a thriving practice that specializes in thyroid and hormonal health. He has written many books, but these are the four that I have read. Each of them presents case studies from his clinical practice along with the science behind the topics discussed. I learned a lot about iodine and thyroid health from his books.

Toxic Superfoods by Sally Norton, MPH

Norton is the queen of oxalates and did a ton of deep research to put this book together. Most people don't even know what oxalate is—I know I didn't. This is an essential read for anyone who has eaten a large amount of plant foods and wants to know the impact of plant toxins on their metabolic health.

MEDICAL SCIENCE AND RESEARCH

Burn by Herman Pontzer, PhD

In this fascinating read, Pontzer shows how human metabolism really works in order to help you improve your metabolic health and manage your weight. It turns out that exercise doesn't do much to improve metabolism, but it does help keep your body functioning optimally. Regardless of activity level, you burn about 3,000 calories per day. Pontzer's thought-provoking research just might change the way you think about calories, food, and exercise.

Lies My Doctor Told Me: Medical Myths That Can Harm Your Health by Ken D. Berry, MD

Dr. Berry is considered the king of carnivore. In this book, he dives into common myths in the medical and nutritional fields and gives no-nonsense, easy-to-understand information that everyone needs to know.

Nature Wants Us to Be Fat by Richard J. Johnson, MD

Dr. Johnson has been researching obesity and diabetes for over twenty years and is specifically interested in the roles that fructose and uric acid play in these debilitating conditions. This book discusses a fructose-powered "survival switch" that seems to be the metabolic pathway for fat storage. Interesting research and excellent reading.

Stay Off My Operating Table by Philip Ovadia, MD

Dr. Ovadia is a heart surgeon who is sick of people dying from a preventable disease. In his book, he discusses the current state of metabolic health in the US and gives actionable steps to improve yours. He shows you how to eat in a metabolically healthy way using five different dietary lifestyles and talks about myths and FAQs when it comes to heart health.

HEART DISEASE THEORIES AND RESEARCH

The Clot Thickens by Dr. Malcolm Kendrick

Dr. Kendrick puts forth several alternative theories for the true causes of heart disease in this easy-to-read, well-written book. I really like his sense of humor and ability to make a difficult topic more accessible.

Fat and Cholesterol Don't Cause Heart Attacks and Statins Are Not the Solution by THINCS (The International Network of Cholesterol Skeptics)

This collection of articles disputes the dogma that dietary fat and cholesterol cause heart disease. Other topics include the dangers of statins and low-fat diets and the role that infections, nutrient deficiencies, and other factors play in the formation of cardiovascular disease.

Lipid Lunacy: Diet Delusions and What Really Causes Heart Disease by THINCS (The International Network of Cholesterol Skeptics)

The second collection of articles from THINCS discusses more theories about the true causes of heart disease. It addresses a multitude of topics, including saturated fat and the diet-heart hypothesis.

REGENERATIVE AGRICULTURE AND SUSTAINABILITY

A Bold Return to Giving a Damn by Will Harris

Harris is the owner of White Oak Pastures, a regenerative ranch and farm in Georgia. In this book, he shares his journey from conventional farmer and cattleman to regenerative farmer and steward of his land and animals. Harris is a salt-of-the-earth, no-nonsense man, and this book has excellent insights into restoring the land, caring for domesticated animals, and reinvigorating a community.

Sacred Cow: The Case for Better Meat by Diana Rodgers, RD, and Robb Wolf

This book makes a nutritional, environmental, and ethical case for better meat. There is a companion documentary film. Regenerative agriculture and ethically raised meat can do amazing things for metabolic health and the environment, and this book lays out the science behind it all.

The Vegetarian Myth: Food, Justice, and Sustainability by Lierre Keith

Keith is a former vegan, and this book dispels the myths that a plant-based diet is better for your health, the environment, and animals. Keith writes from a creative perspective, and this book got me to think of certain topics from a different angle.

FASTING

The Complete Guide to Fasting: Heal Your Body Through Intermittent, Alternate-Day, and Extended Fasting by Dr. Jason Fung

Dr. Fung is the guy you want to listen to about fasting. He has been using various forms of fasting in his clinical practice for years, and this book will teach you how to fast effectively.

The Protein-Sparing Modified Fast Method: Over 120 Recipes to Accelerate Weight Loss & Improve Healing by Maria Emmerich and Craig Emmerich

While this book isn't about the carnivore diet, it does have high-quality information about protein-sparing modified fasting, which focuses on preserving muscle while losing body fat. This fasting method can be highly effective for overweight and obese people and is worth taking a look at. The Emmeriches have been in the low-carb/keto space for over twenty years, and all of their books are excellent.

MISCELLANEOUS

The Daily Stoic, The Obstacle is the Way, Stillness is the Key, and Ego is the Enemy by Ryan Holiday

I have learned so much from Ryan Holiday's many inspiring books on Stoicism. I would start with these four titles for a good overview of the philosophy.

Discourses by Epictetus

Often seen as one of the more challenging books on Stoicism, but full of insights, Holiday recommends the Penguin translations as the most reader friendly.

The Five Minute Journal by Intelligent Change

I love this little journal. It allows me to practice gratitude and plan my day while taking only a few minutes to complete.

Letters of a Stoic by Seneca

This book is a collection of personal letters written by the Roman philosopher Seneca to his friend Lucilius. The letters give advice on how to live a more virtuous and meaningful life, always through a Stoic lens.

Meditations by Marcus Aurelius

If you are diving into Stoicism, you must read the definitive Meditations. Holiday references it often in his work, and he recommends the Gregory Hays translation because it is written in modern English and is much easier to read than others.

INDEX

A

A1c, 69, 163, 167
abstainers, 61
accuracy, of DEXA scans, 176
acid reflux, as a physical symptom, 131
adiponectin, 125, 126
Air Fryer Brined Turkey Breast recipe, 308–309
Air Fryer Egg Bites recipe, 232–233
Air Fryer Sausage Rosemary Cream Cheese Bites recipe, 248–249
alcohol, 79, 144
Alfredo Sauce recipe, 351
  Carnivore White Pizza, 282–285
  Turkey Alfredo, 310–311
Ali, Nadir, 126
all meat, seafood, eggs, and butter version of carnivore, 57, 58–59
all meat, seafood, eggs, butter, and high-fat dairy version of carnivore, 57, 59–60
all meat and all seafood version of carnivore, 57, 58–59
allulose
  Carnivore Cinnamon Rolls, 240–241
  Carnivore Ice Cream, 334–335
  Carnivore Ice Cream Sandwiches—Two Ways, 336–337
  Cloud Bread Loaf or Buns, 372–373
  Mini Cheesecakes, 338–339
  Pumpkin Spice Cheesecake, 314–315
  Sweet Cream Cheese-Filled Crepes, 238–239
  Whipped Cream & Mascarpone, 340–341
ALT, 167
American cheese
  Extreme Double Bacon Cheeseburger, 268–269
American Diabetes Association, 44, 155
American Kajmak recipe, 357
  Ćevaps (Serbian Sausages), 224–225
  Pljeskavica (Serbian Burgers), 222–223
amino acids, 32
andouille sausage
  Hearty Meat Soup, 264–265
animal fats, 33, 74
animal proteins, 32
animal-based diets, used in medicine, 43–44
anxiety, as a physical symptom, 129
artificial sweeteners, 77, 143
Asiago cheese
  Garlicky Smothered Brussels Sprouts, 322–323
  Garlicky Smothered Green Beans, 328–329
AST, 167
athletes, carnivore diet for, 48, 151
Atkins, Robert, 14, 57
Atkins diet, 14, 57
Aurelius, Marcus, *Meditations*, 383
autoimmunity, 133

B

B vitamins, 172
B12 vitamin, 163, 168, 174
bacon
  Air Fryer Egg Bites, 232–233
  Bacon, Egg & Cheese Sandwich, 242–243
  Bacon & Cheese Cloud Bread Loaf/Buns, 372–373
  Bacon Mayonnaise, 352–353
  Beefy Bacon-Wrapped Stuffed Onion Rings, 320–321
  Burgers with Benefits, 208–209
  Carnivore Mac & Cheese Casserole, 278–281

Chicken Sliders with Spicy Mayo, 250–251
Deviled Eggs, 252–253
Extreme Double Bacon Cheeseburger, 268–269
Garlicky Smothered Brussels Sprouts, 322–323
Garlicky Smothered Green Beans, 328–329
Jalapeño Poppers, 318–319
Meat Lover's Pizza Roll-Ups, 254–255
overview, 75
Soufflé Omelet, 230–231
Spicy Bacon-Wrapped Chorizo Dogs, 286–287
Spicy Chicken Sandwiches, 272–273
Turkey Sandwich, 312–313
Wedge Salad, 324–325
Bacon, Egg & Cheese Sandwich recipe, 242–243
Bacon & Cheese Cloud Bread Loaf/Buns recipe, 372–373
Extreme Double Bacon Cheeseburger, 268–269
Bacon Mayonnaise recipe, 352–353
Bacon, Egg & Cheese Sandwich, 242–243
Crab Cakes with Rémoulade, 292–293
Deviled Eggs, 252–253
Extreme Double Bacon Cheeseburger, 268–269
Pot Roast Sandwich, 270–271
Turkey Sandwich, 312–313
bad breath, 149
Baker, Shawn, 20, 99
The Carnivore Diet, 14, 379
banana peppers
Pljeskavica (Serbian Burgers), 222–223
Barbieri, Angus, 122
bare minimum items, for carnivore kitchen, 73
bariatric surgery, 63, 113, 135
baseline measurements, 68–70
Basted Ribeye recipe, 196–197
BBQ Spice Rub recipe, 347
Brisket, 206–207
beef
Air Fryer Egg Bites, 232–233
Basted Ribeye, 196–197
Beef Stroganoff, 276–277
Beefy Bacon-Wrapped Stuffed Onion Rings, 320–321
Breakfast Casserole, 228–229
Burgers with Benefits, 208–209
Carnivore Tacos, 288–289
Ćevaps (Serbian Sausages), 224–225
Chili Cheese Dog Meatballs, 290–291
Dehydrated Ground Meat, 212–213
Extreme Double Bacon Cheeseburger, 268–269
Fajita Wrap, 266–267
for carnivore kitchen, 73
grass-fed vs. grain-fed, 75, 141
Ground Beef & Eggs, 234–235
Hearty Meat Soup, 264–265
overview, 75
Pljeskavica (Serbian Burgers), 222–223
Prime Rib, 198–199
Reuben Roll-Ups, 326–327
Slow Cooker Pot Roast, 218–219
Spicy Bacon-Wrapped Chorizo Dogs, 286–287
Taco Balls, 294–295
beef, salt, and water version of carnivore, 57, 58
beef bone broth
Beef Stroganoff, 276–277
beef fat
Rendered Tallow, 194–195
beef feet
Pihtije (Meat Jelly), 258–259
beef gelatin powder
Carnivore Crepes/Noodles, 364–365
Carnivore Gravy, 306–307
beef marrow bones
Roasted Bone Marrow, 204–205
Beef Stroganoff recipe, 276–277
beef tallow
Whipped Tallow Bites, 342–343

Beefy Bacon-Wrapped Stuffed Onion Rings recipe, 320–321
BelGioiso, 323
Berry, Ken D., 19, 99
Lies My Doctor Told Me: Medical Myths That Can Harm Your Health, 381
beverages, 78–79, 140–146
Big Tobacco, 10
The Big Fat Surprise (Teicholz), 379
Bikman, Benjamin, *Why We Get Sick*, 379
BillyDoe Meats, 134
bioavailability, 32–34
birds/waterfowl, for carnivore kitchen, 74
blood glucose, 36
blood sugar markers, 167, 172
blood testing, 185
blood work, 162–174
blue cheese
Burgers with Benefits, 208–209
Wedge Salad, 324–325
Wings, 220–221
Blue Zones, 109
body composition
history in DEXA scans, 177
trending report in DEXA scans, 180
body odor, 149
A Bold Return to Giving a Damn (Harris), 382
bone broth
Beef Stroganoff, 276–277
Carnivore Gravy, 306–307
Egg Pudding, 214–215
Bone Marrow Butter recipe, 358–359
Marrownaise, 354–355
bowel movements, 148
Brain Energy (Palmer), 59
Breakfast Casserole recipe, 228–229
breakfast sausage
Soufflé Omelet, 230–231
breath testing, 185
Breeze, Anita, 132
Bright, Elizabeth, *Good Fat Is Good for Women: Menopause and Eating Good Fat Is Good for Girls: Puberty and Adolescence*, 379–380
Brined Spatchcocked Turkey recipe, 300–303
Carnivore Gravy, 306–307
Brisket recipe, 206–207
Bristol Stool Chart, 130
Brownstein, David, 171, 186
Iodine: Why You Need It, Why You Can't Live Without It, 187, 380
The Miracle of Natural Hormones, 380
Overcoming Thyroid Disorders, 380
Salt Your Way to Health, 380
Brussels sprouts
Garlicky Smothered Brussels Sprouts, 322–323
budgets
carnivore diet on, 79–80, 140
limited, 52
Buffalo sauce
Wings, 220–221
BUN/creatinine ratio, 167
Burgers with Benefits recipe, 208–209
Burn (Pontzer), 381
butter, 75, 143
Butter Bites recipe, 332–333
Buttermilk Ranch Dressing recipe, 360–361
Air Fryer Sausage Rosemary Cream Cheese Bites, 248–249
Beefy Bacon-Wrapped Stuffed Onion Rings, 320–321
Cheesy Pepperoni Chips, 246–247
Meat Lover's Pizza Roll-Ups, 254–255
Wedge Salad, 324–325
Wings, 220–221
Buxton, Jayne, *The Great Plant-Based Con*, 155, 379

C

cacao powder
Carnivore Ice Cream Sandwiches—Two Ways, 336–337
Mini Cheesecakes, 338–339

Cajun Seasoning recipe, 345–346
Crab Cakes with Rémoulade, 292–293
Fajita Wrap, 266–267
Spiced Pumpkin-Shaped Cheese Ball, 304–305
calories, requirements for, 92–93
Campbell-McBride, Natasha, *Gut and Physiology Syndrome*, 133, 380
cancer, 44, 50, 156
carbohydrates
four-week gradual carbohydrate reduction, 84–87
ketosis and, 186
overview, 31, 60
requirements for, 155
Carnivore Cinnamon Rolls recipe, 240–241
Carnivore Crepes/Noodles recipe, 364–365
Beef Stroganoff, 276–277
Carnivore Cinnamon Rolls, 240–241
Sweet Cream Cheese-Filled Crepes, 238–239
Turkey Alfredo, 310–311
carnivore diet
ancestral origins of, 37–43
benefits of, 45
on a budget, 79–80
cold turkey or easing into, 60–62
compared with other diets, 46
Day 1 worksheet, 55
determining your whys, 56, 62
in hospitals, 146
kitchen prep for, 72–82
mental preparation for, 65–71
myths, 154–160
overeating, 121
overview, 13–14, 31, 54
recommended reading for, 379–380
reservations about, 49–52
special considerations, 62–64
troubleshooting, 116–138
versions, 57–60
while traveling, 145
who it's for, 47–48, 151, 152
why it works, 32–36
Carnivore Flatbread recipe, 366–367
Carnivore Quesadilla, 296–297
Carnivore Gravy recipe, 306–307
Carnivore Ice Cream recipe, 334–335
Carnivore Ice Cream Sandwiches—Two Ways, 336–337
Carnivore Ice Cream Sandwiches—Two Ways recipe, 336–337
Carnivore in the Kitchen (Luna), 379
Carnivore Mac & Cheese Casserole recipe, 278–281
Carnivore Quesadilla recipe, 296–297
Carnivore Tacos recipe, 288–289
Carnivore White Pizza recipe, 282–285
The Carnivore Code (Cho), 379
The Carnivore Diet (Baker), 14, 379
Ćevaps (Serbian Sausages) recipe, 224–225
Chaffee, Anthony, 88
Chaffles recipe, 368–369
Bacon, Egg & Cheese Sandwich, 242–243
Turkey Sandwich, 312–313
Change Your Diet, Change Your Mind (Ede), 59, 110, 379
charred meat, 142
cheating, 145–146
cheddar cheese
Air Fryer Egg Bites, 232–233
Bacon, Egg & Cheese Sandwich, 242–243
Bacon & Cheese Cloud Bread Loaf/Buns, 372–373
Breakfast Casserole, 228–229
Burgers with Benefits, 208–209
Carnivore Mac & Cheese Casserole, 278–281
Carnivore Tacos, 288–289
Chaffles, 368–369
Cheddar Cheese Cloud Bread Loaf/Buns, 372–373
Cheesy Pepperoni Chips, 246–247
Chicken Sliders with Spicy Mayo, 250–251
Chili Cheese Dog Meatballs, 290–291

cheddar cheese *(continued)*
Extreme Double Bacon Cheeseburger, 268–269
Jalapeño Poppers, 318–319
Spiced Pumpkin-Shaped Cheese Ball, 304–305
Taco Balls, 294–295
Cheddar Cheese Cloud Bread Loaf/Buns recipe, 372–373
cheese. *See also specific types*
Pljeskavica (Serbian Burgers), 222–223
Cheesy Pepperoni Chips recipe, 246–247
chicken
Carnivore Mac & Cheese Casserole, 278–281
Carnivore Quesadilla, 296–297
Carnivore Tacos, 288–289
Carnivore White Pizza, 282–285
Chicken Sliders with Spicy Mayo, 250–251
Chicken Soup, 262–263
Crispy Baked Chicken Thighs & Drumsticks, 210–211
Dehydrated Ground Meat, 212–213
for carnivore kitchen, 73
Hearty Meat Soup, 264–265
overview, 75
Spicy Chicken Sandwiches, 272–273
Wings, 220–221
chicken bone broth
Carnivore Gravy, 306–307
Chicken & Pork Seasoning recipe, 348
Crispy Baked Chicken Thighs & Drumsticks, 210–211
Spicy Chicken Sandwiches, 272–273
Chicken Sliders with Spicy Mayo recipe, 250–251
Chicken Soup recipe, 262–263
children, carnivore diet for, 47–48, 152
Chili Cheese Dog Meatballs recipe, 290–291
chili peppers
Pljeskavica (Serbian Burgers), 222–223
Chili Spice Seasoning recipe, 349
Chili Cheese Dog Meatballs, 290–291
Cho, Judy, 20
The Carnivore Code, 379
cholesterol
lipid panel, 166
myths about, 156–158
overview, 50–51, 147
chorizo
Carnivore Quesadilla, 296–297
Spicy Bacon-Wrapped Chorizo Dogs, 286–287
Chris Cooking Nashville, 132
chronic cardio, 103
chronic inflammatory response syndrome (CIRS), 113, 118
chronic kidney disease (CKD), 49, 148, 156
chuck roast
Slow Cooker Pot Roast, 218–219
cinnamon
Carnivore Cinnamon Rolls, 240–241
Carnivore Ice Cream, 334–335
Carnivore Ice Cream Sandwiches—Two Ways, 336–337
circadian rhythm, 104, 105
circadian training, 108
Citizen Science Foundation, 50–51
The Clot Thickens (Kendrick), 381
Cloud Bread Loaf or Buns recipe, 372–373
Bacon, Egg & Cheese Sandwich, 242–243
Burgers with Benefits, 208–209
Pot Roast Sandwich, 270–271
Roasted Bone Marrow, 204–205
Spicy Chicken Sandwiches, 272–273
Turkey Sandwich, 312–313
coffee, 78
cold turkey, 60–62
Collaborative Science Conference, 51
community, importance of, 109
comparing yourself, to others, 65
complete proteins, 32
The Complete Guide to Fasting: Heal Your Body Through Intermittent, Alternate-Day, and Extended Fasting (Fung), 122, 382

comprehensive metabolic panel, 69, 163
constipation, as a physical symptom, 130
continuous glucose monitoring (CGM), 181–183
continuous ketone monitoring, 185
corned beef
    Reuben Roll-Ups, 326–327
Cornish Hen recipe, 216–217
coronary artery calcium (CAC) scan, 188–189
coronary computed tomography angiography (CCTA), 189
cortisol, 103
cost
    of continuous glucose monitors, 181–182
    of DEXA scans, 175
Cotija cheese
    Carnivore Mac & Cheese Casserole, 278–281
    Taco Balls, 294–295
cottage cheese
    Carnivore Ice Cream Sandwiches—Two Ways, 336–337
    Cottage Cheese Flatbread, 370–371
    Cottage Cheese Flatbread Rounds, 370–371
Cottage Cheese Flatbread recipe, 370–371
    Carnivore Quesadilla, 296–297
    Chicken Sliders with Spicy Mayo, 250–251
    Fajita Wrap, 266–267
Cottage Cheese Flatbread Rounds recipe, 370–371
Crab Cakes with Rémoulade recipe, 292–293
cream cheese
    Air Fryer Sausage Rosemary Cream Cheese Bites, 248–249
    American Kajmak, 357
    Beef Stroganoff, 276–277
    Carnivore Cinnamon Rolls, 240–241
    Jalapeño Poppers, 318–319
    Mini Cheesecakes, 338–339
    Pumpkin Spice Cheesecake, 314–315
    Spiced Pumpkin-Shaped Cheese Ball, 304–305
    Sweet Cream Cheese-Filled Crepes, 238–239
    Taco Balls, 294–295
Crispy Baked Chicken Thighs & Drumsticks recipe, 210–211
Cvarci (Serbian Pork Cracklings) recipe, 256–257

D

Dahhaj, Zaid, 108
The Daily Stoic (Holiday), 383
dairy
    for carnivore kitchen, 74
    overeating, 121
Dark Calories: How Vegetable Oils Destroy Our Health and How We Can Get It Back (Shanahan), 380
Dehydrated Ground Meat recipe, 212–213
beef tallow, 342–343
delegation, as a stress management skill, 106
Deviled Eggs recipe, 252–253
DEXA scans, 69, 175–180
diabetes, 43, 155
diarrhea, as a physical symptom, 129
Dietary Guidelines for Americans, 146
dietary issues, 133–135
digestive system, 39–40
dill pickles
    Crab Cakes with Rémoulade, 292–293
    Reuben Roll-Ups, 326–327
    Spicy Chicken Sandwiches, 272–273
dill weed
    Buttermilk Ranch Dressing, 360–361
Discourses (Epictetus), 383
Dowdell, Erin, 23–24
drinks, 78–79, 140–146
dual-energy X-ray absorptiometry (DEXA) scans. *See* DEXA scans

E

Ede, Georgia, *Change Your Diet, Change Your Mind*, 59, 110, 379
eGFR, 167
Egg Pudding recipe, 214–215

eggs
- Air Fryer Egg Bites, 232–233
- Bacon, Egg & Cheese Sandwich, 242–243
- Bacon Mayonnaise, 352–353
- Breakfast Casserole, 228–229
- Carnivore Crepes/Noodles, 364–365
- Carnivore Flatbread, 366–367
- Carnivore Ice Cream, 334–335
- Carnivore Ice Cream Sandwiches—Two Ways, 336–337
- Carnivore Mac & Cheese Casserole, 278–281
- Carnivore Tacos, 288–289
- Carnivore White Pizza, 282–285
- Chaffles, 368–369
- Chicken Sliders with Spicy Mayo, 250–251
- Cloud Bread Loaf or Buns, 372–373
- Cottage Cheese Flatbread, 370–371
- Cottage Cheese Flatbread Rounds, 370–371
- Crab Cakes with Rémoulade, 292–293
- Deviled Eggs, 252–253
- Egg Pudding, 214–215
- Ground Beef & Eggs, 234–235
- Hard-Boiled Eggs, 236–237
- Marrownaise, 354–355
- Mini Cheesecakes, 338–339
- overview, 75
- Pumpkin Spice Cheesecake, 314–315
- Soft-Boiled Eggs, 236–237
- Soufflé Omelet, 230–231
- Wedge Salad, 324–325

Ego is the Enemy (Holiday), 383

electrolytes
- Butter Bites, 332–333
- overview, 117

Emmerich, Maria and Craig, *The Protein-Sparing Modified Fast Method: Over 120 Recipes to Accelerate Weight Loss & Improve Healing*, 382

energy, low, as a physical symptom, 128–129

environment
- importance of, 114
- myths about, 154–155

Environmental Protection Agency (EPA), 34

Epictetus, *Discourses*, 383

epilepsy, 44

expectations, managing, 65, 66–68, 116–117

extended fasting, 122

Extreme Double Bacon Cheeseburger recipe, 268–269

F

Fajita Wrap recipe, 266–267

FAQ, 140–152

fasting
- for DEXA scans, 175–176
- etiquette for, 164
- importance of, 111–112
- overview, 44, 96, 122–123
- recommended reading for, 382

fasting glucose, 125, 126, 167

fasting insulin, 69, 125, 126, 163, 167

fat adapted, 150

Fat and Cholesterol Don't Cause Heart Attacks and Statins Are Not the Solution (THINCS), 381

fats
- overview, 75, 90–91
- requirements for, 95, 117

fat-to-protein ratio, 90–91

Feldman, Dave, 50

ferritin, 163, 168, 173

feta cheese
- Carnivore Mac & Cheese Casserole, 278–281

fiber, 148, 155

fibrinogen, 157

fish and seafood
- Crab Cakes with Rémoulade, 292–293
- for carnivore kitchen, 74
- King Crab, 202–203
- overview, 75
- Walleye, 200–201

Fisher, Erin, 24–25

The Five Minute Journal (Intelligent Change), 110, 383

folate, 163, 168, 174
food boredom, 132
food science, recommended reading for, 380
foods
  amounts of, 116
  FAQ, 140–146
  fried, 145
  reintroducing, 100
  tracking, 120
Foster, Russell, *Life Time*, 105
four-week gradual carbohydrate reduction, 84–87
free T3, 164, 171
free T4, 164, 171
frequency
  of DEXA scans, 175
  of meals, 96
fried food, 145
fruits
  low-oxalate, low-lectin, lower-carb, 85
  myths about, 159
Fung, Jason, *The Complete Guide to Fasting: Heal Your Body Through Intermittent, Alternate-Day, and Extended Fasting*, 122, 382

G

gallbladder, 64, 134
gallstones, 132
garlic
  Bone Marrow Butter, 358–359
  Brined Spatchcocked Turkey, 300–303
  Buttermilk Ranch Dressing, 360–361
  Cornish Hen, 216–217
  Garlicky Smothered Brussels Sprouts, 322–323
  Garlicky Smothered Green Beans, 328–329
Garlicky Smothered Brussels Sprouts recipe, 322–323
Garlicky Smothered Green Beans recipe, 328–329
gas, 149
gelatin powder
  Carnivore Crepes/Noodles, 364–365
  Carnivore Gravy, 306–307
genetic testing, for mutations, 188
GGT, 69, 163, 167
GLP-1 receptor agonists, 12, 64
glucose, optimal levels for, 182
glycocalyx, 157
glyphosate (Roundup), 34
goal-setting, 66–68
Good Fat Is Good for Women: Menopause and Eating Good Fat Is Good for Girls: Puberty and Adolescence (Bright), 379–380
Gouda cheese
  Spicy Bacon-Wrapped Chorizo Dogs, 286–287
Gould Steve, 27
grain-fed vs. grass-fed beef, 75, 141
The Great Plant-Based Con (Buxton), 155, 379
Greek yogurt
  Carnivore Flatbread, 366–367
green beans
  Garlicky Smothered Green Beans, 328–329
green onions
  Garlicky Smothered Green Beans, 328–329
  Wedge Salad, 324–325
grocery shopping, guidelines for, 75
ground beef
  Air Fryer Egg Bites, 232–233
  Beef Stroganoff, 276–277
  Beefy Bacon-Wrapped Stuffed Onion Rings, 320–321
  Breakfast Casserole, 228–229
  Burgers with Benefits, 208–209
  Carnivore Tacos, 288–289
  Ćevaps (Serbian Sausages), 224–225
  Chili Cheese Dog Meatballs, 290–291
  Dehydrated Ground Meat, 212–213
  Extreme Double Bacon Cheeseburger, 268–269
  Ground Beef & Eggs, 234–235
  Hearty Meat Soup, 264–265

ground beef *(continued)*
- overview, 75
- Pljeskavica (Serbian Burgers), 222–223
- Spicy Bacon-Wrapped Chorizo Dogs, 286–287
- Taco Balls, 294–295

Ground Beef & Eggs recipe, 234–235
ground chicken/turkey
- Dehydrated Ground Meat, 212–213

ground pork
- Ćevaps (Serbian Sausages), 224–225
- Dehydrated Ground Meat, 212–213
- Pljeskavica (Serbian Burgers), 222–223

Gut and Physiology Syndrome (Campbell-McBride), 133, 380

H

Hagerty, Jo, 25–26
hair loss, 149
Hakala Labs, 187
half-and-half
- Air Fryer Egg Bites, 232–233
- Carnivore Ice Cream, 334–335
- Ground Beef & Eggs, 234–235

ham
- Air Fryer Egg Bites, 232–233
- Burgers with Benefits, 208–209
- Pihtije (Meat Jelly), 258–259

Hard-Boiled Eggs recipe, 236–237
Harris, Will, *A Bold Return to Giving a Damn*, 382
HDL, 125, 126, 147, 165, 166, 169–170
health, pillars of, 102–107
healthy gut, 148
heart disease, 156–158, 381
heart palpitations, as a physical symptom, 129
heart testing, 188–189
Hearty Meat Soup recipe, 264–265
heavy cream
- Alfredo Sauce, 351
- Breakfast Casserole, 228–229
- Carnivore Cinnamon Rolls, 240–241
- Carnivore Gravy, 306–307
- Carnivore Ice Cream, 334–335
- Carnivore Mac & Cheese Casserole, 278–281
- Egg Pudding, 214–215
- Whipped Cream & Mascarpone, 340–341

herbal tea, 78
hierarchy of needs, 109
high-oxalate foods, 61
histamine reactions, 49, 134
Holiday, Ryan, 383
holidays, 137
HOMA-IR, 125, 126
homocysteine, 163, 168, 172, 188
honey, 342–343
hormesis, importance of, 112
Hornaman, Amie, 171
hospitals, carnivore diet in, 146
hot dogs
- Chili Cheese Dog Meatballs, 290–291
- overview, 75
- Spicy Bacon-Wrapped Chorizo Dogs, 286–287

hot sauce
- Carnivore Tacos, 288–289
- Crab Cakes with Rémoulade, 292–293
- Fajita Wrap, 266–267
- Pot Roast Sandwich, 270–271
- Spicy Chicken Sandwiches, 272–273
- Spicy Mayonnaise, 356

hs-CRP, 69, 163, 168, 172
human digestive system, 39–40
hunger cues, 98
hydration, 78, 111, 117
hypothyroidism, 113, 121

I

Ice Age, 39
iceberg lettuce
- Wedge Salad, 324–325

"In-Depth Reference Guide to the Carnivore Diet" video, 20
inflammatory foods, 119

insulin resistance, 124–125
Intelligent Change, 383
intermittent fasting, 96, 111
intuitive eating, 89
iodine testing, 186–187
Iodine: Why You Need It, Why You Can't Live Without It (Brownstein), 187, 380
Italian sausage
  Air Fryer Sausage Rosemary Cream Cheese Bites, 248–249
  Meat Lover's Pizza Roll-Ups, 254–255

J

jalapeño peppers
  Jalapeño Poppers, 318–319
  Pljeskavica (Serbian Burgers), 222–223
Jalapeño Poppers recipe, 318–319
Joe Rogan Experience (podcast), 18
Johnson, Richard J., *Nature Wants Us to Be Fat*, 381

K

Keith, Lierre, *The Vegetarian Myth: Food, Justice, and Sustainability*, 51, 382
Kendrick, Malcolm, *The Clot Thickens*, 381
keto flu, 20, 70–71, 98
ketoacidosis, 185–186
ketogenic diet, 44
ketones, measuring, 184–186
ketosis, 160, 184–186
kidneys
  disease of, 49
  function of, 167
  markers for, 172–173
  meat and, 156
  protein and, 148
Kiehl, Cristie, 22
Kiltz, Robert, 99
King Crab recipe, 202–203
kitchen, preparing for carnivore diet, 72–82
Kruse, Jack, 108

L

lard
  Cvarci (Serbian Pork Cracklings), 256–257
Lascaux cave, 38
LDL, 147, 156–158, 165, 166, 169–170, 171
leaky gut, 133
legumes, low-oxalate, low-lectin, lower-carb, 86
lemons
  Bacon Mayonnaise, 352–353
  Buttermilk Ranch Dressing, 360–361
  Carnivore Mac & Cheese Casserole, 278–281
  Crab Cakes with Rémoulade, 292–293
  King Crab, 202–203
  Marrownaise, 354–355
  Walleye, 200–201
Letters of a Stoic (Seneca), 383
lettuce
  Wedge Salad, 324–325
L-glutamine, 133
Lies My Doctor Told Me: Medical Myths That Can Harm Your Health (Berry), 381
Life Time (Foster), 105
lifestyle shift, 66
limited budgets, 52
lion diet, 57, 58
lipedema, 64
Lipid Lunacy: Diet Delusions and What Really Causes Heart Disease (THINCS), 381
lipid panel, 69, 163, 165, 166
lipids, 171
lipotoxicity, 124–125, 172
liver function, 167
liver markers, 172–173
Living Well After Schizophrenia (West), 110
loose stools, as a physical symptom, 129
Low Carb Down Under conference, 51
low energy, as a physical symptom, 128
Luna, Courtney, 132
  Carnivore in the Kitchen, 379

M

Ma, Bella, 127
Maasai tribe, 41
macrophages, 157
marinara sauce
  Air Fryer Sausage Rosemary Cream Cheese Bites, 248–249
markers, improving, 171–174
Marrownaise recipe, 354–355
  Crab Cakes with Rémoulade, 292–293
mascarpone cheese
  Whipped Cream & Mascarpone, 340–341
Maslow's hierarchy of needs, 109
meal plan, 82
meal prep, 81
meals, frequency/timing of, 96
measurements, baseline, 68–70
meat and fruit diet, 57
Meat Lover's Pizza Roll-Ups recipe, 254–255
meats. *See also specific types*
  Air Fryer Egg Bites, 232–233
  aversions to, 132
  Breakfast Casserole, 228–229
  charred, 142
  kidneys and, 156
  organ, 142
  processed, 76, 141
  raw, 145
medical science and research, recommended reading for, 381
medications
  animal-based diets used in, 43–44
  continuing when on carnivore, 63
Meditations (Aurelius), 383
megafauna, 39
melatonin, 105
mental health, 59, 110
mental preparation, for carnivore diet, 65–71
metabolic health
  decline in, 124–127
  factors for, 108–114
  FAQ, 147–150
Metabolic Mind YouTube channel, 59, 110
methylated, 172
microplastics, 114
Miles, Karen, 27
milk
  Carnivore Mac & Cheese Casserole, 278–281
mindset, 65–66
minerals, 147
Mini Cheesecakes recipe, 338–339
The Miracle of Natural Hormones (Brownstein), 380
miscellaneous health questions, 150–152
Mitich, Jenny
  personal story of, 16–21
  website, 54
moderators, 61
mold exposure, 114, 118
monitoring progress, 162–189
monoculture, 34
month 1 on carnivore, 88–98
month 2 on carnivore, 98
months 3–12 on carnivore, 98–99
Mounjaro, 12
movement, as a pillar of health, 102, 103–104
mozzarella cheese
  Carnivore Flatbread, 366–367
  Carnivore Mac & Cheese Casserole, 278–281
  Carnivore Quesadilla, 296–297
  Carnivore White Pizza, 282–285
  Meat Lover's Pizza Roll-Ups, 254–255
  Soufflé Omelet, 230–231
muscle cramping, as a physical symptom, 128–129
mustard
  Brisket, 206–207
mutations, genetic testing for, 188
myths, 154–160, 182–183

N

natural sugar substitutes, 77
Nature Wants Us to Be Fat (Johnson), 381
Nazon, Raymond, 127

NMR LipoProfile, 163, 169–170
non-ruminant herbivore, 40
nonstick coatings, 145
Norton, Sally, *Toxic Superfoods*, 380
Norwitz, Nick, 51
Not By Bread Alone (Stefansson), 380
nutrient deficiencies, 113
nutrient density, 92
nutrition, as a pillar of health, 102
nuts and seeds, low-oxalate, low-lectin, lower-carb, 86

O

The Obstacle is the Way (Holiday), 383
OmegaCheck, 163, 168–169
one meal a day (OMAD), 82
one year and beyond on carnivore, 99–100
onions
  Beefy Bacon-Wrapped Stuffed Onion Rings, 320–321
  Pljeskavica (Serbian Burgers), 222–223
optimal ranges, for blood work, 165–171
organ meats, 142
orthorexia, 71
Ovadia, Philip, *Stay Off My Operating Table*, 381
Overcoming Thyroid Disorders (Brownstein), 380
overeating
  carnivore foods, 121
  dairy, 121
overnutrition, 49
Own Your Labs, 162
oxalate dumping, 20, 98, 99, 131–132
Ozempic, 12

P

pain tolerance, 62
Palmer, Christopher, *Brain Energy*, 59
Parmesan cheese
  Alfredo Sauce, 351
  Carnivore Mac & Cheese Casserole, 278–281
  Carnivore Tacos, 288–289
  Carnivore White Pizza, 282–285
  Garlicky Smothered Brussels Sprouts, 322–323
  Garlicky Smothered Green Beans, 328–329
Pecorino Romano cheese
  Air Fryer Sausage Rosemary Cream Cheese Bites, 248–249
pepper Jack cheese
  Beefy Bacon-Wrapped Stuffed Onion Rings, 320–321
  Spicy Bacon-Wrapped Chorizo Dogs, 286–287
  Spicy Chicken Sandwiches, 272–273
pepperoni
  Carnivore White Pizza, 282–285
  Cheesy Pepperoni Chips, 246–247
  Meat Lover's Pizza Roll-Ups, 254–255
  overview, 284
pesticides, 34
physical symptoms, 128–132
phytochemicals, 34
Pihtije (Meat Jelly) recipe, 258–259
plant fats, 33
Pljeskavica (Serbian Burgers) recipe, 222–223
Pontzer, Herman, *Burn*, 381
pork
  Ćevaps (Serbian Sausages), 224–225
  Dehydrated Ground Meat, 212–213
  for carnivore kitchen, 73
  overview, 75
  Pljeskavica (Serbian Burgers), 222–223
pork belly
  Cvarci (Serbian Pork Cracklings), 256–257
pork feet
  Pihtije (Meat Jelly), 258–259
pork rinds
  Carnivore Mac & Cheese Casserole, 278–281
  Carnivore Tacos, 288–289
  Carnivore White Pizza, 282–285
positive affirmations/thinking, 66
positivity, 65–66

Pot Roast Sandwich recipe, 270–271
"Primal Blueprint" (Sisson), 18
Prime Rib recipe, 198–199
priming, 127
processed foods, 36
processed meats, 74, 76, 141
progress monitoring
- basics of ketosis, 184–186
- blood work, 162–174
- continuous glucose monitoring (CGM), 181–183
- DEXA, 175–180
- genetic testing for mutations, 188
- heart testing, 188–189
- iodine testing, 186–187
- measuring ketones, 184–186
- overview, 162

protein
- kidneys and, 148
- overview, 90–91
- requirements for, 93–94

protein powder
- Cloud Bread Loaf or Buns, 372–373
- overview, 144

protein-sparing modified fast (PSMF), 123
The Protein-Sparing Modified Fast Method: Over 120 Recipes to Accelerate Weight Loss & Improve Healing (Emmerich and Emmerich), 382
Pumpkin Spice Cheesecake recipe, 314–315
pushers, 138

R

rabbit digestive system, 39–40
racing heart, as a physical symptom, 129
radiation levels, from DEXA scans, 175
randomized controlled trial (RCT), 376
raw meat, 145
reading, recommended, 378–383
recommended daily allowances (RDAs), 113–114
recommended reading, 378–383
red meat
- cancer and, 156
- diabetes and, 155
- for carnivore kitchen, 73

regenerative agriculture, recommended reading for, 382
reintroducing foods, 100
religious fasting, 123
religious restrictions, 52
Rendered Tallow recipe, 194–195
requirements, nutrition, 89
Reuben Roll-Ups recipe, 326–327
reverse dieting, 120, 127
reverse T3, 164, 171
ribeye steak
- Basted Ribeye, 196–197

Roasted Bone Marrow recipe, 204–205
Rodgers, Diana, *Sacred Cow: The Case for Better Meat*, 382
Rogers, Curtis, 22–23
Rollo, John, 43
Romano cheese
- Garlicky Smothered Brussels Sprouts, 322–323
- Garlicky Smothered Green Beans, 328–329

rosemary
- Air Fryer Brined Turkey Breast, 308–309
- Air Fryer Sausage Rosemary Cream Cheese Bites, 248–249
- Bone Marrow Butter, 358–359
- Brined Spatchcocked Turkey, 300–303
- Chicken Soup, 262–263
- Cornish Hen, 216–217
- Hearty Meat Soup, 264–265

ruminant animals version of carnivore, 57
ruminant herbivore, 40

S

Sacred Cow: The Case for Better Meat (Rodgers), 382
safety myths, 154

sage
  Brined Spatchcocked Turkey, 300–303
Saladino, Paul, 20
salt, 142
Salt Your Way to Health (Brownstein), 380
sardine fasting, 122
sauces, 142–143
sauerkraut
  Reuben Roll-Ups, 326–327
sausage
  Air Fryer Egg Bites, 232–233
  Air Fryer Sausage Rosemary Cream Cheese Bites, 248–249
  Hearty Meat Soup, 264–265
  Meat Lover's Pizza Roll-Ups, 254–255
  overview, 75
  Soufflé Omelet, 230–231
saying no, as a stress management skill, 107
scientific papers, evaluating, 374–378
scurvy, 158
seafood. *See* fish and seafood
seasonings. *See* spices and seasonings
seeds. *See* nuts and seeds
Seneca, *Letters of a Stoic*, 383
Shanahan, Catherine, *Dark Calories: How Vegetable Oils Destroy Our Health and How We Can Get It Back*, 380
sherry
  Brined Spatchcocked Turkey, 300–303
sickness, eating carnivore during, 150
Sisson, Mark, 18
skin conditions, 132
sleep, as a pillar of health, 102, 104–105
Slow Cooker Pot Roast recipe, 218–219
  Pot Roast Sandwich, 270–271
snacking, 96–97, 121
Society of Metabolic Health Practitioners, 50
Soft-Boiled Eggs recipe, 236–237
soil health, 34–35
Soto-Mota, Adrian, 51
Soufflé Omelet recipe, 230–231
soups
  Chicken Soup, 262–263
  Hearty Meat Soup, 264–265
sour cream
  Air Fryer Egg Bites, 232–233
  Buttermilk Ranch Dressing, 360–361
  Carnivore Quesadilla, 296–297
  Carnivore Tacos, 288–289
  Fajita Wrap, 266–267
  Mini Cheesecakes, 338–339
  Pumpkin Spice Cheesecake, 314–315
  Taco Balls, 294–295
special health issues/considerations, 62–64, 133–135
Spiced Pumpkin-Shaped Cheese Ball recipe, 304–305
spices and seasonings
  BBQ Spice Rub, 347
  Cajun Seasoning, 346
  Chicken & Pork Seasoning, 348
  Chili Spice Seasoning, 349
  Taco Seasoning, 350
  use on carnivore, 77, 142–143
Spicy Bacon-Wrapped Chorizo Dogs recipe, 286–287
Spicy Chicken Sandwiches recipe, 272–273
Spicy Mayonnaise recipe, 356
  Chicken Sliders with Spicy Mayo, 250–251
  Spicy Bacon-Wrapped Chorizo Dogs, 286–287
  Spicy Chicken Sandwiches, 272–273
sprinting, 103
Standard American Diet (SAD), 11, 60
standard lipid panel, 69
Stay Off My Operating Table (Ovadia), 381
steaks, 75
Stefansson, Vilhjalmur, 41
  Not by Bread Alone, 380
stools, loose, as a physical symptom, 129
strength training, 103
stress, as a pillar of health, 102, 106–107

strip steak
  Fajita Wrap, 266–267
sugar, 36
sugar cravings, 98
sugar substitutes
  Carnivore Cinnamon Rolls, 240–241
  Carnivore Ice Cream, 334–335
  Carnivore Ice Cream Sandwiches—Two Ways, 336–337
  overview, 143
  Pumpkin Spice Cheesecake, 314–315
  Sweet Cream Cheese-Filled Crepes, 238–239
sunlight, importance of, 108–109
sunscreen, 152
supplementation, 113–114
supplies, kitchen, 81
support, getting, 70
sustainability, recommended reading for, 382
Sweet Cream Cheese-Filled Crepes recipe, 238–239
Swiss cheese
  Reuben Roll-Ups, 326–327
Symposium for Metabolic Health, 51

T

Taco Balls recipe, 294–295
Taco Seasoning recipe, 350
  Carnivore Tacos, 288–289
  Taco Balls, 294–295
talking to others about carnivore, 136–138
Teicholz, Nina, *The Big Fat Surprise*, 379
telogen effluvium, 149
testimonials, 22–27
TG/GDL ratio, 125, 126
Thanksgiving menu, 301
therapeutic ketogenic diet, 44
The International Network of Cholesterol Skeptics (THINCS), 381
thyme
  Bone Marrow Butter, 358–359
  Brined Spatchcocked Turkey, 300–303
thyroglobulin antibodies, 164, 171
thyroid issues, 121
thyroid markers, 171, 174
thyroid-stimulating hormone (TSH), 121, 164, 171
time constraints, 62
timeline
  four-week gradual carbohydrate reduction, 84–87
  month 1, 88–98
  month 2, 98
  months 3–12, 98–99
  one year and beyond, 99–100
timing
  meal, 96
  sleep, 104
tomatoes
  Wedge Salad, 324–325
tools, kitchen, 81
total body bone density report, in DEXA scans, 179
total daily energy expenditure (TDEE), 120
Toxic Superfoods (Norton), 380
TPO antibodies, 164, 171
tracking food, 120
traveling, carnivore diet while, 145
triglycerides, 125, 126, 147, 165, 166
Tripp, Jonathan, 26–27
troubleshooting
  common mistakes, 116–117
  food boredom, 132
  meat aversions, 132
  metabolic health declining, 124–127
  no weight loss, 124–127
  physical symptoms, 128–132
  special health/dietary issues, 133–135
  talking to others, 136–138
  weight-loss stalls, 118–123

turkey
    Air Fryer Brined Turkey Breast, 308–309
    Brined Spatchcocked Turkey, 300–303
    Carnivore Gravy, 306–307
    Dehydrated Ground Meat, 212–213
    Turkey Alfredo, 310–311
    Turkey Sandwich, 312–313
Turkey Alfredo recipe, 310–311
Turkey Sandwich recipe, 312–313
2020–2025 USDA Dietary Guidelines for Americans, 9–10
2022 National Healthcare Quality and Disparities Report, 9
type 1 diabetes, 43, 155
type 2 diabetes, 155

U

Ulta Lab Tests, 162
ultra-processed foods, 36, 66, 148
undereating, 120
uric acid, 163, 168, 173
urine hydration scale, 78
urine testing, 185
UVA/UVB exposure, 105, 152

V

veal
    Pihtije (Meat Jelly), 258–259
vegans, 51
vegetables
    Fajita Wrap, 266–267
    low-oxalate, low-lectin, lower-carb, 86
    myths about, 159
vegetarians, 51
The Vegetarian Myth: Food, Justice, and Sustainability (Keith), 51, 382
versions, of carnivore diet, 57–60
visceral adipose tissue (VAT), in DEXA scans, 178
visceral fat accumulation, 125, 126
visioning, 66
vitamin C, 113–114, 147, 158
vitamin D, 69, 105, 108–109, 113, 147, 173–174
vitamin D 25, 147, 163, 168
VLDL, 165

W

Walk-In Lab, 162
Walleye recipe, 200–201
water, 78, 111
water fasting, 111–112
waterfowl, for carnivore kitchen, 74
websites
    Citizen Science Foundation, 51
    Collaborative Science Conference, 51
    Low Carb Down Under, 51
    Mitich, Jenny, 54
    Symposium for Metabolic Health, 51
Wedge Salad recipe, 324–325
weight gain, 61
weight loss, 65, 118–127
Wentz, Isabella, 171
West, Lauren Kennedy, *Living Well After Schizophrenia*, 110
Whipped Cream & Mascarpone recipe, 340–341
Whipped Tallow Bites recipe, 342–343
whole-food diet, 60
Why We Get Sick (Bikman), 379
Whys, determining your, 56
Wilder, Russell Morse, 44
Wings recipe, 220–221
work-related activities, staying carnivore during, 137

Y–Z

yogurt
    Carnivore Flatbread, 366–367
Zeroing In On Health forum, 14